This photograph of Kayla Itsines was taken in the Flinders Ranges region of South Australia, approximately 450 km from Adelaide.

THE BIKINI BODY MOTIVATION & HABITS GUIDE

KAYLA ITSINES

THE BIKINI BODY MOTIVATION & HABITS GUIDE

St. Martin's Griffin   New York

THE BIKINI BODY MOTIVATION & HABITS GUIDE. Text copyright © 2017 by Kayla Itsines. Photographs copyright © Jeremy Simons. All rights reserved. Printed in the United States of America. For information, address St. Martin's Press, 175 Fifth Avenue, New York, N.Y. 10010

www.stmartins.com

Photography by Jeremy Simons
Photography assistance by Joshua Witheford
Prop and food styling by Michelle Noerianto
Food preparation by Tammi Kwok
Editing by Rachel Carter and Ariane Durkin
Props kindly supplied by Bison Home
Colour and reproduction by Splitting Image Colour Studio
Production Manager: Adriana Coada

The Library of Congress Cataloging-in-Publication Data is available upon request.

ISBN 978-1-250-13761-6 (paper over board)
ISBN 978-1-250-13762-3 (ebook)

Our books may be purchased in bulk for promotional, educational, or business use. Please contact your local bookseller or the Macmillan Corporate and Premium Sales Department at 1-800-221-7945, extension 5442, or by email at MacmillanSpecialMarkets@macmillan.com.

First published 2017 by Pan Macmillan Australia Pty Limited
1 Market Street, Sydney, New South Wales, Australia 2000

First U.S. Edition: December 2017

10 9 8 7 6 5 4 3 2 1

CONTENTS

- -

DOWNLOADABLES

To assist you in developing and keeping good habits, I have included some planners and checklists in this book. You can find these items on the pages below or you can download a copy at **kaylaitsines.com/28dayguide/book2**

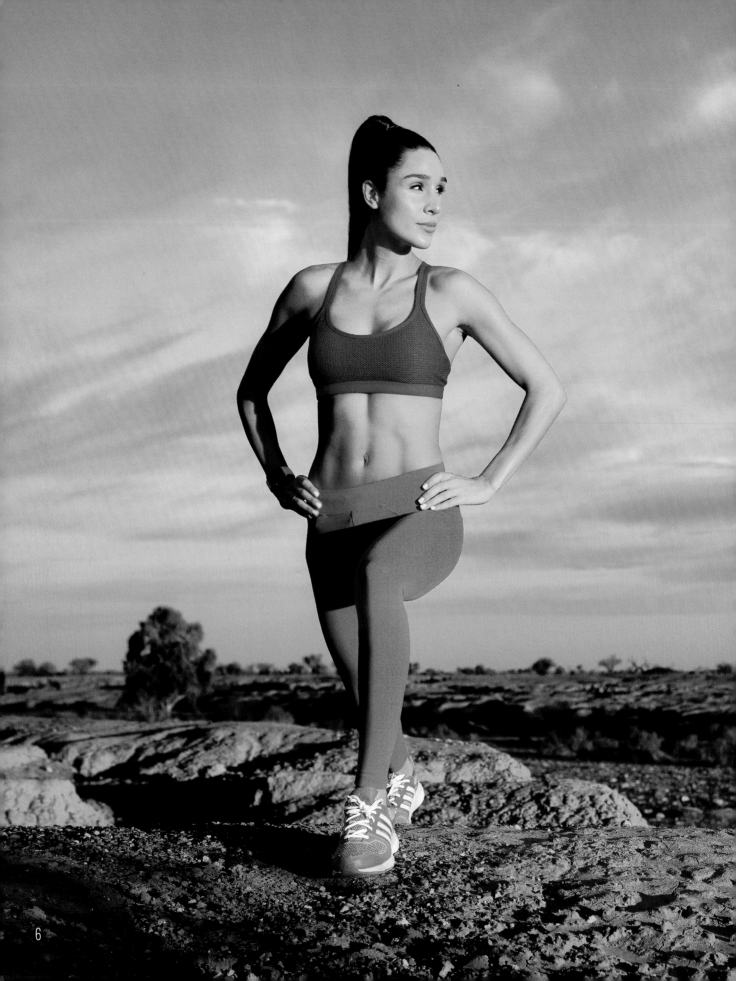

NOTE FROM KAYLA

Throughout my years of personal training, I've educated and supported millions of women just like you to improve your health and fitness—and your life! My first book, *The Bikini Body 28-Day Healthy Eating & Lifestyle Guide,* and my Bikini Body Guides (BBG) have helped women around the world make permanent and sustainable changes to both their mindset and lifestyle. I've made it my mission to help as many women as possible achieve their ideal body and feel more confident and happy.

The global fitness community my partner, Tobi, and I established has now grown to 20 million women, and just keeps on growing. Through this community, I have learned a lot about what makes women want to change their lives for the better. And more often than not, the reasons women decide to make a change—and whether or not they are successful—involve two key factors: motivation and good habits. To try and get a picture of what's really happening in the lives of those in our fitness community, Tobi and I put together a survey that was completed by almost 40,000 women.

We asked them questions like:

- Do you feel insecure?
- Are you happy with your body?
- Are you more concerned about your face, the shape of your body, or the size of your body?
- Which body part are you most concerned about?
- Have you ever felt demotivated?
- Does being insecure demotivate you?
- If so, have you chosen not to train because of that insecurity?

The answers to our survey were very revealing. They confirmed many things we thought already and we learned many things we didn't know or expect. Here's a rundown:

Lots of women like to work out. In fact, some countries say that more than half the members of any gym are women!

But 98% of women surveyed said they felt insecure at some point.

Not only are we a little insecure, but fewer than 1 in 3 of us are happy with our body.

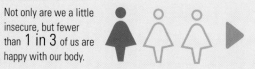

80% of us are completely "absessed," with abs being the body part we are most insecure about, and the body part we focus on the most when it comes to training.

It's actually not our face or the shape of our body we are most concerned with: 85% of women surveyed are most concerned about the SIZE of their bodies.

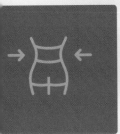

I would've thought that if we were feeling insecure and wanted to change our bodies, we would take steps to work on this, yet insecurity demotivates almost half of us, stopping us from continuing with training or living a healthier lifestyle.

We feel so demotivated sometimes that more than 56% choose NOT to train because of how we feel about our body.

▼

Wait...
so when we feel bad about our body, we don't want to train to try to feel better?

3 in 5 of us quit training because we feel demotivated.

◀

More than 3 in 5 of us lose motivation mostly from not noticing results.

▼

Yet 3 in 5 of us also don't complete all of our workouts each week!

So, we don't want to train when we feel bad about our body. If we finally do get the courage up to actually work out, we rarely do what the programs say, and then we lose motivation because we're not seeing results.

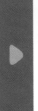

If this many women are affected by motivation issues, then let's figure out how to not only get motivated, but stay motivated, and create good habits for life!

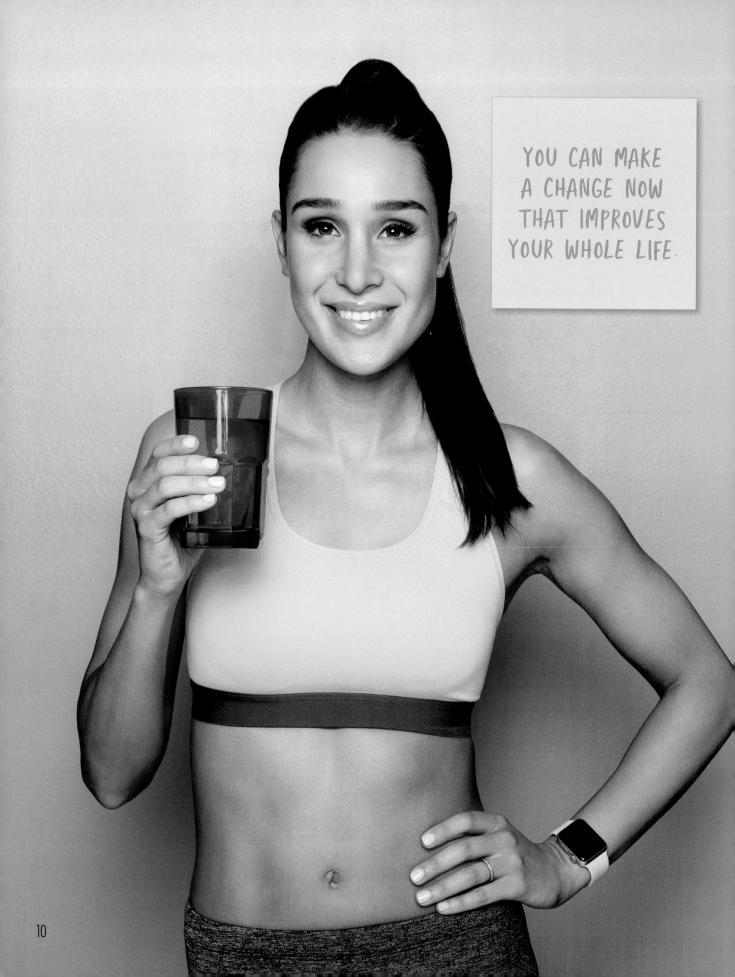

YOU CAN MAKE
A CHANGE NOW
THAT IMPROVES
YOUR WHOLE LIFE.

INTRODUCTION

In my first book, I wrote mostly about "what" to do to make a healthy lifestyle change. I focused on:

- Educational content
- A 28-day workout and meal plan
- More than 200 recipes

This information was the perfect start to guide you through your lifestyle change. I wanted to provide as much information as I could and to make the information as flexible as possible. This way it would fit YOU and your lifestyle easily, and form a great foundation and plan for health from a holistic perspective.

I want to provide you with the keys to making sure your healthy lifestyle sticks and you achieve YOUR goals. Once you finish reading this book you will know how to motivate yourself and how to use your motivation to create habits that will stick. By following these steps, you can get the results you have been wanting.

In this second book, you'll gain:

- Important knowledge about motivation
  How and why you feel motivated
  How you can control and leverage
  (i.e. use) that motivation to get you started
- An understanding of habits
  What are habits?
  How can you stop bad habits?
  How can you create new ones?
- A 28-day extension of the workout and meal plan
- Another 200+ recipes.

I've always been an advocate for using education to help women understand why you should make the effort with your health. My books provide a pathway to success in health for women of all ages, shapes, and sizes. Collectively, this information covers the "what and how" in relation to workouts and nutrition, to enable you to achieve your ideal confidence, health, and happiness.

Part of my responsibility as a personal trainer is to essentially "make you do what you need to do" in order to achieve the best results. Since I can't physically control your actions, part of that responsibility is to understand how to motivate you and educate you to create positive habits.

To learn as much as possible about these topics, Tobi and I have undertaken some research. This involved an analysis of the behaviour of women, in particular with regards to physical fitness goals. We were able to do this by providing a survey to 40,000 women, from all over the world. The survey focused on understanding women's insecurities, what motivates us, how we manage motivation for workouts and diets, and more.

In this second book, the chapters on motivation and habit will give YOU and other members of the global women's fitness community the "why." Why do you feel motivated (or not motivated) to do things to change your lifestyle? With a true understanding of how you can use motivation to help create new and healthy habits, you can expect success. You will be able to create and sustain a better, healthier lifestyle to help you achieve the confidence that you deserve.

Ultimately, my goal is to help more women just like YOU start and finish a workout or nutrition program with habits that lay the foundation for a new, sustainable and healthy lifestyle.

Giving you the tools

My intention is to help more women just like YOU to feel your most confident. I believe feeling physically strong and confident in your ability is a great place to start. I want to give you the mental tools to not just motivate you, but to help you form good habits relating to your well-being. This can be the basis for a sustainable, healthy lifestyle.

To me, the idea of a "bikini body" isn't a certain body shape. It's a state of mind where you feel confident, healthy, and strong. It is when you feel good about yourself.

You are one of a kind. There is no one else who has your smile, your laugh, your personality. And you should celebrate the things that make you unique, rather than wishing you looked like someone else. By being kind to yourself, you can learn to be grateful for all of the wonderful things that your body and mind can do.

My goal is to help you build confidence by overcoming challenges you experience with your healthy lifestyle. The first step towards achieving this is clearly identifying what it is you want to achieve. From my experience, most women want to become a stronger version of themselves. You want to be the most confident, strong, and positive person possible, and you can achieve that through following a healthy lifestyle.

unique

adjective being the only one of its kind; unlike anything else.

If you have read my first book, you are probably aware that I believe these are the most important tools anyone can have.

Health
To me, good health relates to many aspects of your day-to-day life. It's not just about having toned arms or glowing skin. Your mindset can also have a big impact on your life. Do you feel as though you're in a good place physically, emotionally, and socially?

Confidence
Confidence has a lot to do with your attitude, particularly when it comes to your well-being. Do you feel as though you can tackle anything life throws at you? Do you feel happy in your own skin? Confidence is often a sign of good health.

Strength
Again, this is not just about your physical strength. Mentally, do you feel strong? If you've had a bad day, can you pick yourself up? How positive are your thoughts when it comes to your health, mind, and body?

My belief is that health, confidence, and strength—through regular exercise, good nutrition, and positive goal setting—is the best way to achieve happiness.

The long-term approach to forming good habits

At some point in your life, you have probably known someone, or you may have even tried yourself to kick-start a new lifestyle with fad diets or by overtraining. You might have noticed quick results to begin with, but those changes probably didn't stick around for the long term. My approach doesn't include quick fixes. To me, good health is about focusing on how you feel.

As I have learned with many of my clients, for a healthy lifestyle to stick, there are three important considerations: balance, flexibility, and simplicity. You need to be able to balance your diet, workouts, and me-time to help yourself stay on track. The same goes for flexibility: your healthy lifestyle should still be able to accommodate some of the things you want to do (such as going out for dinner with friends), or else you may feel overwhelmed or deprived and want to give it up. Finally, if your training and eating plans are not simple enough for you to understand, it can make it very hard for you to follow them correctly.

I am a big believer that you should do something every day to feel good about yourself. Taking a small step, such as learning more about healthy foods, can make a big difference, particularly if you build on this with more small steps. Eventually these steps lead to good habits of looking after yourself physically and emotionally.

It's no surprise that motivation levels can change frequently with your mood or environment. Many women ask me how I stay so motivated to work out and eat healthily. My honest answer to this question is always the same: I don't. It's true—there are times when I don't feel motivated to train or eat well but because I've developed good habits over a long period of time, my discipline kicks in and I can get over these feelings of low motivation.

I want to help educate you and women just like you to understand HOW to form these good habits. I understand that for many of you, it can be hard to know where to begin, or what is right for you. My first book focused on the basics of diet and nutrition education, to empower you with the knowledge to make good decisions. In this book, I will teach you how to focus on your goals and how to get results by understanding what motivates you and how to form good health habits.

MY METHOD

In my first book, I introduced you to the main principles that I believe are the foundations for a healthy lifestyle. In this book, I want to help you understand how you can utilise that knowledge, as well as how to use motivation to build good habits that support your healthy lifestyle choices.

My BBG program focuses on key areas: nutrition, training, and lifestyle. Let me give you a little refresher.

NUTRITION

Healthy eating is essential for everyone, and monitoring your food intake is important if you are committing to a healthy lifestyle. I have devised a food group distribution method (in collaboration with dietitians) that helps to make meal planning simple. Using this method allows you to easily substitute meals or foods based on your preferences, while still helping you to meet your recommended calorie and nutrition requirements each day.

TRAINING

Regular physical activity, including some form of resistance, is key to a healthy lifestyle.

Physical activity helps to stimulate your muscles, increase bone density, improve cardiovascular health, and reduce the risk of injury from an inactive lifestyle.

My training plans consist of two to four cardio sessions (of varying intensity) and three resistance circuit training sessions per week. Resistance training involves using some form of resistance to increase the difficulty of different types of muscle movements. The resistance can come from your own body weight (as with squats or push-ups), or external weights such as dumbbells. My resistance workouts include a mix of plyometric (jump), body-weight, and strength-building exercises, which have been incorporated into high-intensity circuits. Cardio is any form of aerobic exercise, such as walking, running, swimming, or cycling. I recommend two types of cardio. The first is Low-Intensity Steady State (or "LISS"), which is equivalent to 30–45 minutes of walking or any other form of low-intensity cardio. The second is High-Intensity Interval Training (or "HIIT"), which is equivalent to a 30-second sprint (defined as "work"), followed by a 30-second walk (defined as "rest"). These "work" and "rest" periods are then repeated for a designated amount of time, usually 10–15 minutes.

LIFESTYLE

By lifestyle, I mean achieving a balance between work and play. While it's important for you to eat a balanced diet and follow a training plan to help you reach your goals, you need time to dedicate to the things that make you happy as well. How you feel each day can be impacted by work, stress, the amount of sleep you've had, and many other factors. Trying to balance all of these areas can be difficult.

Support from friends and family can make this delicate balancing act a little easier. Surround yourself with people who support your health goals and you should have a much better chance of achieving them.

Check out the Instagram hashtags #sweatwithkayla, #bbgcommunity and #kaylaitsines to connect with millions of women around the world who can support and encourage you.

KNOWLEDGE = POWER

I believe education is very important when managing your health and fitness. Understanding the basic principles of nutrition and exercise can help you to make educated and positive choices regarding your health, as you understand WHY they are good choices. This understanding also allows for adaptations in your meal planning, particularly if you have a sensitivity to or intolerance for a particular food. This knowledge can lead to a more flexible, healthier, and happier lifestyle.

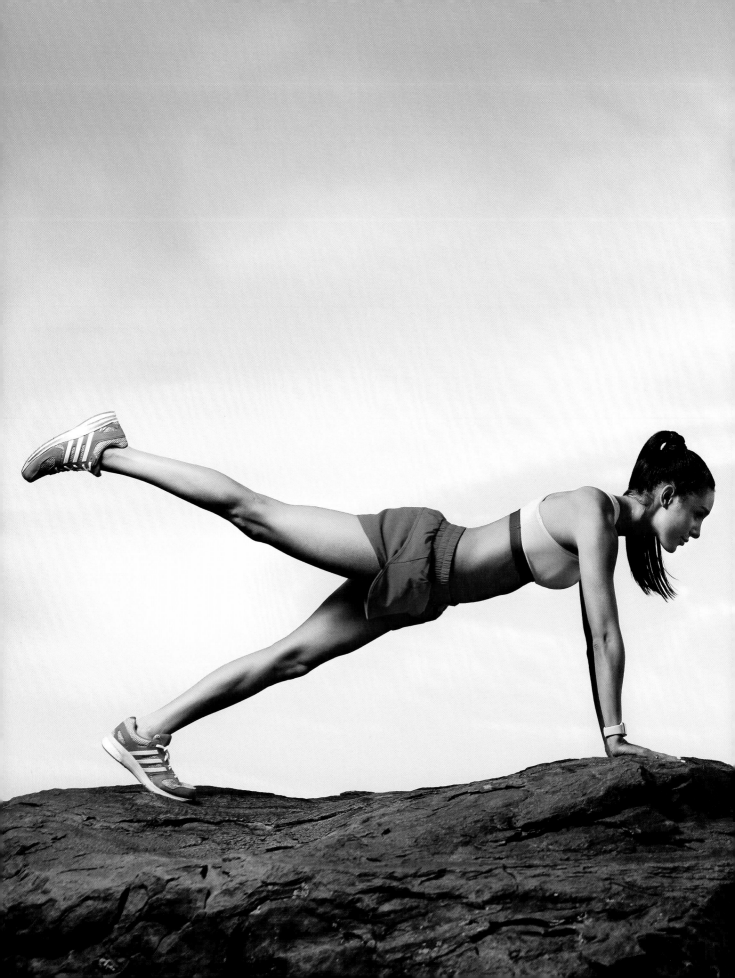

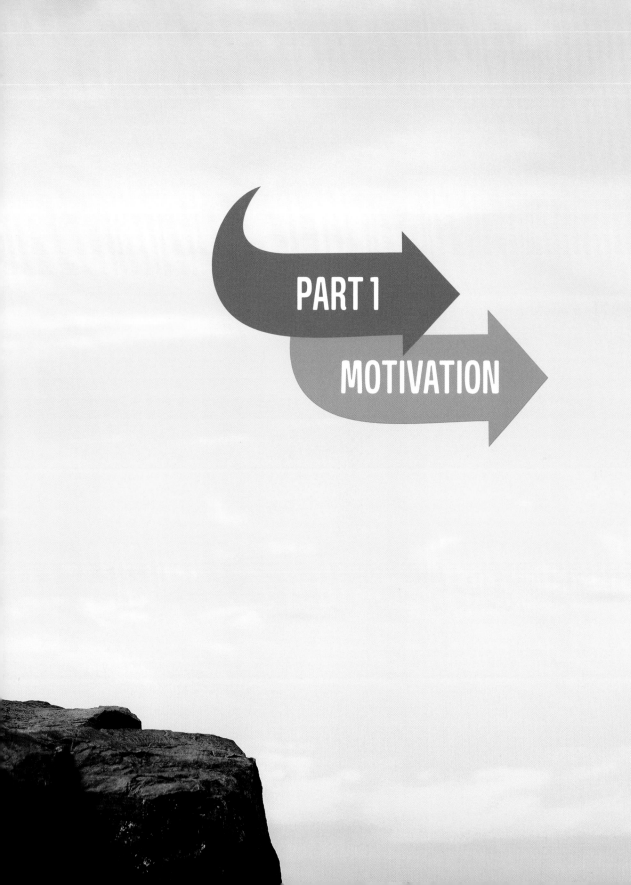

PART 1

MOTIVATION

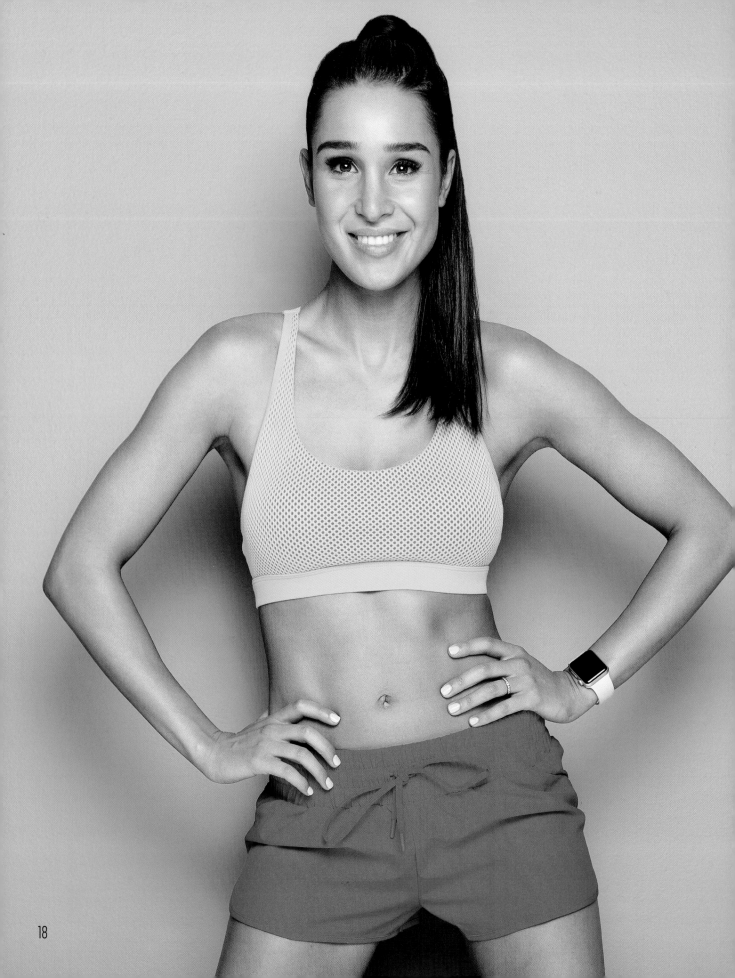

MY MISSION

My mission is to help as many women as possible achieve their ideal body, confidence, and happiness.

In order for me to do that, and to help my clients perform well, I need to maintain a solid understanding of the reasons many women decide to change their lives and the struggles they have in reaching their goals.

During my many years of experience as a personal trainer, my clients have often told me of the roller coaster they feel they're on (or have been on) when it comes to their motivation. Sometimes they feel highly motivated and then life, study, work, or something unexpected or unplanned gets in the way and they're off-track. In these times, when our motivation is down, it often affects our desire to exercise, our capacity to stick to workout and nutrition regimes and, ultimately, our ability to succeed long term. This was confirmed in the survey Tobi and I did, which identified a staggering 95% of us feel demotivated at some point during our health and fitness journey.

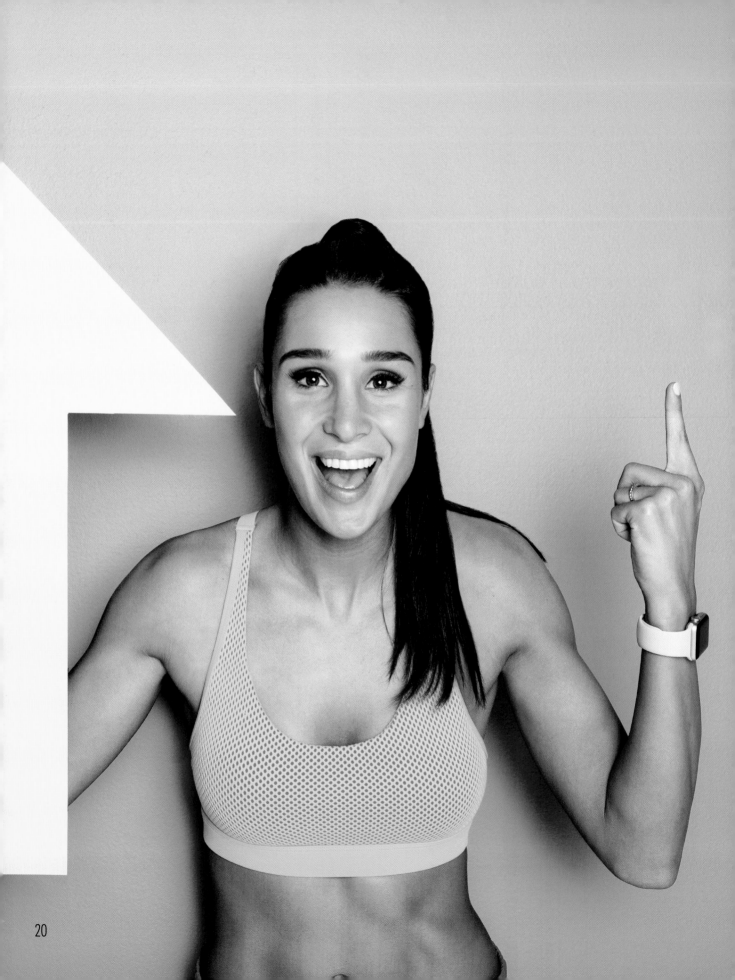

Their journey looks
something like this,
which you might also
be able to relate to.

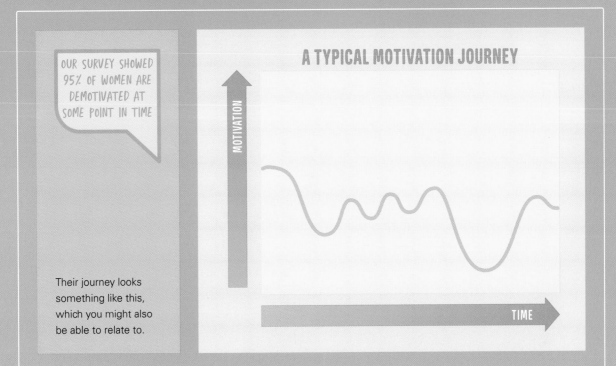

A TYPICAL MOTIVATION JOURNEY

MOTIVATION

TIME

My goal in the following pages of this book is to help you understand
what motivation really is and to give you the secret formula.

Although motivation
is continuously
fluctuating, once you
understand and apply
this knowledge, you
can not only increase
your motivation levels
BUT you can also
stabilise them for
a longer period of
time (see graph to
the right). This is the
real key that all my
successful clients
understand.

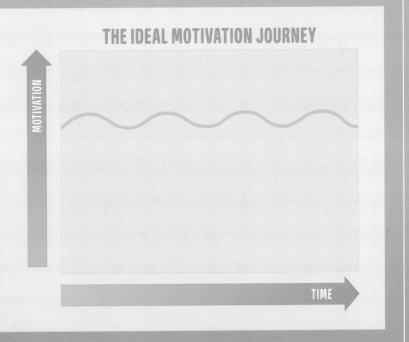

THE IDEAL MOTIVATION JOURNEY

MOTIVATION

TIME

MOTIVATION

If motivation is defined as the reason for acting a particular way, this means our behaviour is directly linked to us wanting to achieve or acquire something. In other words, action equals outcome.

motivation

noun, singular   reason or reasons for acting or behaving in a particular way.

Here's a simple example all of us can relate to. A proposed pay raise at work motivates you to work harder than ever before a big presentation.

Hard work = effort
Motivation = reward of a pay rise

At some point in your life, you've probably felt motivated to do something. A question I am regularly asked is:

> "Why then don't I feel motivated to work out or eat healthily?"

Simply put, you probably *do* feel motivated to work out at times. Think back to the last time you felt really motivated to work on yourself. Were you able to put that motivation to use? And if you did, were you then able to commit to those changes on a long-term basis? I know that for many women, sticking to those lifestyle changes for a longer period of time is the biggest problem.

When it comes to achieving your goals, motivation isn't always enough. In order to work towards your goals, motivation needs to be high, and your goals need to be a priority. Being motivated to achieve your goals takes a lot of energy, as your mind can only focus on so many things at once. That's why it is important to decide on your priorities and to understand what impacts your level of motivation.

The level of your motivation to do or get something is usually equal to your "perceived value" for that object.

For example, the greater the reward, the more motivated you are. How you define the value and the likelihood of success is actually the key to determining the extent of your motivation.

How do we measure motivation?

In order for us to measure motivation, we need to be clear about the simple formula defining it. Understanding this can help you make better life decisions, especially complex ones related to your health and fitness, as they continually change and evolve over time.

We can break down our motivation level into two compounding factors: value and expectancy. Basically, this means if our value for something is high, but our expectancy for success is low, we won't be highly motivated to achieve that goal. This also applies the opposite way: if our expectancy of achieving something is high, yet we don't value the goal enough, our motivation will also be low. In order for us to understand how to feel more motivated and how to leverage that motivation (i.e. how to use that motivation effectively), we need to understand the concepts of value and expectancy.

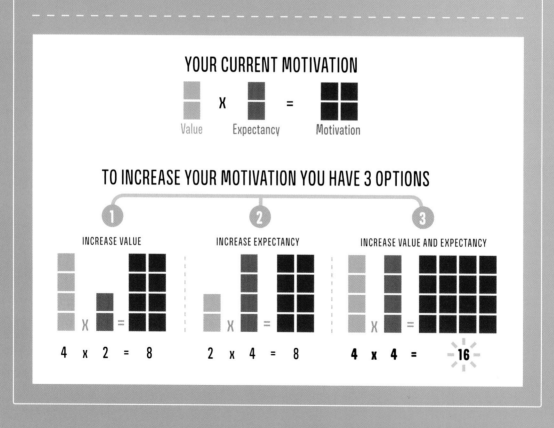

YOUR CURRENT MOTIVATION

Value X Expectancy = Motivation

TO INCREASE YOUR MOTIVATION YOU HAVE 3 OPTIONS

1 INCREASE VALUE

2 INCREASE EXPECTANCY

3 INCREASE VALUE AND EXPECTANCY

4 x 2 = 8

2 x 4 = 8

4 x 4 = 16

VALUE x EXPECTANCY = MOTIVATION

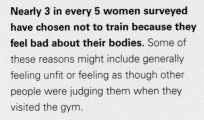

Nearly 3 in every 5 women surveyed have chosen not to train because they feel bad about their bodies. Some of these reasons might include generally feeling unfit or feeling as though other people were judging them when they visited the gym.

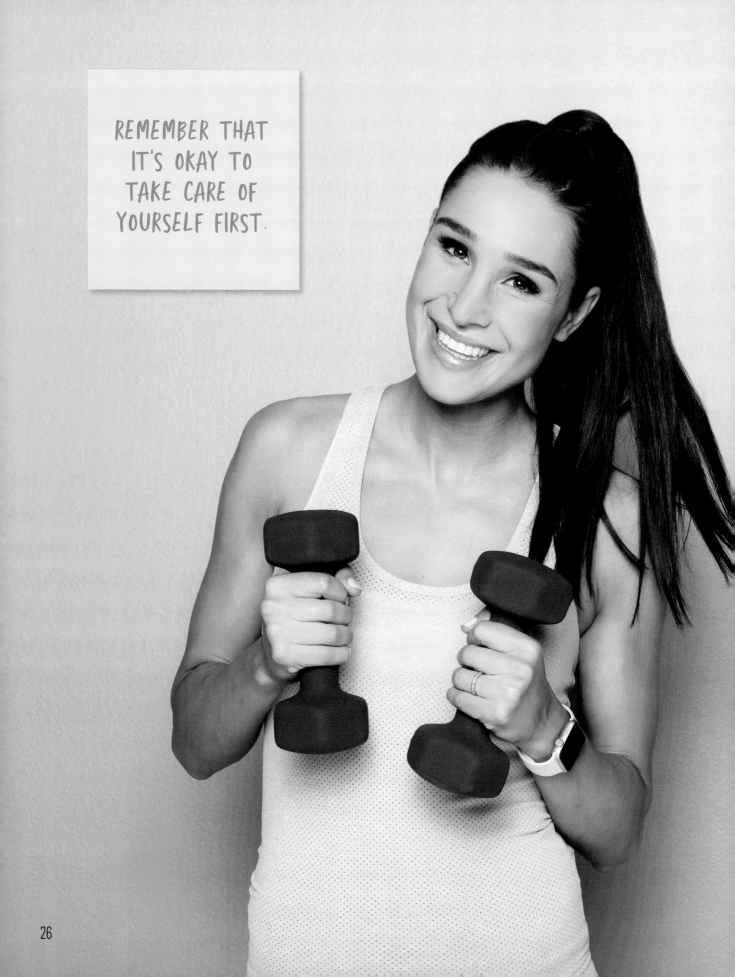

REMEMBER THAT
IT'S OKAY TO
TAKE CARE OF
YOURSELF FIRST.

26

VALUE

Value is one of two contributing factors to motivation. When we talk about value, we're not referring to the price. The word "value" really means how important something is to us. Not everything has a monetary price, but everything has a value. The value you place on something depends on many things, including your preferences, habits, environment, cultural background, experiences, and more.

value
noun
the regard that something is held to deserve; the importance, worth, or usefulness of something.

Not only is the value of something influenced by the changing criteria above, but each person values things differently. While you may value something highly, it doesn't mean that everyone else does. This is called *relative* or *perceived* value, and it basically means that while something may be the same "price," it may be worth more or less to two different people.

High Value

For example, your grandmother (or yiayia for me) might give you an old bracelet. To any other person, it may be just a bracelet, but to you it's the bracelet that your grandmother wore to her wedding, which has been passed down for two generations. It has a huge amount of value to you, but not to many other people. Your perceived value for this bracelet is higher than that of another bracelet.

Low Value

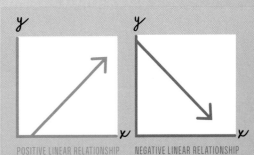

POSITIVE LINEAR RELATIONSHIP   NEGATIVE LINEAR RELATIONSHIP

x **= Value**
y **= Motivation**

As you would've seen in the motivation formula, value is only one of two elements for measuring motivation. Therefore if expectancy remains the same, as our value for something increases, our overall motivation level increases. This is an extremely important point, because if we can harness ways to increase our perceived value for something it means we can also increase our motivation. I will touch on how to increase value, and, therefore, motivation, later in the book.

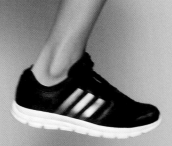

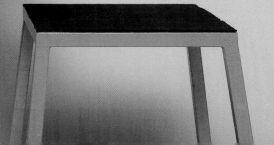

EXPECTANCY

The concept of value begs the question: if we value a goal or outcome highly enough, why doesn't this increase our motivation? The answer is simple—we need to believe we can achieve it. We might believe this goal is THE most important thing for us to do right now, but in order to be motivated we need to believe we can achieve it: this is expectancy. If we are not confident that we can actually achieve our goal, our motivation decreases and, therefore, our action and effort does too.

expectancy

noun the state of thinking or hoping that something, especially something good, will happen.

Expectancy can be defined as your level of confidence in completing a particular task or project. In other words, your level of confidence for success. I am sure you can relate to this: as things get more difficult or you're less competent and experienced, your expectancy typically decreases because this introduces stress and a higher chance of failure.

Why don't we believe we can succeed?

■ **We get concerned about what we don't know.**

■ **We fear what we can't see.**

■ **We are cautious of what we aren't competent or experienced in.**

In order to maximise our expectancy, or feeling of confidence to succeed, we need to know why we believe we will or won't succeed, specifically in relation to health and fitness. When training, I often hear clients say "I just can't do it" for their last few push-ups. We fear uncertainty.

For example, you might be scared about trying a box jump, because you have never jumped that high before and you don't know if you can make it. As your fear sets in, your expectancy for success decreases. As I've explained, when expectancy goes down, so can our motivation to do the jump.

More than half of the women surveyed have chosen not to train because of a lack of motivation relating to their insecurities. Have you ever stopped a workout because you didn't think you could keep going, or finish?

You are not alone.

Nearly a third of the women surveyed admit to feeling demotivated and stopping a workout because it feels too hard.

In my experience most workouts are designed to be achievable, however, when it gets challenging we start losing confidence in our ability to succeed. As I've explained, if expectancy decreases, so does your motivation.

Something that is often overlooked or misunderstood is competency and the effect it has on our confidence and expectancy. By competence, I mean having the necessary knowledge, skill, or ability to do something. A great way to think of competence is as follows:

High competency ⇨ High confidence ⇨ High expectancy

Low competency ⇨ Low confidence ⇨ Low expectancy

As you can see above, an increase in competency has a positive effect on your confidence and, therefore, your expectancy.

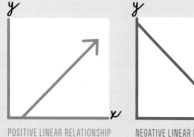
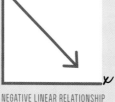

POSITIVE LINEAR RELATIONSHIP   NEGATIVE LINEAR RELATIONSHIP

x = **Expectancy**

y = **Motivation**

Expectancy is the second of two factors that impact your motivation. Therefore, if value remains the same, as your expectancy increases, your overall motivation level increases too. If we can harness ways to increase our expectancy for something, it means we can also increase our motivation. I will touch more on how to increase expectancy and, therefore, motivation later in the book. To put it simply, we feel most confident about things we know well, have done before, are competent at, and that are clearly defined.

Expectancy is how confident you are that you can succeed at something and can influence your level of motivation. The more confident you are that you can achieve something, the more motivated you feel to do so. Understanding the formula for motivation is key to your success.

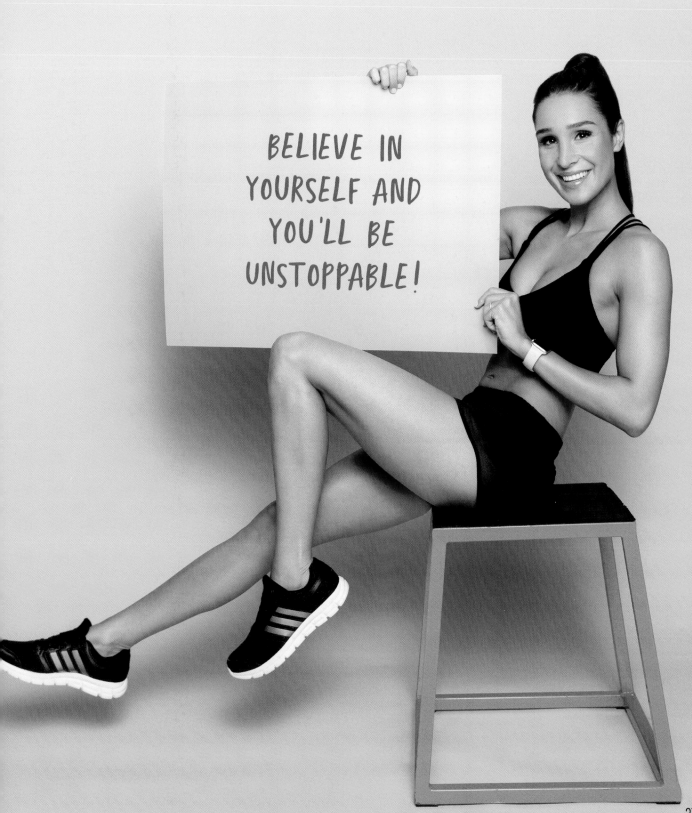

BELIEVE IN
YOURSELF AND
YOU'LL BE
UNSTOPPABLE!

THE PROBLEM

When we talk about motivation, we are referring to doing something. In relation to health and fitness, that something is typically setting a goal related to a specific outcome. There are many different goals that can relate to lifestyle and health, so the process of setting these goals will vary from person to person.

What are some of our health and fitness goals?

I have listed some of the most common goals below, and also included some of the reasons why we wish to achieve them.

GOAL	WHY?
To lose weight	Wedding
	Formal event
	Children and family
	Feel more body confident
Get fitter and stronger	Sickness or disease recovery
	Feel better physically and mentally
	Children and family
Recover from an injury	Pain relief
	Perform better
	Allow more training

As we know, if you are highly motivated you are more likely to make a significant commitment to your goal. Of course, you become highly motivated by increasing the two criteria, value and expectancy. To commit to your goals, they need to be important to you, and you need to believe you can succeed.

Why is our motivation for health and fitness goals different?

Women often tell me they find it hard to motivate themselves to achieve their health and fitness goals. As a part of our survey, we asked women some questions about what they find demotivating. The number one reason was that women just like you felt they didn't see results. In fact, 2 in 3 women said that they lose motivation to work out because they don't see enough results, or feel progress fast enough. However, as I said earlier, 3 in 5 women surveyed aren't actually following their entire weekly program, and more than half didn't complete the program.

IT'S A NEGATIVE LOOP

1. DON'T FOLLOW WORKOUT PROGRAMS
2. DON'T SEE RESULTS
3. GET DEMOTIVATED
4. RESTART

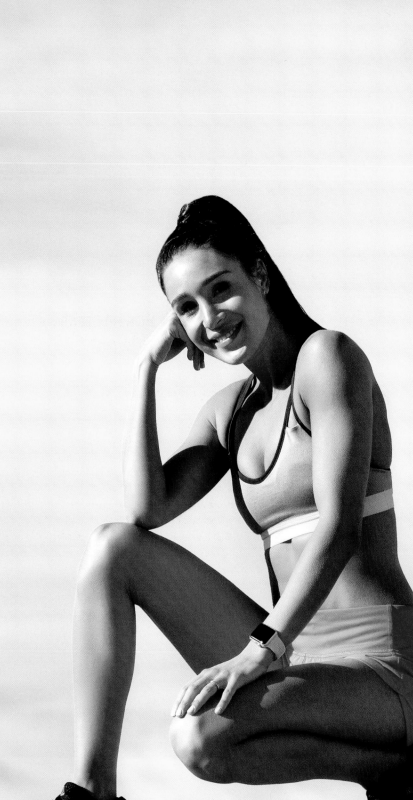

BBG STORIES

"I've always been self-conscious about going to the gym or training in a group where I may be compared to other people or judged. Usually I do not follow plans as I get unmotivated and say I'll just do it later or I'm too busy. Currently I'm on week 6 of your 12-week challenge and love it. I've never stuck something out for so long in terms of fitness. I love that I can feel my body changing already. I do this whilst working full-time and also studying at night school. I have not missed a resistance training session yet but may not always get the chance to do all my cardio workouts. I don't follow the meal plan, however, I do make healthy choices. My family told me I wouldn't be able to do it, it is a sham, just go to the gym. I am prepared to prove them wrong."

Typically when we don't understand why we should do something, we simply don't do it. By not eating the right balance of foods or skipping workouts, *we aren't actually giving ourselves a chance to get the best results possible.* This is ironic, because the data from our survey showed that 63% of women are demotivated when they don't get the results they want.

> Not getting the results they want is the single biggest demotivating factor for women, and only 1 in 3 women say they get the results they expected from a workout program.

One of the main reasons we lose motivation to work out is because it isn't clear to us why doing just one workout a week isn't the same as doing three. Without this understanding, the value of the advice diminishes and we can lose motivation to continue following the plan.

> We can't value something if we don't understand its purpose, and if we don't value it, we are far less motivated to do it.

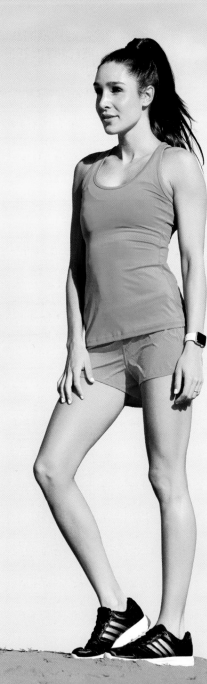

There are four key reasons why we might find it difficult to remain motivated to achieve our health and fitness goals. ① ② ③ ④

FITNESS GOALS ARE HARD TO VALUE BECAUSE THEY CAN'T BE SEEN OR TOUCHED

If you apply the motivation formula (see page 25) to health and fitness goals, you will see some clear reasons why it is hard to achieve and sustain motivation throughout your health and fitness journey. If we look at the value category, you will see some things are easier than others to define a value for.

EASY TO DEFINE VALUE	DIFFICULT TO DEFINE VALUE
Goals associated with:	*Goals associated with:*
1. Injury rehabilitation	1. Feeling better
2. Disease and illness recovery	2. Looking better
3. Pain relief	3. Performing better

Items in the first column are easier to value because they have a defined outcome. If you are sick, injured, or in pain, your outcome is recovery, which is clearly defined as no longer experiencing these issues. However, it is difficult to define a value for feeling better or performing better, because these are less quantifiable. What if we don't look or feel the way we expected? So our key issue here is that it is hard to define a true value for many goals, such as feeling better or being happier. Without a clearly definable value, you can be on a direct path to disappointment as your lack of motivation quickly becomes crippling.

WE FIND IT DIFFICULT TO TRUST THE INFORMATION WE ARE PROVIDED WITH

Although your goals may be clearly defined, the process of achieving them may not be. Most of us have a limited understanding of the human body and the concepts associated with weight loss or rehabilitation, such as how fat loss works, exercise methodologies, nutrition, and dieting. Because of this, most of us try to seek advice online, where there can be many differing opinions, many of which are not based on science.

As a result of this poor-quality information, many failed attempts at weight loss (and other goals associated with health and fitness) are publicly voiced, and this disappointment can cause a loss of faith in the industry as a whole.

In 2015, when I did my first world boot camp tour, the one piece of feedback I continually heard from women after each workout was: "I can't believe your program actually works." My workout and nutrition plans are certainly not the only ones that work, but the women who have used my program voiced a clear lack of faith or understanding in other information available online or from other personal trainers. This lack of knowledge is the exact reason why all my books, eBooks, and my app have such a strong focus on education.

3 OFTEN WHEN YOU EMBARK ON A FITNESS JOURNEY, IT'S SOMETHING YOU HAVEN'T DONE BEFORE

Looking at the concept of expectancy, there are a number of different issues that can affect your fitness journey. As I explained earlier, we are most confident about things we know well, have done before (think competency again), and that are clearly defined.

When you try something new, like following a meal plan or starting a new workout program, it can feel overwhelming because you aren't familiar with it. Once you have a better understanding of the steps on your fitness journey, it can feel less daunting to follow them.

Most of the women surveyed haven't had to undergo rehabilitation after an injury; some have never tried to lose weight before. It is especially easy to see how women who haven't done these things before may feel some anxiety and begin to doubt their ability to succeed.

4 IT IS DIFFICULT TO MEASURE SUCCESS, ESPECIALLY IF SUCCESS IS A FEELING

Although we can measure goals like weight loss or improved physical appearance on the scales or in photos, it can still be difficult to determine progress. As I explained in my previous book, the weight on the scales can go up and down daily, without any actual reduction in fat. This can be a result of changes in your hydration level, food intake, or other factors. Visual progress is quite similar—it can also be subject to the time of day or day of the week. Even bodily functions like your period may impact your visual appearance temporarily; however you may have actually lost a lot of weight prior.

Other goals such as "feeling better" or "being more energetic" are even more difficult to measure because when you feel better it's hard to imagine not feeling the way you do right now. If you can't accurately remember "how you felt" before, it can be difficult for you to compare it to how you're feeling now and measure this improvement.

What this all means

Overall, motivation is often low when it comes to personal health and fitness goals. These goals often don't have finish lines; they can be complicated and based on information we don't trust or completely understand, experiences we haven't had or feelings we can't define. In relation to the motivation formula, this means we don't have a clearly defined set of values for the goal, and we don't have a lot of confidence in our ability to succeed (expectancy). Because both factors that make up motivation are low, our motivation is diminished and this can ultimately result in failure. The positive we can take from this is that we have identified areas of confusion and weakness, which means we can look for a solution that can help improve our motivation and, therefore, our results.

I know this idea can feel a little overwhelming, but now you have a better understanding of how motivation works and you can use this to your advantage. You can become more motivated, stay motivated, and ultimately use this motivation to get better long-term results.

YOUR MIND KNOWS
WHEN IT'S TIME
TO MAKE A
CHANGE. TRUST
YOURSELF.

In the previous section I discussed the issues around maintaining your motivation when it comes to your health and fitness goals. Now that we have identified these problems, we can work towards finding solutions to help improve your motivation levels. This is known as "leveraging your motivation."

In the table below, you will see I have outlined some of the key focus areas and how they can motivate us. I have included examples to help you see how you can use value and expectancy to achieve your goals.

EDUCATION AND KNOWLEDGE

FOCUS AREAS	IMPACTS ON		HOW THIS MOTIVATES US	HOW YOU CAN ACHIEVE THIS
	VALUE	EXPECTANCY		
(a) Why our health is important	V	E	Recognising that our bodies function at their best when healthy, and how this enables us to live a more fulfilled and active life.	Immerse yourself in knowledge. Read my blog articles, watch documentaries, or listen to podcasts about health, fitness, nutrition, and lifestyle.
(b) Basic nutrition and weight loss	V	E	Understanding the fundamentals of good nutrition and how weight loss can contribute to overall good health.	Apply your acquired knowledge about nutrition and weight loss to optimise your diet.
(c) Workout expectations	V	E	An awareness of our body's response to exercise and the positive effects that regular exercise has on our physical and mental state.	The hard work has been done for you here—use my app to structure your workouts through a combination of cardio, resistance, recovery, and rest.

How education can help

The first key focus area outlined previously is education, which is so important to help you make long-term changes to your lifestyle. When we look at the motivation formula, value and expectancy can improve with education.

Value: Being educated about something, such as your health, can make it feel more valuable to you because you understand its purpose. The decisions you make relating to your health are based on the knowledge you have. Without this knowledge, your decisions would be little more than a guess.

Expectancy: The more educated you are about a particular topic, the more confident you feel. If you are educated about health and fitness, weight loss, or rehabilitation, you expect to get better results and feel more confident in your ability to succeed. Perhaps most important, you actually know what to expect.

Let's look at it this way—if someone prescribes to you a certain style of eating and a certain amount of workouts each week, it's fair to say you may not always follow their advice. Of course, there are lots of factors involved, such as your desire, dedication, or energy. But if you have a clear understanding of WHY you are doing these things, based on the knowledge you have gained, you are often more likely to do them because you understand the value they present.

Understanding basic health principles as simple as why we need to eat a certain amount of food justifies why we should eat it. The idea of understanding exercise output requirements makes the concept of working out a goal, not a chore. This awareness relates to your health and fitness goals or health and fitness activities.

PLANNING

FOCUS AREAS	IMPACTS ON		HOW THIS MOTIVATES US	HOW YOU CAN ACHIEVE THIS
	VALUE	EXPECTANCY		
(a) Define your goals	V		Defining what you want to achieve by simply writing it down or verbalising it will make it real for you and attach value to it.	Create a mood board for inspiration, then sit down and reflect on where you are now and where you want to be—then write this all down!
(b) Define your "why?"	V		Understanding why you wish to achieve something will give it significance and increase its value to you. Try to focus on the emotional benefit most.	Under each of your goals, write the "why." Then ask yourself: am I doing this for ME? Or am I doing it to make OTHER people happy? Delete any goals that are not serving YOU well!
(c) Ensure that it is achievable		E	Having realistic goals that you KNOW are achievable can help put you in a positive mindframe and can increase your expectancy.	From your list of goals remaining, prioritise them and then reflect on whether you can do them all in your current schedule.
(d) Set a timeframe	V		Having a goal which has a defined end point gives you something to strive for.	Will your goal be achieved in 3, 6, or 12 months? Remember that you need to be patient with yourself and allow time to see progress.
(e) Break it down and define your deliverables ▪ *How many workouts?* ▪ *Which foods?* ▪ *How much sleep?*		E	Breaking down a big goal gives you clarity on where to start and the best way to manage the process.	Break your goal down into small, manageable steps (i.e. what are you going to do each week/fortnight to help you achieve your goal?) In my app, I break down my programs into 12 individual weeks. Each week I specify how many and what type of workouts you need to complete, plus provide food recommendations for you to get the most out of my program.

FOCUS AREAS	IMPACTS ON		HOW THIS MOTIVATES US	HOW YOU CAN ACHIEVE THIS
	VALUE	EXPECTANCY		
(f) Set mini goals and milestones ▪ *A number of workouts* ▪ *Meal preparation*		E	Having a few milestones (i.e. checkpoints) along the way can help you verify that you are on the right track or whether you need to modify your strategy for the remaining weeks.	Think about ways you can measure progress and write these down. It is good to focus on how you are feeling inside as well—for example, whether you have more energy or are feeling happier. In my program, I recommend that women take a progress photo every 4 weeks so they can see physical improvements over a period of time.
(g) Make an accountability calendar ▪ *Remind yourself to check in*		E	An accountability calendar can help you stay on track with your goals. Seeing each workout planned out is a good reminder, which helps you to build habits.	Using the information in (e) and (f), draw a calendar that has all your workouts and meal prep days mapped out. Placing this calendar in a highly visible area like on your fridge will remind you and may also be a talking point with family members who can help keep you accountable. It's also rewarding to tick or cross off your workouts as you'll be able to see progress, adding to your sense of accomplishment for the week.
(h) Reduce distractions		E	Identifying the factors which prevent us from achieving our goals allows us to implement strategies to help keep us on track.	You might need to make some sacrifices in order to achieve your goals—for example, you might need to cut out some TV time each night.
(i) Celebrate each mini goal (and of course the big goals)	V		Giving yourself something to look forward to can help keep you going when your motivation wanes.	Think about a little reward you can give yourself—a massage or a pamper day is always nice!

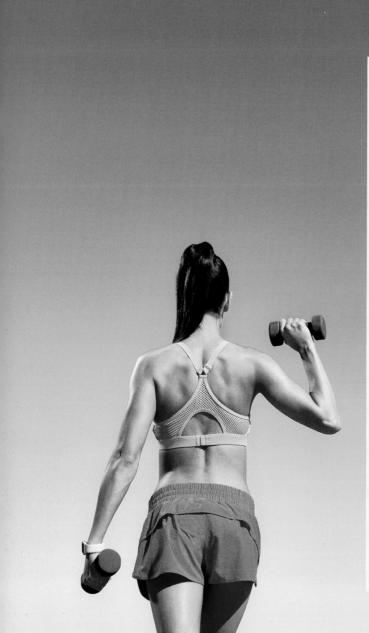

Planning for success

The second key focus area is planning. Once you have acquired the knowledge you need, the next step is to build a plan that optimises your chances of success.

Here are the four elements of effective planning:

1. Set accountability goals
2. Track yourself
3. Divide into tasks and get small wins
4. Reduce distractions or direct negativity

I have always found creating lists hugely beneficial, and many of my clients also find this to be the case. On the next page, I have provided a checklist you can use (or download online) to fill in when you need a motivation lift. It is important that you fill out the entire checklist, and be sure to refer to the table on the previous page to see examples of how you can increase your value or expectancy. The checklist is designed to help you focus on ways to make yourself motivated, and stay motivated. As you know, while your motivation is high, you are more likely to succeed.

I fill in my checklist then set a 2-week reminder to check in on it and update it where necessary. If I start becoming demotivated, it can be as simple as swapping some items in and out to refresh my motivation level.

PLANNING YOUR GOALS CHECKLIST

Below is a checklist that can help you to build a plan for reaching your goals. You can download a copy of this checklist by visiting kaylaitsines.com/28dayguide/book2/goals

What is your goal?	I want to feel better and lose some weight. I think losing 7 pounds will help me to feel better about myself.
What are two things you will do to increase your value? (See the previous tables)	Learn more about the positive effects exercise has on my body, which I can use to remind myself why I am doing this, and that it will work. Celebrate my achievements by having a massage.
What are two things you will do to increase your expectancy? (See the previous tables)	Understand how many workouts and recovery sessions I should be doing each week. Plan my weekly workouts and slot them into my calendar.
How will you measure success?	I want to feel and look better, therefore I will take progress photos and waist measurements, and weigh myself.
How often will you check progress?	Every 14 days.
When do you want to achieve the goal?	After 10 weeks.
What do you need to do to put yourself in the best position to achieve this goal?	Follow my weekly workout and diet guidelines.

SUMMING UP MOTIVATION

1 Motivation is affected by how much you value a goal and how confident you are that you can succeed.

2 We often have low motivation for health and fitness goals because these goals are complex, difficult to measure, and full of processes and experiences that are foreign.

3 With more knowledge about a given activity, we can be more motivated because we understand the process and value the outcome more.

4 Through some strategic planning and answering some important questions you can significantly increase your motivation and in turn the likelihood for success.

5 With these strategies you can expect to get the results you deserve.

6 Relying on only motivation to maintain your health can be unreliable, as your motivations may change over time.

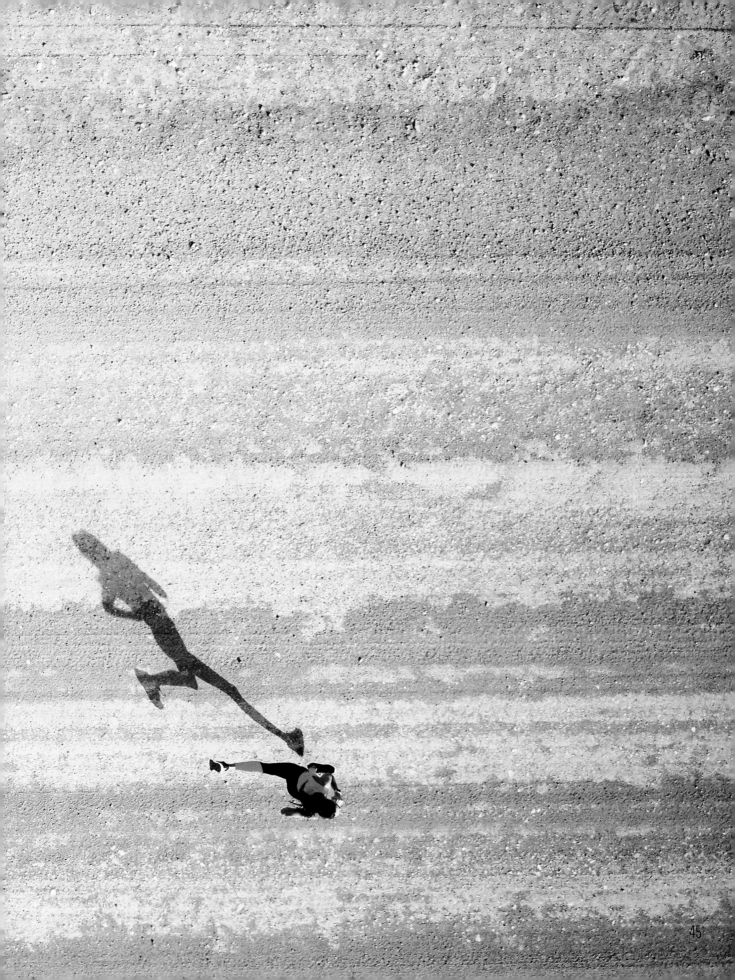

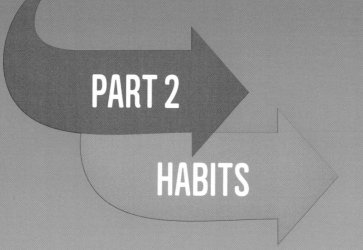

PART 2

HABITS

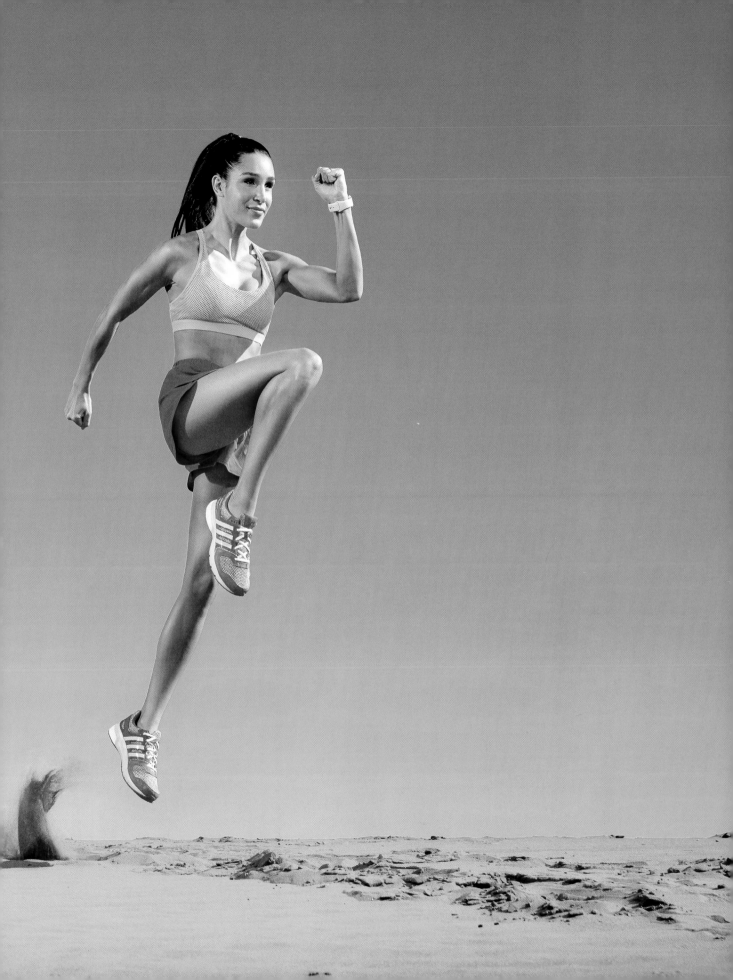

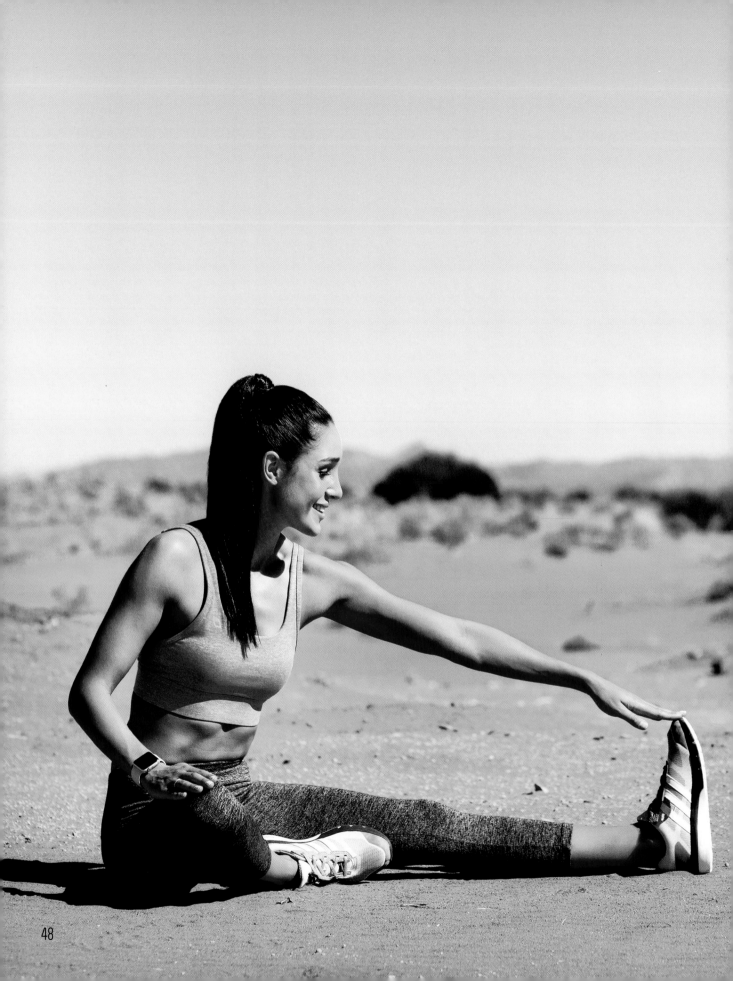

HABITS

I want to help as many women as possible achieve their ideal body, confidence, and happiness, for life.

You'll notice that I've added "for life." As I said earlier, I want long-term life-changing results for women. While motivation is an integral part of success in any area of life, I think that to ultimately obtain long-term success, motivation needs to be combined with good habits and discipline. The discipline of good habits can help you keep going during times when your motivation wavers.

THE MOTIVATION AND HABIT JOURNEY

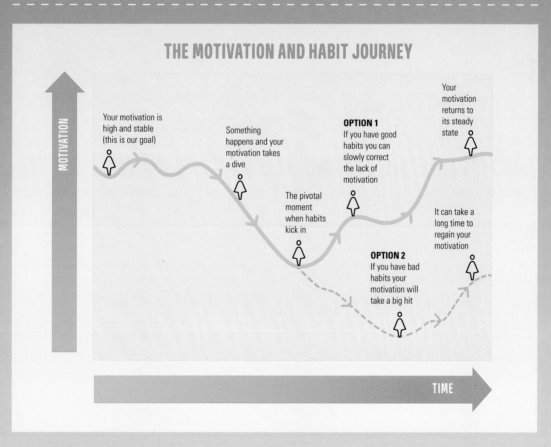

MOTIVATION

Your motivation is high and stable (this is our goal)

Something happens and your motivation takes a dive

The pivotal moment when habits kick in

OPTION 1
If you have good habits you can slowly correct the lack of motivation

Your motivation returns to its steady state

It can take a long time to regain your motivation

OPTION 2
If you have bad habits your motivation will take a big hit

TIME

In order for me to expand my skills as a personal trainer, on top of motivation, I have spent a lot of time learning about habits. Most important, how you can create good habits, and how *you can fix bad ones*.

The impact habits have on your life is huge and undeniable. It is likely you often move, act, and react in very habitual ways without even realising it. It has been fundamental to my success as a trainer that I was able to help other women, just like you, to understand how and why you are habitual and how to leverage this behaviour for your benefit.

MAKE AN EFFORT TO CREATE BETTER HABITS FOR YOURSELF. TODAY. TOMORROW. EVERY DAY.

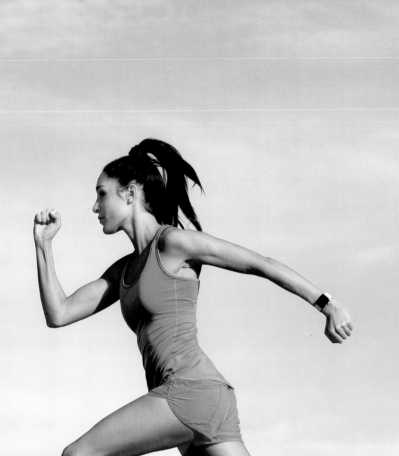

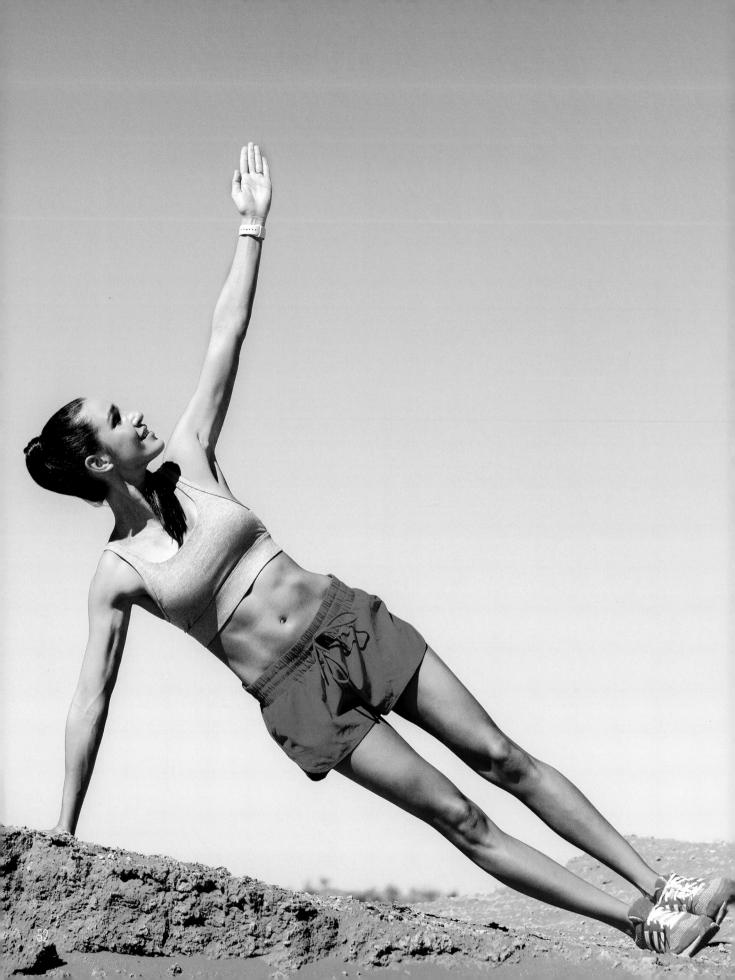

habit

noun

a settled or regular tendency or practice, especially one that is hard to give up.

A habit is a clearly defined set of events or actions that you take based on a certain cue and reward. This is typically an unconscious process, meaning that you aren't properly aware you are doing it. The process of recognising the cue, and reacting to it, is usually automatic.

Habits can be very useful behavioural mechanisms because they make you a little predictable and consistent. When you have the right habits, they can automate positive behaviour, which can influence your life in a very beneficial way.

The habit loop is a good example:

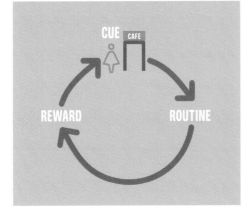

The **cue**, or trigger, is something that initiates the habitual behaviour or routine. Some examples of cues can be:

- A location
- A time of the day
- An emotional state
- A thought
- A belief
- Other people

The **routine**, or habitual behaviour, is what you do as a result of the cue. Examples include:

- Setting an alarm for the morning when you get into bed each night
- Taking the stairs instead of the escalator or lift
- Drinking water instead of soft drink

The **reward** is the positive feeling that generates the automation of our behaviour, which creates the loop. This positive feeling could be associated with many things and can be as simple as:

- Having more time because you decided to wake up earlier using an alarm
- Being fitter from being more physically active
- Feeling more energetic from meal prepping and eating healthier food

Being able to break the structure of habits down into three key elements is a fundamental step to success. You can use your new understanding of these three elements to help recognise faults in your existing behaviour and habits, analyse opportunities to improve existing habits, and create new healthy habits for your future.

Why are habits important?

Habits are an important part of our daily behaviour and can fundamentally alter the outcome, for better or worse, of most things we commit time to. This includes our health and lifestyle choices. Our habitual behaviour is triggered by cues in our environment and our personality. Because of this our habits automate a significant portion of our behaviour. Whether it be putting a jacket on when we are cold, or eating chocolate when we feel sad, we are creatures of habit through and through. The good thing about this is because you can leverage habits (i.e., influence or control them), you can provide yourself a structure for consistency which can help to create positive results.

A collection of habits can work together to form a healthy living system. Think of it as a system to manage your lifestyle. My many years' experience working with women just like you has taught me a lot of things.

One positive lesson I've learned is once you create your system, it is very easy to maintain. You can use a collection of cues and triggers to automate, and most important, sustain your positive behaviour.

It is very common for women to associate emotions with habits—for example, reaching for "comfort food" if you are upset after having an argument with a loved one. Obviously this emotional association can go both ways—it can be good for good habits and bad for bad habits. If you are proactive, and make your habits deliberately, having an emotional attachment to things can be a very positive and powerful tool. All you need now is a great reason to get started. When my clients tell me, "I just don't know how to get started," I tell them:

THE ONLY
LIMITATIONS
ARE THOSE
YOU PLACE ON
YOURSELF.

How can we break bad habits?

The great thing about understanding how habits work is knowing that they can be leveraged. You can understand your good and bad habits, and you can get rid of the bad ones, improve the good ones, and start to create new habits. Before forming any new habits, I think the best first step is to identify what your existing bad habits are and understand the underlying cause. Three ways to identify your bad habits are:

1. CREATE A NOTE FILE TO IDENTIFY YOUR HABITS

When training clients face-to-face, I've found identifying bad habits is very helpful for making behaviour changes. Most of us have phones on us during the day. Create a new note file in your phone and write down different behaviours or moments during the day that make you feel negatively about your health, your physical appearance, your confidence, or lifestyle. As you note each one down, try to identify what the trigger was.

See the example on the opposite page; this table is also available online.

Your triggers will be easy to identify, and sometimes surprising because they are usually quite obvious. Maybe you read a certain magazine and instantly feel overwhelmingly insecure about your body. Maybe your friend (who seems to eat whatever she wants and still maintain her health and body) eats a chocolate bar, so you feel irritated and eat one too. Or maybe while waiting in line at the supermarket, you impulse-buy an unhealthy snack.

Almost all psychologists, personal trainers, and life coaches will tell you the same thing: in order to overcome a bad habit, a negative emotion or similar, you need to understand WHY it has become a habit. Using this table and the simple concept of taking notes will help you identify your bad habits and the cues that trigger them.

2. REMIND YOURSELF TO TRACK HOW REGULARLY IT HAPPENS

It is important to track how regularly this behaviour occurs, like a tally, because the more frequently this behaviour occurs, the more notes you take. Taking those notes regularly places the issue at the front of your mind. Becoming more and more aware of those habits is a big part of taking steps to deal with them and replacing them with better thoughts and behaviour.

Even though you may commit to taking notes, you might forget, because taking notes is a habit in itself too. The best way to avoid forgetting is to give yourself a reminder. So, in your daily calendar, add reminders to take some time to reflect on what has happened during the day. If anything comes to mind that you think was negative and you can avoid, or was something you would deem a bad habit, add it to your notes.

Taking five minutes out of your day to note these behaviours will place them at the front of your mind, which can make this sort of thinking stick. It may be just what you need to remember to start changing those habits, and avoiding those triggers. This puts you on the road to success!

3. REMOVE THE CUE OR TRIGGER

Now that you are regularly identifying and noting bad habits and what makes you feel insecure, the path to feeling better is simple. These habits and issues will now be at the front of your mind and you already know how to remove or alter the cue, or prepare for it.

The easiest way to avoid getting burnt is by not touching the fire. But when you go shopping, you can't avoid the checkout. In situations where the environment is the trigger, but it's unavoidable, you simply need to be aware of it. For example, with the shopping scenario, you could go at quieter times so you spend less time waiting at the checkout. If you can't go at a quieter time, only take enough money with you for the exact items that you need. You can't spend what you don't have on you.

UNDERSTANDING YOUR HABITS

To help you identify and understand some of your habits, answer the questions in the below table.
You can download this table at kaylaitsines.com/28dayguide/book2/habits

What happened and how did you feel?	How often does this happen?	What triggered it? What were you doing at the time? (activity, environment, people, object)
1. Late-night snacking is making me frustrated because I am working out hard during the day and feel like I ruin it each night by eating chocolate or lollies in bed.	Three nights this week.	I find myself snacking late at night while I watch Suits in bed with my boyfriend. We often find we're reaching for unhealthy snacks during the ad breaks.
2. I feel annoyed that I impulse-bought a cupcake while grabbing a coffee before my meeting. I should have had a healthy snack ready instead.	Once this week.	I bought the cupcake because I didn't bring any healthy snacks with me and I knew I would get hungry. I was stressed about the meeting and didn't take the time to look for a healthier option. I wasn't organised and prepared.
3.		
4.		
5.		

COMMON HABITS

To help kickstart improving your habits, I want to show you some that are very common among women. Chances are you may relate to some of these situations or feelings. If you do, add them to your list of notes and track them.

NUTRITION HABITS

HABIT	TRIGGER	REALITY
Not drinking enough water	Reaching for soft drinks or juices instead of water, or not carrying water with you.	Being dehydrated is one of the most common forms of discomfort. Try to carry a water bottle with you each day and sip continually throughout the day. Simple reminders a few times a day can help you. The Sweat app has a tracker for this.
Binge-eating	Feeling stressed or anxious, or feeling bored.	Binge-eating is more often associated with emotions than hunger. Try to find a way to distract yourself, such as going for a quick walk, talking to a friend or having a cup of tea. Practise self-care habits (such as yoga or meditation) to help you deal with stress or anxiety.
Skipping breakfast	Sleeping in and not having time to prepare and eat breakfast, or not feeling hungry when you wake.	This may be linked to sleep; make sure you are waking up with enough time to have breakfast. You may not feel hungry when you first get up, so try making something healthy to take with you to eat once you feel ready. Have breakfast foods at home and try to choose simple ones (at least 2–3 different types means you can switch it up so you don't get bored).
Snacking on unhealthy foods	Feeling stressed and reaching for comfort foods, or not having enough time to prepare healthy snacks, or impulse-buying.	If you prep and eat healthy meals and snacks, you should find yourself feeling less hungry. If you still like grazing, pack healthy snacks to take with you wherever you go, so you won't feel tempted by unhealthy snacks.
Eating a lot of fast food	Not planning meals in advance. Waiting until you are hungry to eat. Not food-shopping on a regular basis.	Fast food is almost always eaten as a convenience food so the easiest way to fix this is to not have the need to conveniently eat. Try to work on being organised and prep healthy meals and snacks in advance so you always have suitable healthy options. Packing healthy snacks can help you avoid reaching for fast food.
Ordering unhealthy food when dining out	Being distracted and not reviewing the menu for healthy options. Not wanting to be singled out for choosing healthier dining options.	Eating out doesn't have to mean high-fat fast food. This can be a really good opportunity to taste and learn new healthy dishes you can make at home. If dining out is your only form of indulging, then still make use of it for that purpose, but don't go over the top. Try and keep it balanced with a good mix of protein, carbs, fats, etc.

EXERCISE HABITS

HABIT	TRIGGER	REALITY
Not training because you are tired	Not allowing adequate rest time during the week, having a busy schedule or feeling mentally tired due to stress.	You know your body best, and whether you are physically tired or using it as an excuse. Be disciplined about your decisions. Rest time is important if you are unwell or your body is fatigued; you are in the best position to judge that. Remember that exercise can be helpful for managing stress, and the rush of endorphins (feel-good chemicals released by your brain) can make a big difference to your mood and how you are feeling. Following a healthy, balanced diet can provide sufficient energy and nutrients to help your body perform at its peak.
Not resting enough between workouts	Feeling the need to make up on missed training sessions or thinking you'll get better results with more.	One of the fastest ways to get an injury or to slow down progress is to overtrain; it puts extra stress on your body. Use a weekly workout planner and follow it to make sure you aren't putting excess strain on your body. Allocated rest and recovery time in your planner is a reminder to give your body time to repair itself.
Not working out when you get your period	Feeling discomfort or bloating, mood changes, tiredness, or period pain.	You may still be able to train when your period starts, even if it is a gentle walk. Listen to your body; if you feel as though you can't physically train, a rest day is okay. Don't use it as an excuse though; YOU know your body best and know when you physically aren't able to do your normal workout. Try gentler exercises instead, such as going for a walk, yoga, or pilates. For some women, periods can be debilitating, making it hard to work out. It may be wise to speak with a healthcare professional about exercising safely.

LIFESTYLE HABITS

HABIT	TRIGGER	REALITY
Not getting enough sleep	Feeling anxious or overwhelmed, having a busy schedule, or working irregular hours.	Getting enough sleep is a must for a healthy lifestyle, so you will need to prioritise sleep over other things (for example, watching late-night TV shows or playing with your phone in bed). Where possible, follow a regular routine before bed to prepare your body for sleep. Use an alarm for both going to bed AND waking up. Try to find ways to help manage your stress or anxiety, such as getting regular exercise, practising meditation, or keeping a journal.
Social over-drinking	Socialising with friends over drinks, or trying to keep up with friends who drink regularly.	I don't personally drink alcohol but understand and respect that a lot of women do. The issue isn't necessarily drinking, but often "overdrinking." To prevent this, set yourself a limit prior to going out. Once you reach your limit, replace alcoholic drinks with water or infused sparkling water (fruit juice or low-sugar soft drinks may also be okay in moderation).
Overusing pain relief	Injuring yourself, or not spending time on recovery or resting to give your body the chance to repair itself.	When you are injured or sick, pain relief can be helpful. However, it can quickly become something people rely on. Pain relief can sometimes be used as a form of mental relief, rather than for physical pain, which can be a bad habit. If you have persistent pain or a recurring injury, it is best to see a healthcare professional to diagnose and get help managing the problem.

Having bad habits shouldn't make you feel as though anything is hopeless. Using the process outlined in the previous table, you can clearly identify and track your bad habits. Once you find the cue or trigger for the behaviour, you can work on breaking the habit by becoming accountable.

BBG STORIES

"I've struggled for a long time to get motivated to lose weight. Ever since I was 12, I would tell myself, "Okay this summer you're going to work out!" Then when summer came all I would do is pig out on food, and then the endless cycle of telling myself I'd try again that summer would begin. I've finally realised I don't need to wait till summer to begin my journey, and since I started in January I've lost 12 pounds. Now it's not a lot, but it's a really good start for me. Some days I get frustrated because I don't see the results I'm looking for, but that's okay because I know it's a weight-loss journey not a race! This is the beginning of a whole new lifestyle change."

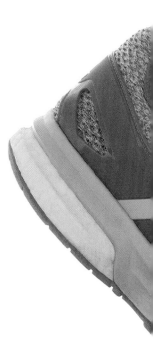

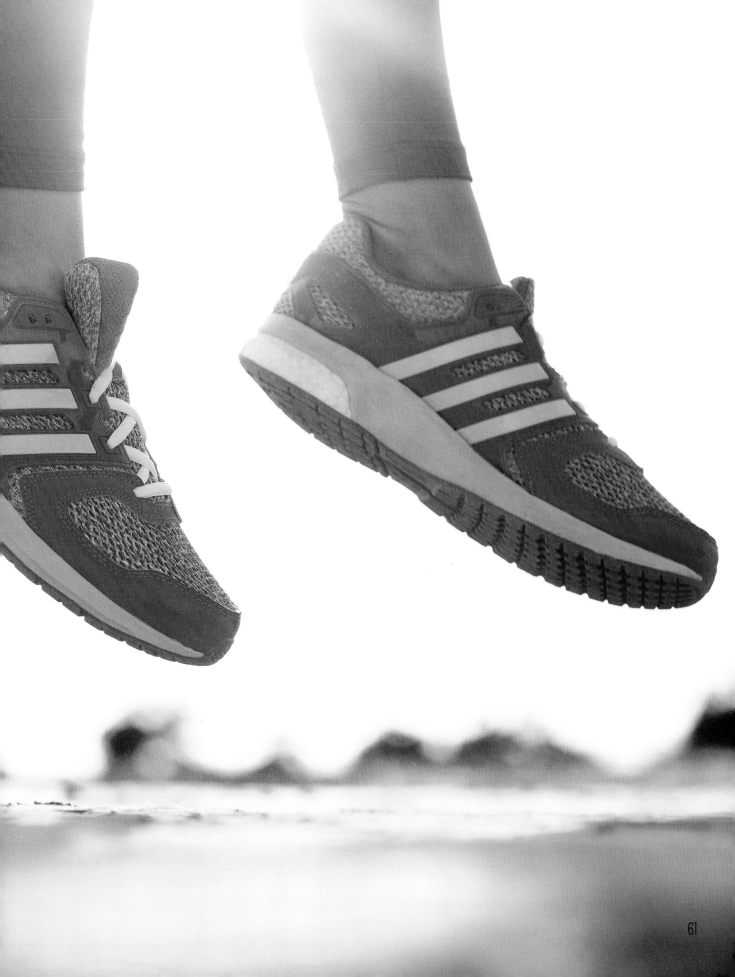

How can we form new habits?

In the same way you can break old or bad habits, you can also deliberately create new and effective ones to improve your health. However, before doing so it is very important to make sure the new behaviours you are attempting to learn are ones you actually want to keep. The easiest way to figure out the right habits to build is to identify the ones that will have the biggest impact on the success of your health journey. Whether your goal is improved fitness, weight loss, increased strength, or just feeling better in general through improved health, all of the following will apply, and, therefore, I think it is best if you focus on making habits surrounding these key areas. For me, these are probably three of the most important habits that exist in these areas.

1. REST: SLEEP SCHEDULE ⇨ GETTING ENOUGH SLEEP

Part of allowing yourself to do the things you want to do is having the energy to do so, which largely comes from being rested. I have found having a sleep schedule really helps remind me to try and ensure I get 7 to 8 hours of quality sleep. For me, this is as simple as using alarms to keep a consistent bedtime and waking time. However, other useful strategies you should consider include: reducing screen time at night, reducing your alcohol intake, creating a nighttime ritual to wind down, and removing distractions from your bedroom. Prioritising sleep is important for overall well-being, and sleep trackers can help you identify whether you are truly getting enough quality sleep.

2. NUTRITION: MEAL PREP ⇨ EATING THE RIGHT TYPES AND AMOUNTS OF FOODS

Along with getting enough sleep, a good diet is a fundamental factor when considering your energy levels, as well as many other areas of your health. In my experience, regardless of the diet you "follow," if you don't observe the principles of the eating plan, it can affect your ability to reach the desired outcome. For most women, the first step to consistent healthy eating is learning about the importance of meal prep. When you prepare meals in advance, you are committing to eating whatever it is you make the next day. As you make a continual effort to eat the healthy meals you prepare, you actually follow the diet. This means you are consistently eating nutritious meals that provide you with energy.

In order for meal prep to work, you will need to organise yourself in a way that best suits your personal circumstances. For example, do you want to meal prep for the entire week (where you will freeze some portions)? Or perhaps you only want to meal prep for 2–3 days of the week when you know your schedule is crazy and you need to have healthy meals ready to go. Once you have worked this out you can establish how many portions you need to create of your recipe(s) and then write a shopping list (see pages 101–107 and my downloadables). I also recommend that you allocate time for shopping and cooking in your schedule to ensure success.

3. FITNESS: WORKOUT PLANNING ⇨ MAKING TIME FOR WORKOUTS AND RECOVERY

Finally, if you have all the energy you need, and are well rested, you can work out. I bet after reading the first two points you can probably guess I am going to say "create a workout schedule." As silly as it may sound, it's true! My recommendation is that you book time in your week, every week, to exercise. A lot of people say, "I know what I need to do, I will get my workouts in, trust me." But the truth is actually that 60% of women surveyed mentioned they don't end up getting the results they desire, and 60% of women also confess to not completing all of the workouts suggested in their workout guides. I bet you can also guess the biggest reason why women aren't getting all their workouts in: because of "no time." More often than not, "having no time" really just translates to "you didn't make time."

Forming healthy habits

HABIT	TRIGGER	OTHER TIPS
To walk more during the day	Add reminders. Use a step counter or step tracker to see how much you actually walk throughout the day.	Challenge friends to use step trackers with you. Find alternative routes to work or college.
Eat breakfast daily	Use a food logger to see your food intake throughout each day. Add reminders to prepare the night before and wake up on time.	Have multiple different breakfast options at home. Prepare what you can the night before.
Drink more water	Use a water tracker to see how much you actually drink each day. Add reminders to check progress during and at the end of the day.	Don't just drink water; try alternatives such as tea, aminos, and more. Try adding slices of fruit to your water for extra flavour. Eat water-rich foods to increase your hydration levels too, such as cucumber, watermelon, and lettuce.
Eat healthy snacks	Use a food logger to monitor your food intake. Add reminders to prepare snacks the night before.	Find healthy snack ideas to try (see the recipe chapter on page 108 for mine!). Swap recipes or snack ideas with friends. Add snack preparation into your meal prep routine. Keep some healthy snacks at work or in your bag to eat on the go.
Spending time on recovery	Add stretching and foam-rolling to your workout planner. Stretch before and after each workout.	Keep your foam roller nearby so you can use it anytime.
Develop a bedtime routine	Set reminders to get to bed at a regular time.	Spend a few minutes before bed making a note of your to-do list. Try to eat a few hours before going to bed so you are not sleeping on a full stomach. Try meditation to calm your mind before bed if you find it hard to wind down.

SUMMING UP HABITS

 1 Habits are a clearly defined set of behaviours that take place based on a certain cue and a proposed reward.

 2 Habits help to automate your behaviour (whether good or bad), provide a structure for consistency, and can be the reason you keep doing things.

3 Understanding habits allows you to work on decreasing your negative behaviours and increasing your positive habits.

 4 You can form new habits if you break things down and make yourself accountable.

5 Habits can be the foundation for your sustained success with health.

6 For your best chance at success you should focus on creating habits around sleep, food, and exercise.

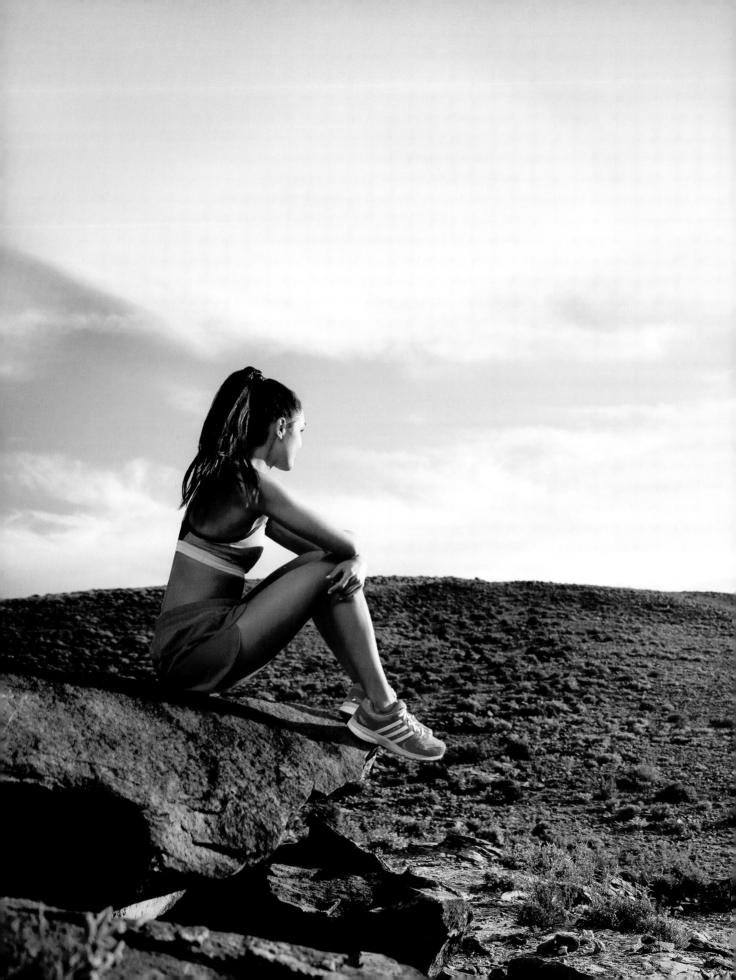

PART 3

NUTRITION

AND MEAL PLANS

"GOOD" NUTRITION

"Good" nutrition means eating a wide variety of healthy foods from all of the six main food groups. Each of these food groups has its own unique set of nutrients and it is important to eat foods from all of these groups (except in cases where there is an allergy or intolerance), and in the right amounts. They can provide you with enough energy to fuel your lifestyle, plus the amounts of vitamins and minerals needed to allow your body to function at its best.

GRAINS

6 RECOMMENDED
DAILY SERVINGS

Grain-based foods such as rice, quinoa, oats, muesli, breads, and cereals are your body's primary source of carbohydrates and preferred source of energy. These foods also provide other key nutrients, including protein, fibre, B group vitamins, and minerals such as iron, zinc, and magnesium.

VEGETABLES AND LEGUMES

5 RECOMMENDED
DAILY SERVINGS

Vegetables are nutrient-dense and relatively low in energy. This means they contain lots of good stuff but don't provide many calories, which is great if you have a big appetite. What makes them particularly beneficial is that they contain an abundance of vitamins and minerals, fibre, and a range of phytochemicals (chemicals naturally found in plants that can help your body combat disease). Legumes, such as chickpeas and lentils, are a valuable source of protein.

LEAN MEAT, SEAFOOD, EGGS, AND MEAT ALTERNATIVES

2½ RECOMMENDED
DAILY SERVINGS

This food group typically includes red meat (beef, lamb), poultry (chicken and turkey), seafood, eggs, and legumes. These foods are your body's best source of protein. They also provide you with a long list of minerals (including iodine, iron, and zinc), vitamins, and healthy fats. For vegetarians or vegans, this group primarily consists of eggs, legumes, tofu, and tempeh.

DAIRY PRODUCTS AND ALTERNATIVES

2½ RECOMMENDED
DAILY SERVINGS

Milk, cheese, and yoghurt, and their dairy-free alternatives, are particularly rich in calcium, a mineral that is important for bone and muscle health. These foods also provide your body with protein, iodine, vitamin A, vitamin D, riboflavin (vitamin B2), vitamin B12, and zinc.

FRUIT

2 RECOMMENDED
DAILY SERVINGS

Fruit is a rich source of vitamins, including vitamin C and folate. It also provides you with potassium, fibre, and carbohydrates in the form of natural sugars. Fruit skins (the edible ones) are especially high in fibre.

HEALTHY FATS

2 RECOMMENDED
DAILY SERVINGS

Foods such as avocados, nuts, and seeds provide you with essential fatty acids the body cannot produce on its own. These fatty acids supply the body with energy and contribute to the overall structure and function of your cells.

Nutrients: the building blocks to good health

We all need adequate nutrients to keep our bodies working optimally, and a well-balanced diet provides this. However, many people don't get the right amounts of nutrients, and there can be many reasons for this. You might prefer to eat processed foods, you might have an intolerance to wheat or dairy, or you might choose to follow a vegetarian diet. Any of these things can cause malnutrition (i.e. poor nutrition) and it is important to make adjustments to ensure that a good balance of nutrients is maintained.

My meal plans use the amounts recommended by the Australian Guide to Healthy Eating at eatforhealth.gov.au, allowing you to eat a delicious range of foods knowing that you are comfortably meeting your energy and nutrient requirements. (Other countries will have their own healthy eating guidelines and if outside of Australia you should consult your local authority.)

The nutrients found in whole foods play a massive part in keeping your body strong and performing at its best. Over the next pages I'll explain the main players. Once you're familiar with these and the role they play in keeping your body functioning optimally, you'll have a whole new appreciation of what's in your food.

AT ANY TIME,
YOU CAN MAKE A
CHANGE FOR THE
BETTER. JUST
START WHERE
YOU ARE.

MACRONUTRIENTS

"Macro" means large, and macronutrients are those your body needs in large amounts. Carbohydrates, protein, fats and fibre are the macronutrients that we need to consume every day in large amounts in order to stay healthy. These macronutrients provide your body with the fundamentals it needs for growth, metabolism and healthy body function. They also provide you with energy (calories), although in differing amounts (see below).

As well as this, each macronutrient has different effects on satiety (the feeling of "fullness" you get after a meal). Protein has the strongest effect on satiety, followed by carbohydrates and fats respectively. In other words, if you were to eat exactly the same amount of protein, carbs, and fats, it's the protein food that would make you feel fuller for longer. However, as you'll see, each of these macronutrients plays an important role in the overall functioning of your body.

ONE GRAM OF:

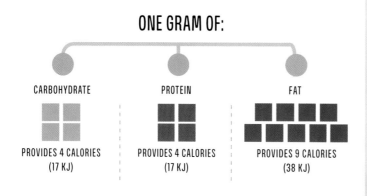

CARBOHYDRATE	PROTEIN	FAT
PROVIDES 4 CALORIES (17 KJ)	PROVIDES 4 CALORIES (17 KJ)	PROVIDES 9 CALORIES (38 KJ)

FAD DIETS

Women who follow extreme (very low fat or very low carb) diets or "fad" diets, which restrict the intake of one or more macronutrients, can find this may have detrimental effects on their health. Although these diets may cause you to lose weight to begin with, this is not always sustainable because of the impact they have on your overall health. I have found that women who follow these types of diets often end up giving up and eventually regain most (if not all) of the weight that they previously lost.

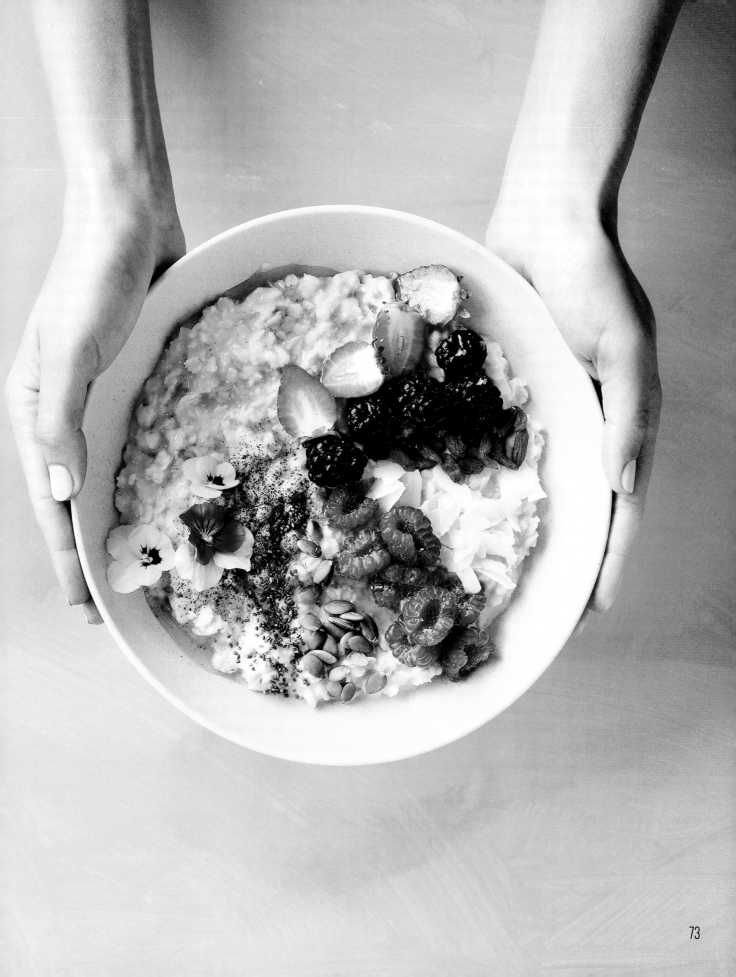

CARBOHYDRATES

Carbohydrates provide your body with glucose, the preferred source of energy for your brain and muscles. The best sources of carbohydrates are grain-based foods such as bread, oats, muesli, rice, and quinoa (whole wheat or whole grain versions are even more beneficial as they are broken down slowly by the body and provide you with longer-lasting energy). Other sources of carbohydrates include fruits, vegetables, legumes, and dairy. Foods rich in carbohydrates also contain generous quantities of essential vitamins and minerals.

PROTEIN

Protein is important for the growth, maintenance, and repair of the body's cells, and provides the building blocks for a number of structures within the human body. Proteins are made up of chains of smaller units called amino acids and there are nine amino acids that can only be obtained from your diet. Animal foods such as red meat, poultry, fish, milk, and eggs naturally contain all nine essential amino acids and are considered complete proteins. Plant foods such as beans, peas, and lentils also contain protein, but they are considered incomplete proteins because they lack one or more of the essential amino acids.

As mentioned previously, protein generally leaves us more satisfied than carbohydrates or fats, which means that including protein foods at every meal may help reduce hunger and snacking. When choosing sources of protein to include in your meals, I recommend ones that are low in saturated and trans fats.

Protein powder should not be used to replace protein foods, but as an optional addition to meals and snacks to boost protein intake.

FATS

Fats play a number of important roles in our body. They help cushion our organs, contribute to the structure of cells, promote growth and development, and allow the body to absorb essential vitamins (A, D, E, and K). In recent decades, fats have acquired a bad reputation, but they have an essential role to play in our diets. Not all fats are created equal though, and we categorise them as "good" fats and "bad" fats. It is important that you consume the right types of fats and in the right proportions.

"Good" fats are monounsaturated and polyunsaturated fats, and are found in vegetables, nuts, seeds, and fish. They are important for reducing LDL (bad) cholesterol, lowering the risk of heart disease and stroke, and promoting a healthy brain and joints. It is recommended that you incorporate "good" fats in your allowable daily fat intake limit.

"Bad" fats are trans and saturated fats, and it is recommended that you limit your intake of these. Trans fats are of particular concern because they elevate LDL (bad) cholesterol and reduce HDL (good) cholesterol levels, which together can increase your risk of heart attack or stroke. Trans fats do not naturally occur in many foods, but can be produced during food manufacturing and processing, so you can avoid them by steering clear of processed foods and choosing wholefoods instead. Saturated fats are most commonly found in meat and dairy foods. These fats are also believed to increase our risk of heart disease by increasing our levels of LDL (bad) cholesterol, so it is recommended that you limit your intake by choosing lean cuts of meat and reduced-fat dairy products.

FIBRE

Fibre is an indigestible form of carbohydrate that has an important role in keeping the digestive system healthy. While it doesn't provide your body with a lot of energy in the same way as carbohydrates, proteins, and fats do, there is a lot of research to suggest that a diet rich in fibre can help protect you against a number of lifestyle diseases, such as cancer, heart disease, obesity, and type 2 diabetes.

Fibre has a cleansing effect and helps food move through our digestive system, preventing the gut wall from being exposed to harmful substances, which can reduce the risk of digestive diseases, such as colon cancer. Fibre can also help to eliminate excess cholesterol via the digestive system, which can help reduce your risk of heart disease. As fibre has quite a complex structure, good bacteria (yes, bacteria can be good!) in your digestive system are needed to help break it down. By consuming fibre regularly, you can help to promote the growth of good bacteria, which play an important role in maintaining digestive and overall health. It also helps regulate the release of insulin after you have eaten. This helps you feel full between meals, preventing overeating and unhealthy snacking, which ultimately helps you maintain a healthy weight.

The National Health and Medical Research Council (NHMRC) of Australia recommends that women eat a minimum of 1 ounce of fibre every day. This can quite easily be achieved by eating a diet that is rich in fruits, vegetables, and cereal grains (particularly wholegrain versions), which is reflected in my meal plans. However, if you eat a high-fibre diet, it's also important that you drink lots of water too, as this will help the fibre work its magic within your digestive system!

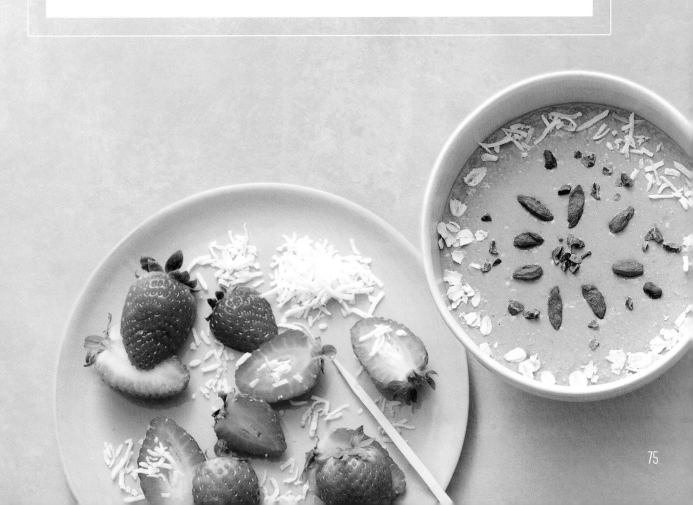

MICRONUTRIENTS

Vitamins and minerals are considered micronutrients. When compared to macronutrients, these are required by the the body in smaller amounts, but are still very important to your overall health. Vitamins are substances that are produced by plants or animals, while minerals are substances found within the soil that are then absorbed by plants or eaten by animals.

- -

IRON

Iron is a mineral whose main role is to act as a key component of haemoglobin, the substance which transports oxygen around the body. Iron deficiency is common in women, as much of our body's iron is found in the blood and we do lose a small amount once a month with our period. As iron is important for energy and delivery of oxygen, it is particularly important for women who get heavy periods to have a steady intake of iron from food sources.

If you don't receive enough iron, in the long term it can result in the gradual depletion of the body's ferritin stores. Once these stores have run out, your body's ability to produce haemoglobin can begin to decrease. Low levels of haemoglobin are usually a sign of late-stage iron deficiency, which is also known as anaemia. The first signs of anaemia may include headaches, tiredness, lack of energy, poor concentration, and frequent infections.

There are two types of iron found in foods: haem iron and non-haem iron. Haem iron is found in red meat and poultry (red meat contains the most haem iron, but is also higher in saturated fats, so it is important to select leaner cuts where possible). Liver and kidney are also rich in iron, but are not necessarily the most popular choices! Non-haem iron can be found in eggs and plant foods, such as breads and cereals, leafy green vegetables, legumes, nuts and nut pastes.

Haem iron is absorbed more readily, which is why you need to eat far more non-haem iron in order to reach the same recommended requirements. The amount of iron you absorb from your food will depend on your body's needs—if you are lacking in iron, your body will generally absorb more.

When trying to incorporate foods that are rich in iron into your diet, it is important to be aware of the way other foods affect your body's ability to absorb it. For example, eating foods high in vitamin C in the same meal can increase absorption of non-haem iron. Some examples of vitamin C–rich foods include citrus fruits, berries, bell peppers, and green vegetables such as broccoli and kale. On the other hand, dairy foods and tannins naturally found in black tea may interfere with the absorption of iron. If you drink black tea regularly, I recommend that you avoid drinking it at meal times and, where possible, make weaker tea or replace with herbal teas. Once again, following the recommended number of servings from each food group can help ensure that you are receiving enough iron from your diet.

CALCIUM

Calcium is an important mineral for the development of healthy bones and teeth. It also plays a role in blood clotting and allows your muscles and nerves to function. The best sources of calcium are dairy products such as milk, cheese, and yoghurt. Small amounts of calcium can also be found in plant foods such as broccoli, chickpeas, dried fruit, and nuts, such as almonds and brazil nuts. If you can't consume dairy products because of an allergy or intolerance, see page 85 for more information on good non-dairy alternatives.

MAGNESIUM

Magnesium is an essential mineral for healthy bones, muscles, and nerves. While calcium is needed to help muscles contract, magnesium helps them relax. This is why magnesium supplements are sometimes used to help reduce headaches that are caused by muscle tension. Magnesium can also help alleviate period symptoms, such as cramps. The best sources of magnesium include leafy green vegetables, legumes, cereals, and nuts. These foods are also high in fibre, so it's a win-win!

VITAMINS

While there are a number of individual vitamins, these can be grouped together based on the role they play in our bodies. For example:

A group vitamins can help maintain eyesight and strengthen your immune system. Sources include eggs, dairy foods, and yellow, orange and green vegetables such as pumpkin, carrot, kale, and spinach.

B group vitamins can help your body convert food into energy, help support your nervous and digestive systems, and aid the production of red blood cells. Sources include meat, fish, poultry, eggs, dairy products, legumes, leafy green vegetables, and some fruits.

Vitamin C is a very powerful antioxidant and can help to strengthen your immune system. It also promotes iron absorption and the production of collagen, which keeps our skin feeling firm and youthful. Sources include citrus fruits, berries, peppers, and green vegetables such as broccoli and kale.

Vitamin D can help our body absorb calcium and phosphorus, two minerals crucial to maintaining bone health. Vitamin D can also help strengthen our immune system and improve mood. While you can get small amounts by eating oily fish and eggs, exposure to sunlight is the best natural source of vitamin D.

Vitamin E is also a powerful antioxidant that helps reduce free-radical damage and inflammation within your body. It can also help promote healthy hair and skin. Some of the best food sources of vitamin E are nuts, seeds, and oils.

Vitamin K plays an important role in blood clotting and maintaining bone health. Sources include leafy green vegetables and fermented foods (such as sauerkraut).

Multivitamin supplements are not the best substitute for a healthy whole food diet, as it is the balanced interplay between the nutrients (both macro and micro) in whole foods that provides the most benefit.

Supplements should only be used to complement a healthy, balanced diet. There may be some cases where using supplements is necessary because your body is lacking in certain nutrients and isn't able to get them from food alone. However, in these cases it is best to speak with your healthcare professional to ensure this is correctly implemented and managed.

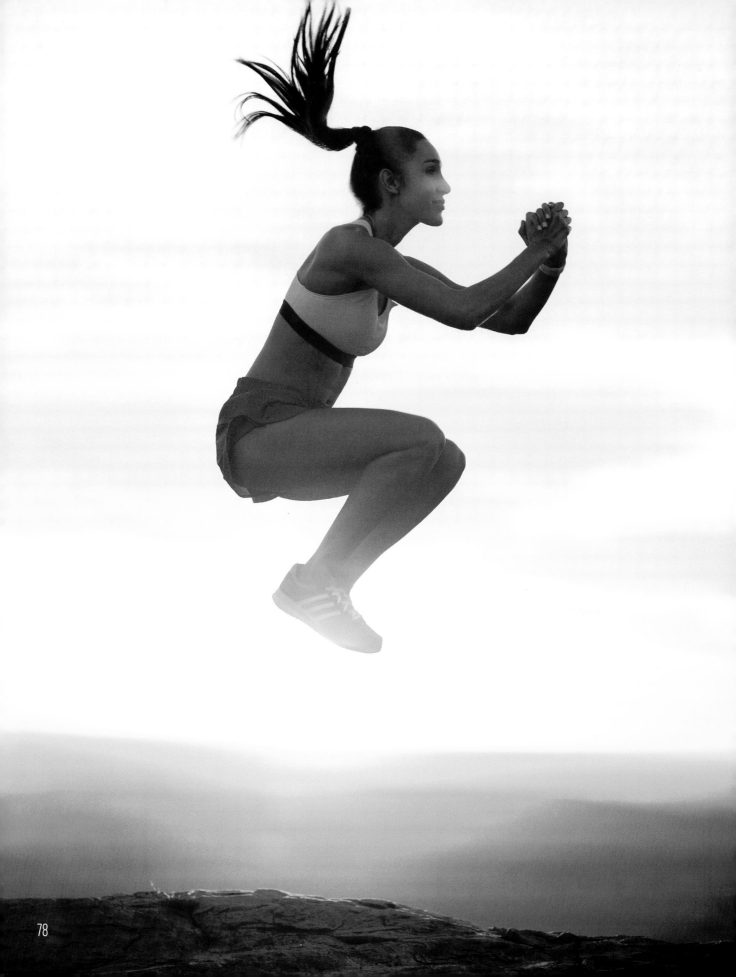

Getting the energy balance right

As well as providing us with nutrients, our food gives us the energy we need to function every day. The amount of energy found in food can be measured in either calories or kilojoules (1 calorie = 4.2 kilojoules). The number of calories you need each day depends on your age, height, weight, gender, how physically active you are, and your health and fitness goals.

The effects of energy intake on body weight can be understood using the simple "calories in–calories out" concept. "Calories in" refers to all the energy that you receive from food each day, whereas "calories out" is the energy that is used by the body to fuel basic functions such as breathing and blinking (often referred to as your Basal Metabolic Rate or BMR), as well as physical activity that you do during the day.

- When you eat the same number of calories that you burn (calories in = calories out), this generally means your weight will remain the same.

- When you eat a lot more calories than you burn (calories in > calories out), the excess energy can be stored within the body for use later and may result in weight or fat gain.

- Eating fewer calories than you burn (calories in < calories out) can potentially result in weight or fat loss.

So, if your goal is to maintain your weight, then you may get the best results by consuming around the same number of calories that you burn. Alternatively, if your goal is to lose weight or fat, then you may need to burn more calories than you consume.

How do I achieve optimal energy balance for fat or weight loss?

Generally speaking, women aged between 16 and 25 who do a moderate amount of exercise and weigh about 120 pounds or more need to eat approximately 2100 calories per day in order to maintain their weight. This is called the maintenance requirement.

Eating fewer calories than we use creates a calorie deficit, meaning the body has to burn existing energy stores (usually fat) to meet its energy needs. Of course, weight/fat loss is quite a complex process and can be influenced by many other variables, but in general if you consume around 500 calories less than your maintenance requirement, and do a moderate amount of exercise, you can expect a 1 pound weight (or fat) loss per week. This is because 1 pound of human fat is equivalent to approximately 3500 calories. So, seven days of a 500-calorie deficit can result in a weekly deficit of 3500 calories. For this reason, the meal plans that I have provided for healthy weight loss are based on a daily calorie intake of approximately 1600–1800 calories.

In simple terms, if you consume 1600 calories a day but burn 2100, your body needs to source energy in order to bridge this 500-calorie gap. This will generally come from energy stores that already exist in your body, such as fat.

Remember though, even if your goal is to lose weight or fat, it is important to provide your body with enough food for it to function at its best and to meet all of your nutrient requirements.

What is the difference between weight loss and fat loss?

When my clients are embarking on a new health and fitness journey, I always tell them not to get caught up with the number on the scales. This is because scales cannot distinguish between different masses in your body, such as water, muscle, and fat. For example, if the scales are showing that you have lost 7 pounds, it is possible that this is from a combination of body masses. And as we know, our weight can also fluctuate slightly throughout the day. Fat loss, on the other hand, generally leads to better muscle definition and tone. You've probably heard the phrase "muscle weighs more than fat," but it is important to understand that while muscle may be heavier than fat, it also takes up less space within the body. This explains why many women begin to see noticeable changes in the mirror, but their weight on the scales is the same or even a little bit higher as a result of their training.

An overview of food allergies and intolerances

Food allergies and intolerances are adverse reactions that occur after eating a certain food or nutrient. A food allergy occurs when your immune system reacts to the consumption of a certain food, responding with a rash or hives, swelling, or even life-threatening reactions such as anaphylaxis. Food intolerances are physical reactions, such as bloating or an upset stomach, that do not involve the immune system.

Allergies or intolerances to food can make it difficult to provide your body with the full range of vitamins and minerals that it needs. Food substitutions are the best way to make your daily food choices easier. In my meal plans, you will see that I have provided some suggestions so that you can be a little bit flexible, without missing out on vital nutrients. Below, I will cover some of the common allergies and intolerances that can impact your food choices.

LACTOSE INTOLERANCE occurs when the body cannot digest or absorb lactose, a type of sugar found in dairy foods. To reduce symptoms, such as bloating or diarrhoea, it is recommended to limit the amount of dairy in your diet. Suitable replacements, such as non-dairy or lactose-free dairy products, can help you make sure you are getting sufficient calcium in your diet.

PEANUT AND TREE NUT ALLERGIES trigger an adverse reaction in the immune system, caused by the proteins found in these foods. Symptoms can occur quickly and may vary from stomach discomfort and skin reactions through to swelling around the mouth and throat. In some cases, the reaction may be severe (such as anaphylaxis). If you have an allergy, always check food labels for traces of nuts or peanuts, and ask restaurant staff if you are eating out.

GLUTEN INTOLERANCE is an adverse reaction to foods containing gluten, such as wheat, barley, and rye. Symptoms include bloating or altered bowel motions after eating foods containing gluten, such as bread, wraps, pasta, and oats.

CELIAC DISEASE is a condition where the immune system reacts to gluten. It may prevent your body from absorbing nutrients properly, potentially leading to nutritional deficiencies or malnutrition, or even damage to your small intestine. Celiac disease is managed through a strict gluten-free diet, such as making the switch to gluten-free breads, wraps, pasta, and oats. Naturally gluten-free foods such as brown rice, quinoa, rice flakes, and quinoa flakes can also be substituted.

Exploring vegetarian and vegan diets

While I myself am not a vegetarian or vegan, I am an advocate for good nutrition. This section will help you to understand how the importance of a balanced, nutritious diet fits in with different eating preferences.

Vegetarian and vegan diets have become increasingly common in recent years. With new research showing the potential associated nutritional and health benefits, along with increased awareness and media attention regarding animal cruelty and ethics, more and more people have transitioned or are open to transitioning to a vegetarian or vegan lifestyle.

The women we surveyed cover a number of dietary preferences:

- Conventional = 83.6%
- Vegetarian = 7.1%
- Pescetarian = 4.7%
- Vegan = 4.6%

I understand that choosing a vegetarian or vegan lifestyle can mean different things to different people and it can be a sensitive subject for some. As a personal trainer, my focus isn't on what your eating preferences are, or why you are choosing them, but more so how you are managing it. This means ensuring you are getting all the nutrients you need on a day-to-day basis to train properly and lead a healthy lifestyle.

As in many other parts of this book, education is one of the fundamentals for creating healthy and lasting habits, irrespective of whether you are currently a vegetarian/vegan or if you are considering transitioning. In the following pages I will touch on some variants of these diets, and highlight that there is not one meal plan or set of recommendations that will suit all individuals who have adopted the lifestyle.

"Between 2012 and 2016, the number of Australian adults whose diet is all or almost all vegetarian has risen from 1.7 million people (or 9.7% of the population) to almost 2.1 million (11.2%)."

roymorgan.com/findings/
vegetarianisms-slow-
but-steady-rise-in-
australia-201608151105

What does being vegetarian mean?

As you now know, a vegetarian diet is often not as simple as just leaving meat off the plate. Defining vegetarianism can be a little difficult, simply because it can mean different things depending on a person's beliefs, culture, or experiences. There are also various subgroups of a vegetarian diet, which I've listed here:

- **LACTO-OVO-VEGETARIAN** — does not eat meat but consumes eggs and dairy products such as milk, yoghurt, and cheese

- **PESCETARIAN** — does not eat red meat and poultry but consumes seafood and shellfish

- **LACTO-VEGETARIAN** — does not eat meat or eggs but consumes dairy products such as milk, yoghurt, and cheese

- **OVO-VEGETARIAN** — does not eat meat or dairy products but consumes eggs.

A well-planned vegetarian diet of any type can have a number of health benefits, including being high in fibre and low in saturated fat. This can make it easier to control calorie intake and, for some people, weight. Studies* have found vegetarians tend to have lower cholesterol and blood pressure, and may be slightly less prone to cancer, heart disease, and diabetes. The reduced risk of chronic disease can be attributed to a vegetarian diet having a higher intake of fruits, vegetables, whole grains, nuts, soy products, and fibre. However, while vegetables can provide a lot of beneficial nutrients, it is also important that vegetarians consume meat alternatives in order to get all of the macro- and micronutrients that the body needs.

Many vegetarians believe their lifestyle is good for the planet, as fewer resources are needed to produce plant-based proteins than animal products.

vegetarian

noun   a person who does not eat meat or fish, and sometimes other animal products, especially for moral, religious, or health reasons.

While there are many publicised benefits of being a vegetarian, there are also misconceptions. One of the main concerns relates to nutrition, and whether a vegetarian diet can be nutritionally "complete." While your body responds to malnutrition in the same universal way as everyone else regardless of the diet you're following, this can be emphasised when particular foods groups are missing from your diet.

As long as vegetarian and subvarieties of vegetarian diets are properly planned, they can still fulfil your body's nutritional requirements. Essential dietary requirements that may be missing from vegetarian diets include vitamins D and B12, protein, zinc, and iron. Particularly as iron is found in red meat, choosing the right sources as a replacement is essential to ensure your diet is nutritionally balanced. Women are particularly at risk of iron deficiencies, something I have explained in greater detail on page 76. As with any diet, eating a variety of foods is the best way to provide your body with the nutrients it requires.

Further misconceptions relating to vegetarian diets revolve around food preparation and eating. Some myths include the idea that vegetarian meals are more expensive to shop for, meal choices when dining out are limited, and food takes a long time to prepare. Another is that vegetarian diets don't provide enough variety. In fact, plant-based diets can offer many different flavours, and shopping to suit a vegetarian diet can be done within almost any budget. As vegetarianism has grown in recent years, the availability of foods to suit vegetarian diners has never been better.

*Studies   Nutrition Australia, Vegetarian Diets, nutritionaustralia.org/national/frequently-asked-questions/vegetarian-diets

J Am Diet Assoc. 2009 Jul;109(7):1266-82 (Journal of the American Dietetic Association), ncbi.nlm.nih.gov/pubmed/19562864

What does being vegan mean?

Vegans do not eat red meat, fish, poultry, eggs, or dairy products. Instead, they eat only plant foods such as grains, dried peas, beans, lentils, nuts, seeds, soy products, vegetables, and fruit. Many vegans may choose to avoid food produced by animals or animal labour. For example, they may not eat honey (as it is made using the labour of bees), or use any products that are derived from animals, such as leather shoes, fur or leather clothing, and more.

vegan

noun a person who does not eat or use animal products.

Like vegetarianism, people follow a vegan diet for varying reasons, including ethics, health benefits, and religion. Defining a vegan diet can be difficult, as individuals may have slightly different beliefs as to what being a vegan involves.

What does choosing to be vegetarian or vegan mean for your health and lifestyle?

For anyone who hasn't tried a vegan or vegetarian diet before, it can be difficult to understand which foods to substitute. You may also have questions about how it will fit into your lifestyle, how it will impact your health, and other ethical conflicts.

When deciding to change your diet one way or another I think three important questions need to be considered:

- What do you see as being the health benefits or risks associated with this change?

- Are there any significant lifestyle changes that you need to implement to accommodate the change?

- Does the diet align with your personal ethics?

There are a number of myths surrounding veganism, the most common being that vegan diets are extremely limited, difficult to prepare, and more expensive to follow than "traditional" diets. This isn't necessarily accurate. There are numerous affordable and accessible vegan-friendly ingredients, including the basics such as lentils, grains, fresh fruit, and vegetables.

Veganism has long been stuck with the myth that it is lacking in sufficient vitamins. In fact, a well-planned vegan diet can meet all your nutritional requirements. Understanding what makes up a balanced and healthy vegan diet is the key to providing your body with the nutrients it needs for optimal health.

Vegan-friendly food covers a huge range of styles and tastes, so with a little planning, there is no reason why you can't enjoy a varied diet that is rich in flavour and nutritional value.

There are plenty of dairy alternatives available nowadays: dairy-free milk (pictured here), such as rice milk, oat milk, almond milk, soy milk, or quinoa milk; soy or dairy-free yoghurt; and soy or dairy-free cheeses (also pictured here).

Nutritional considerations for vegans and vegetarians

If you choose to be vegan or vegetarian, it is important for you to carefully plan a nutritionally appropriate diet. Here are some of the nutritional considerations to take into account.

PROTEIN

The main food sources of protein are red meat, chicken, fish, eggs, and milk. In a vegetarian diet, protein can be provided by consuming eggs, milk or milk products, legumes, and meat alternatives. There are a wide variety of legumes to choose from that provide an excellent source of protein and micronutrients (see page 76).

B12 VITAMIN DEFICIENCY

Vitamin B12 is vital for blood cell formation and the proper functioning of the nervous system. The best sources of vitamin B12 are animal foods such as meat, fish, poultry, eggs, milk, and milk products. While some plant foods may contain a form of vitamin B12, it is not always able to be absorbed and used by the body. Fortified cereals and soy products are an excellent source of B12 for vegans.

It is possible to have vitamin B12 deficiency when following a vegan diet where no animal products are eaten, or if you are a vegetarian who isn't eating enough eggs or dairy products to meet vitamin B12 needs. If this is the case then it may be necessary to add foods fortified with B12 or to take a supplement to meet this need.*

Symptoms of vitamin B12 deficiency can include: weakness and tiredness, shortness of breath, pale skin, constipation or diarrhea, gas, anaemia, loss of appetite, tingling in hands or feet, muscle weakness, altered vision, poor memory, feeling anxious or depressed.

IRON DEFICIENCY

On page 76 I provided information on why iron is important for your body, the two different sources of iron (haem iron and non-haem iron) and the symptoms you can expect to see if you have an iron deficiency.*

For those following a vegetarian or vegan diet, a high proportion of your iron is likely to come from non-haem sources. This typically means that you will have to consume a larger quantity of food in order to achieve the same required daily intake of iron compared to those who also consume haem iron sources (i.e. meat).

That said, if you are following a vegetarian or vegan diet, it is also important to consider the way in which other foods are able to influence its absorption. For example, eating vitamin C–rich foods as part of the same meal as non-haem iron sources can potentially enhance its absorption, whereas "iron blockers" like tea, coffee, and unprocessed bran can inhibit iron being absorbed by the body.

* It's important to listen to your body and look out for the signs and symptoms of vitamin and mineral deficiencies. A simple blood test done by your GP can confirm your health status. In the event that you find yourself with a deficiency, I'd recommend that you work with your GP and an accredited practising dietitian to help you meet your nutritional requirements by following a healthy, balanced diet rather than relying on supplements.

A note about ethics

Many people choose vegetarianism or veganism not only for health purposes but also for ethical reasons. Animal welfare is a consideration for many people who are aware of the methods used for meat and dairy production. Among other methods, meat and dairy products are often produced using intensive farming practices, the hallmarks of which include deforestation and high levels of methane, which could potentially be environmentally unsustainable. The growing of grain crops to feed animals when many of the human population are without food is another ethical issue taken into consideration. Whatever the reasons, the choice is ultimately a personal one and specific to each individual.

Sources of protein

These portions of seafood, eggs, and meat alternatives provide us with protein and are rich in a number of minerals. The serving sizes are equivalent to 1 serving of protein (see page 293). Depending on whether you are adapting to a vegetarian diet (or a subgroup of vegetarianism) or choosing to go vegan, some of the below foods may be used as replacements for meat.

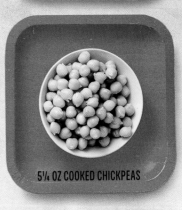
6 OZ TOFU

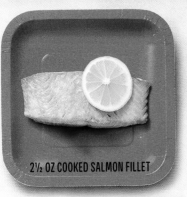
2½ OZ COOKED SALMON FILLET

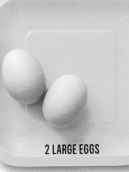
2 LARGE EGGS

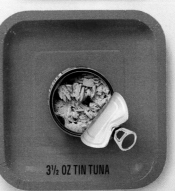
5¼ OZ COOKED CHICKPEAS

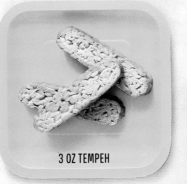
3 OZ TEMPEH

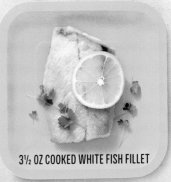
3½ OZ TIN TUNA

3½ OZ COOKED WHITE FISH FILLET

CILANTRO

This is a uniquely flavoured herb that is used widely in Mexican, Indian, and Asian cuisines. Cilantro is great in curries, soups, sauces, and marinades.

MINT

This can be used to make iced or hot tea. Add it to a grain salad with dried fruit and nuts, or toss it with fresh berries for a refreshing and healthy dessert.

PARSLEY

This can be used as a main ingredient in salads, such as tabouli, or as a garnish for a bit of extra flavour. Toss some fresh parsley into brown or wild rice with some lemon juice. Or add it to soups, pasta dishes, eggs, or salads.

DRIED OR FRESH THYME

This is especially tasty when used to season bean or egg dishes. You can sprinkle it with a small amount of olive oil over vegetables, such as potatoes, before roasting them. It also goes well with lemon.

BASIL

This is great for adding flavour to a pasta sauce. Try adding a few fresh basil leaves to your wraps.

DILL

This goes very well with fresh vegetables and fish. It also pairs especially well with cucumbers, making it a great addition to homemade tzatziki.

BOOSTING FLAVOUR

Much like meats, sometimes plant-based, protein-dense foods, such as legumes and other meat alternatives, can be plain and bland if eaten on their own. The addition of herbs and spices can make a huge difference in terms of flavour and overall satisfaction. Here are some of my favourite examples.

HERBS

CHILLI FLAKES

These will add a kick to any dish. Just remember to start with small amounts and then increase to your liking.

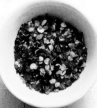

NUTMEG

This can be used in sweet and savoury dishes. A pinch or two in your favourite cookie or cake recipe adds a nice light flavour. It is also delicious paired with pumpkin or sweet potato – add some to your mash.

TURMERIC

This has an earthy flavour and is a great natural food colouring, adding a lovely yellow–orange colour to dishes in Indian and Moroccan cuisine. Turmeric is great to use in curries, stews, relishes, and rice dishes.

CINNAMON

This complements both sweet and savoury dishes. Simply use it to top your toast or low-fat yoghurt, or stir it into your porridge with some toasted nuts. It's great in cooked fruit dishes too. It can also be added to stews and braises in combination with other spices.

CUMIN

Together with chilli powder and garlic, cumin can season vegetables, stews, casseroles, or Mexican-style dishes.

SUMAC

This is a purple-coloured spice that has a tangy lemony flavour. It is commonly used in spice rubs, marinades and dressings, and adds great flavour to eggplant, chickpeas, and lentils.

SPICES

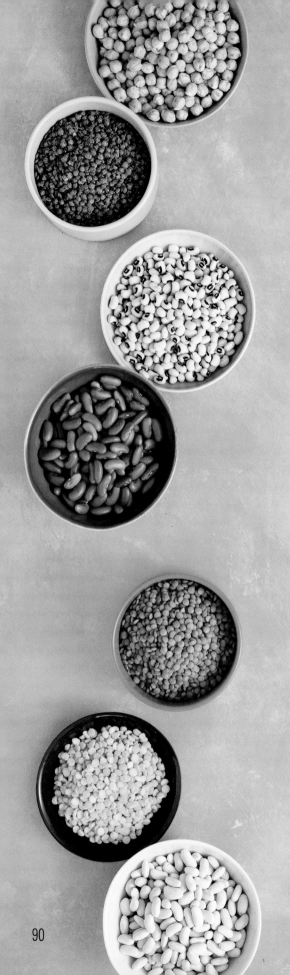

CHICKPEAS

These nutty-tasting, medium-sized peas are the main ingredient in hummus. They also work well in couscous or quinoa dishes, salads, stews, and curries.

PUY LENTILS

These have a unique peppery flavour and hold their shape well after cooking. They are a perfect addition to salads and can add bulk and richness to soups and stews.

BLACK-EYED PEAS

These are medium-sized, cream-coloured beans with a black eye marking. They work well in soups, stews, casseroles, and rice dishes, as well as Vietnamese-style desserts.

RED KIDNEY BEANS

These large, red beans work well in soups, stews, casseroles, salads, and Mexican-style dishes.

LENTILS

These are available in a number of varieties, such as whole red, split red, green, and brown. They are most commonly used in soups, stews, and curries. Red lentils, in particular, tend to break down easily and can take a very short time to cook.

YELLOW SPLIT PEAS

Similar to green split peas, these are high in protein and fibre. Yellow split peas tend to be not as sweet as the green variety and they can be used in the same way, as an addition to soups, stews, and casseroles.

BUTTER BEANS

These large, white beans are a variety of lima bean. They generally have a mild flavour and work well in salads, soups, and casseroles.

LEGUMES

SUPERFOODS

There is no scientific definition of a superfood as such, but they are generally thought of as being nutritionally dense and especially beneficial for our health and well-being. Superfoods naturally have higher amounts of particular nutrients—such as vitamins, minerals, and/or antioxidants. This means superfoods may provide health benefits to your diet; however, that doesn't mean you should eat a diet consisting only of superfoods.

GREENS

These green superfoods contain beneficial vitamins, minerals, and fibre. Wheatgrass contains concentrated amounts of a number of vitamins, minerals, and amino acids. It is sometimes referred to as a "blood builder" as it is believed to increase the production of haemoglobin, the protein within red blood cells that carries oxygen around your body. Barley grass has a similar vitamin and mineral content to wheatgrass and is known for its ability to cleanse and detoxify the body. Kale is a very nutrient-dense vegetable and contains high amounts of some vitamins and minerals that promote healthy skin, hair, and bones. Spinach provides our bodies with similar nutrients to kale, but it does contain more folate—a B vitamin that can help our cells to function and divide properly.

POWDERS

Superfood powders are rich in nutrients and high in antioxidants, and can be great to add to meals to enhance flavour and boost the nutritional value. Cacao is one of the highest plant-based sources of iron. It is also high in magnesium, calcium, and antioxidants. Cacao can also help increase the body's "feel-good" chemicals, serotonin and dopamine. Carob is a great source of vitamins and minerals, as well as gallic acid, known for its antibacterial, antiviral, and antiseptic properties. Maca is jam-packed with vitamins and minerals, and contains a number of unique alkaloids (natural plant-based chemicals) that may help improve the overall functioning of the body's hormonal systems. Spirulina naturally contains all nine essential amino acids and good amounts of iron, which means it can be used to improve the quality of vegetarian or vegan diets.

NUTS AND SEEDS

Nuts and seeds are packed with protein, fatty acids, vitamins, minerals, and fibre, perfect for a superfood! It's important to note they are higher in energy and should be consumed in moderation. Chia seeds contain all nine essential amino acids and omega-3, the good fats known to improve heart health. They contain both soluble and insoluble fibre, which are important for digestive health and increasing feelings of fullness after meals. Pumpkin seeds, also known as pepitas, are a tasty way of obtaining protein, B vitamins, and minerals such as magnesium, iron, and zinc. Walnuts are a good source of protein, fibre, and magnesium. They also have a high level of the brain-boosting omega-3 fatty acid, alpha-linolenic acid. Almonds are rich in vitamin E, calcium, iron, and magnesium, and are one of the lowest calorie options.

GRAINS

Oats, quinoa, buckwheat, and freekeh are four superfood grains that can give you the most nutritional bang for your buck! Oats contain six of the eight B vitamins, which help us to convert food into fuel. Quinoa is gluten-free and one of the only plant foods that contains all nine essential amino acids. Buckwheat is also gluten-free and contains rutin, which can help maintain normal blood flow and blood clotting, and magnesium, which can promote the relaxation of blood vessels and reduce blood pressure—the perfect combination for a healthy cardiovascular system. Freekeh has three times the amount of fibre and protein than brown rice and is high in iron, making it great for vegetarians and vegans. All of these super grains can be quite filling due to their high fibre content, which is perfect for managing your weight.

BERRIES

Berries, such as blueberries, strawberries, raspberries, goji, and acai berries, are considered superfoods because of their naturally high antioxidant content. Anthocyanins, which give berries their vibrant colouring, help protect our cells and DNA from damage. Berries are also high in vitamin C, which can help strengthen the immune system and give our skin a youthful glow, and they contain lots of fibre.

DINING OUT

Much like any change you make to your lifestyle, when you adopt a vegetarian or vegan diet, there is a flow-on effect to other areas of your life. By changing the food you eat, you are likely changing or limiting the flavours you can have, and this can often also affect where or how you can dine out. Vegetarian and vegan dining options are becoming more common, but there are some things to be mindful of:

- Some meat-free dishes rely heavily on carbohydrate-rich foods, which may mean you end up eating more carbs than you would like.

- Beware that although some dishes may claim to be vegetarian, they may in fact contain beef stock or chicken stock (i.e. rice dishes or stews).

- Anyone who follows a vegan diet is probably already aware of how easily non-vegan items can end up on your plate. Dressings, sauces, breads, and oils may contain hidden ingredients that aren't vegan-friendly. For example, fresh pasta is made with eggs, while dried pasta often isn't.

Luckily there are places where you can find delicious vegetarian or vegan meals.

CAFES

- Most will serve eggs or beans with toast, oats, or muesli for breakfast.

- Smashed avocado is a favourite weekend breakfast for many people, and can suit both a vegetarian and vegan diet (provided vegans check for extras, such as butter, first).

- Buckwheat pancakes made with soy milk are a good replacement for traditional pancakes.

- Fruit salad, fresh fruit juice, or a vegetable platter are great snack options.

MEXICAN CUISINE

- Most Mexican dishes can be adapted to be vegetarian, including tacos, fajitas, chimichangas, and burritos.

- Double-check the rice isn't cooked in chicken stock, and, for vegans, ask for no sour cream or cheese. Some bean varieties (such as refried beans) may use pork lard in the cooking process, so double-check this too before eating them.

JAPANESE CUISINE

- Japanese food includes vegetarian dishes such as tofu sushi, tamagoyaki, egg sushi variants, rice and eggplant specialty dishes and tempura vegetables.

- Miso soup, edamame or seaweed salads are great options for starters, and still offer fantastic, authentic flavours. These are a great choice for vegans too as they offer a range of nutrients.

MIDDLE EASTERN CUISINE

- Usually offers a wide range of vegetable curries, lentil and pea dishes (again, ask about preparation methods).

- Falafel or chickpea burgers are a great option for a fast vegetarian or vegan lunch.

- Dolmas, or stuffed grape leaves, offer fantastic variety as the fillings can be easily swapped around.

- Mezze platters are a great share dish. They usually feature hummus, baba ganoush, tabouli, dolmas, olives, and a number of vegetables.

PIZZA

- Most pizza places will have a wide range of vegetarian options, and vegan options (such as those using cheese substitutes) are also becoming more common.

GREEK AND MEDITERRANEAN CUISINES

- Go for the Greek salad, roasted or grilled vegetable platters, or vegetable moussaka.

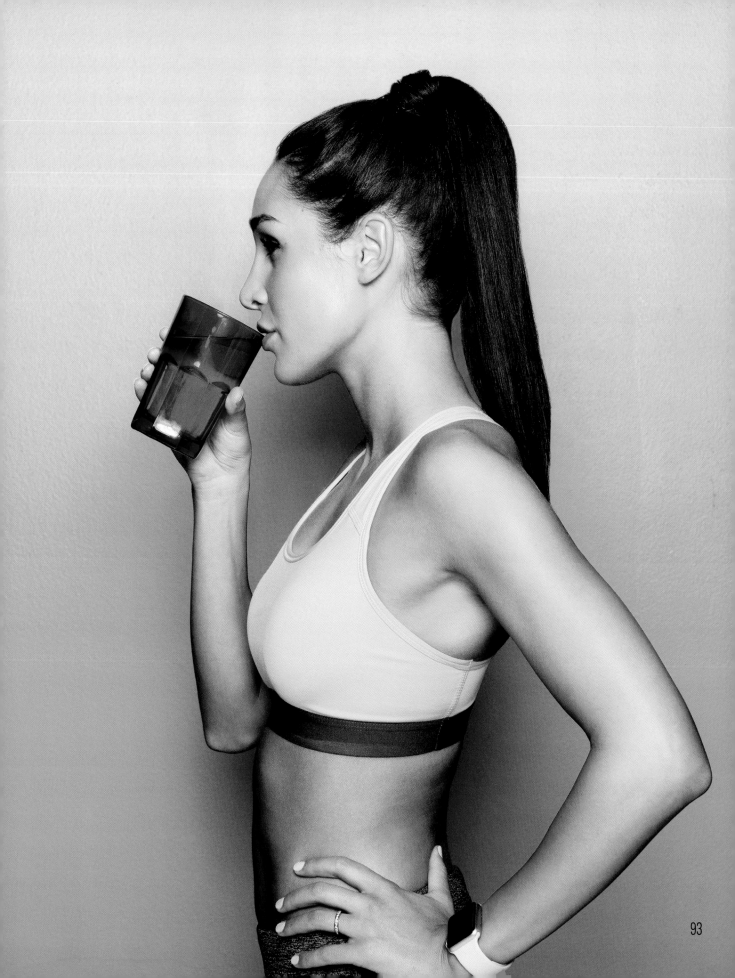

SUMMING UP NUTRITION

1. The basis for good nutrition is a balanced diet containing the right proportions of grains, healthy fats, fruit, vegetables and legumes, dairy products, and lean proteins.

2. Your body needs a balance of macro- and micronutrients in order to function optimally and deficiencies in these may impact your health and well-being.

3. There are different types of vegetarian diets, including pescetarian, lacto-vegetarian, ovo-vegetarian, and lacto-ovo-vegetarian.

4. Vegan diets do not include any animal or animal-based products; vegans may also choose not to eat foods produced by animal labour.

5. Unbalanced vegan or vegetarian diets can be as bad for your health as any other diet that is lacking in nutrients.

6. Following a vegetarian or vegan diet requires planning and an understanding of nutrition in order to meet recommended dietary intakes.

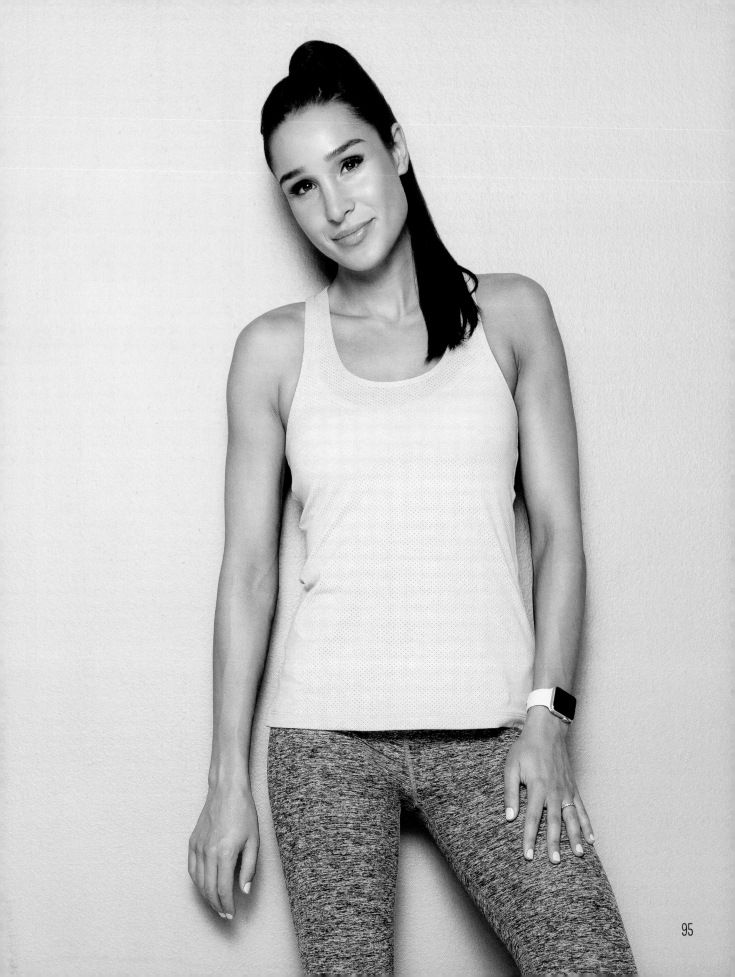

Putting it into action

I believe that eating a healthy diet doesn't have to be complicated. My meal plans are flexible and use a wide variety of foods from all six food groups (see page 68 for an overview of the food groups).

Just as we need nutrients in different amounts, we also need to consume a different number of servings from each of these groups. Here are some examples of sample servings* for common foods in each of the food groups to get you started (see pages 292–295 for a comprehensive list).

* It is important not to confuse "serving size" with "portion size." For example, six servings of grains is not six meals worth of grains, but the total amount of grains that you should be eating every day.

FOOD GROUPS	COMMON FOODS AND SAMPLE SERVINGS
	I have used these food groups to establish a comprehensive 28-day meal plan that provides for all your nutritional needs.
Grains	1 slice whole wheat bread or raisin bread
	½ medium whole wheat roll or whole wheat wrap
	1 oz muesli, rolled oats, or quinoa flakes
	3½ oz cooked quinoa or rice
	3 oz cooked whole wheat pasta
	3½ oz cooked rice vermicelli noodles
	2 whole wheat crispbreads
Vegetables & legumes	NON-STARCHY VEGETABLES
	1 large handful lettuce leaves, baby spinach, arugula, or kale
	1 medium carrot, cucumber, tomato, or zucchini
	1 small onion or beetroot
	½ medium bell pepper or eggplant
	2 celery stalks
	5 oz tinned crushed tomatoes
	STARCHY VEGETABLES & LEGUMES
	½ medium potato or sweet potato
	½ ear of corn or 2 oz tinned or frozen corn kernels
	2¾ oz cooked or tinned legumes (kidney beans, chickpeas, lentils)
Fruit	1 medium apple, banana, orange or mango, or small pear
	6 oz mixed berries or 5¾ oz blueberries or raspberries
	9 oz watermelon or strawberries
	1 large handful grapes (about 25) or cherries (about 20)
	1 oz dried sultanas or 1 oz dried goji berries or cranberries
	½ cup freshly squeezed fruit juice
Dairy products & alternatives	1 cup low-fat milk or calcium-fortified milk
	7 oz low-fat plain yoghurt or soy yoghurt
	1½ oz low-fat hard cheese
	2 oz low-fat salt-reduced feta or 3½ oz low-fat ricotta
	4½ oz low-fat cottage cheese
Lean meat, seafood, eggs & meat alternatives	2⅓ oz cooked lean red meat (beef, lamb)
	2 oz cooked chicken or 3 oz cooked turkey
	3½ oz cooked white fish fillet or tinned tuna
	2½ oz cooked salmon fillet or smoked or tinned salmon
	2 large eggs
	5¼ oz cooked or tinned legumes (kidney beans, chickpeas, lentils)
	6 oz tofu or 3 oz tempeh
Healthy fats	1½ teaspoons monounsaturated or polyunsaturated oil
	⅓ oz nuts or 2 teaspoons nut paste
	1 oz avocado (< ⅛ avocado)

MY MEAL PLANS

If you're already on board with my healthy eating plan, you'll know how simple it is. From page 100 you'll find my delicious meal plans, setting out exactly what you need to eat each and every day for four weeks. This takes away all the hard work of planning, counting calories, or wondering what to cook—I've done it for you! Even better, I've included shopping lists for each week that you can simply download or copy and take with you—no more last-minute scribbling down items, or forgetting that one crucial ingredient. With my shopping lists, the thinking is all done for you, and you can be super organised each week. This simplicity helps make my meal plans easy to follow, making it much more likely that you will stick to healthy eating in the long term.

Added flexibility—it's as easy as A, B, C, D

One thing I've learned from my experience is that everyone's food preferences are different. The beauty of my method is that the meal plans can be adapted to give you plenty of variety.

To help you do this, I have provided four flexible meal variations —**A, B, C & D.**

While each variation contains the same number of meals and the required number of servings from all of the main food groups, they differ in the way these food groups are distributed throughout the day. This means you can have different types of foods at different times of the day during the week to suit your individual lifestyle and preferences.

For example, if you don't like the Chocolate & Mint Smoothie Bowl, a "B" option, you can replace it with the Cherry Smoothie Bowl or Mango Smoothie Bowl, or any other breakfast meal in the book that has the same icon.

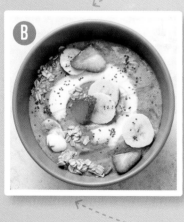

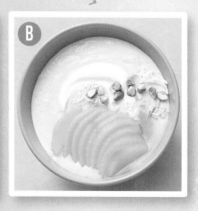

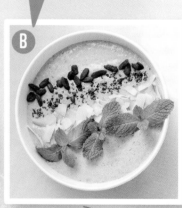

	A	B	C	D
Breakfast	2 servings grains 1 serving fruit 1 serving dairy products & alternatives	1 serving grains 1½ servings fruit ½ serving vegetables & legumes 1½ servings dairy products & alternatives 1 serving healthy fats	2 servings grains ½ serving fruit ¾ serving dairy products & alternatives 1½ servings healthy fats	2 servings grains 1 serving vegetables & legumes ½ serving dairy products & alternatives 1 serving lean meat, seafood, eggs & meat alternatives 1 serving healthy fats
Snack A.M.	1 serving grains 1 serving vegetables & legumes ½ serving lean meat, seafood, eggs & meat alternatives	½ serving fruit 1 serving healthy fats	1 serving grains 1½ servings fruit 1 serving dairy products & alternatives	1 serving grains 1 serving fruit ½ serving dairy products & alternatives
Lunch	1 serving grains 2 servings vegetables & legumes 1 serving lean meat, seafood, eggs & meat alternatives	2 servings grains 1½ servings vegetables & legumes ½ serving dairy products & alternatives 1 serving lean meat, seafood, eggs & meat alternatives	2 servings grains 1½ servings vegetables & legumes 1 serving lean meat, seafood, eggs & meat alternatives	1 serving grains 1½ servings vegetables & legumes ½ serving dairy products & alternatives ½ serving lean meat, seafood, eggs & meat alternatives
Snack P.M.	1 serving fruit 1½ servings dairy products & alternatives	1 serving grains 1 serving vegetables & legumes ½ serving lean meat, seafood, eggs & meat alternatives	1 serving grains ¼ serving dairy products & alternatives	1 serving grains ½ serving vegetables & legumes ½ serving dairy products & alternatives
Dinner	2 servings grains 2 servings vegetables & legumes 1 serving lean meat, seafood, eggs & meat alternatives 2 servings healthy fats	2 servings grains 2 servings vegetables & legumes ½ serving dairy products & alternatives 1 serving lean meat, seafood, eggs & meat alternatives	3½ servings vegetables (1 starchy) ½ serving dairy products & alternatives 1½ servings lean meat, seafood, eggs & meat alternatives ½ serving healthy fats	1 serving grains 2 servings vegetables & legumes 1 serving fruit 1 serving lean meat, seafood, eggs & meat alternatives ½ serving dairy products & alternatives 1 serving healthy fats

For example, each meal in Option D contains a small serving of grains, whereas Option C contains more grain servings earlier in the day, but none at dinner. To keep it convenient and simple, the plan has varying days with varying layouts to suit all meal types.

The upshot is, if you come across a meal within the 28-day meal plan that does not suit your taste preferences, you can replace it with another recipe labelled with the same letter.

While it is important for you to meet all of the recommended food group servings throughout the day, whichever way you do that is up to you!

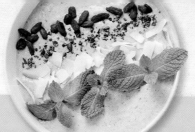

WEEK ONE

	DAY 1	DAY 2	DAY 3	DAY 4	DAY 5	DAY 6	DAY 7
	A	**B**	**C**	**D**	**A**	**B**	**C**
Breakfast	Blueberry Pancakes (page 112)	Chocolate & Mint Smoothie Bowl (page 116)	Avocado, Feta & Pomegranate Toast Topper (page 120)	Tomato & Spinach Frittata (page 124)	Berry Porridge (page 128)	Carrot Smoothie Bowl (page 132)	Banana & Almond Ricotta Toast Topper (page 136)
Snack A.M.	Rice Crackers with Arugula & White Bean Dip (page 112)	Trail Mix (page 116)	Chai & Pear Parfait (page 120)	Matcha Yoghurt & Muesli (page 124)	Salmon & Cucumber on Rice Cakes (page 128)	Banana & Peanut Butter Stack (page 132)	Pine-lime Smoothie (page 136)
Lunch	Lettuce Cups (page 112)	Cajun Chicken Wrap (page 116)	Black Rice Sushi (page 120)	Pumpkin & Feta Bruschetta (page 124)	Open Chicken Burger (page 128)	Roasted Eggplant Pasta Salad (page 132)	Quinoa Tabouli Salad (page 136)
Snack P.M.	Chocolate & Banana Mousse (page 113)	Pita Triangles with Baba Ganoush (page 117)	Flatbread with Cranberry & Cottage Cheese (page 121)	Rice Crackers with Beetroot & Yoghurt Dip (page 125)	Iced Chocolate (page 129)	Pita Triangles with Beetroot Dip (page 133)	Rice Crackers with Minted Yoghurt (page 137)
Dinner	Pistachio-crusted Salmon with Zesty Quinoa (page 113)	Chickpea, Tomato & Kale Soup (page 117)	Healthy Parmigiana & Salad (page 121)	Chopped Salad (page 125)	Beef Pho (page 129)	Seafood Pizza (page 133)	Sweet Potato Spaghetti (page 137)

SHOPPING LIST

While fresh ingredients such as fruit and vegetables are a staple in any healthy-eating plan (including this one), they are generally purchased from week to week because they have a short shelf-life. The pantry staples list below is made up of ingredients that are used often in my meal plan, swap-outs, and naughty-made-nice recipes, but also have a long shelf-life and can be stored easily—whether that be in the pantry, refrigerator, or freezer.

PANTRY STAPLES

apple cider vinegar
arborio rice
baking powder
balsamic vinegar
beef stock, salt-reduced
black beans, tinned
black pepper, ground
bocconcini, baby
bread, whole grain
bread, whole wheat
bread crumbs, panko
brown rice
cacao powder, raw
Cajun seasoning
cannellini beans, tinned
capers
cayenne pepper
chickpeas, tinned
chilli flakes, dried
chilli powder
cinnamon, ground
cinnamon, sticks
cloves, ground
cloves, whole
coconut, flaked
coconut, shredded
coconut milk, light
coconut oil
coffee
cilantro, dried
cilantro, ground
couscous
cumin, ground
curry paste, green
curry powder
eggs, large
fish sauce
four bean mix, tinned
flour, whole wheat
garam masala
ginger, ground
honey
kidney beans, tinned
lasagna sheets, whole wheat
maple syrup

milk, low-fat
mixed berries, frozen
muesli, natural
mustard, Dijon
mustard, whole grain
nutmeg, ground
oil spray
olive oil
oregano, dried
orzo
paprika, smoked
paprika, sweet
pasta, whole wheat
peanut butter, 100% natural
pearl barley
pearl couscous
quinoa
quinoa flakes
quinoa flour
red lentils, dried
red wine vinegar
rice cakes
rice crackers, plain
rice stick noodles
rolled oats
rosemary, dried
rye crispbreads
salmon, tinned
sea salt
star anise
tahini
tamari or soy sauce, salt-reduced
thyme, dried
tomato passata (purée)
tomatoes, tinned crushed
tuna, tinned in springwater
turmeric, ground
vanilla extract, pure
vegetable stock, salt-reduced
vermicelli noodles
water crackers, plain
white vinegar
yoghurt, low-fat plain

GRAINS

2 oz black rice
½ whole wheat lavash
2 whole wheat pita bread
½ medium whole wheat roll
1 whole wheat wrap

FRUIT

4 bananas
7 oz blueberries
5 medjool dates
2 tsp goji berries
1 kiwi fruit
½ medium orange
3 passionfruit
2 small pears
6 oz peeled pineapple
1 pomegranate

VEGETABLES

1 bag arugula leaves
5 asparagus spears
1 bag baby spinach leaves
1 large handful bean sprouts
1½ small beetroots
1¾ oz broccolini
¾ medium red bell pepper
1 medium carrot
½ celery stalk
¾ oz corn kernels
3½ Lebanese cucumbers
¾ medium eggplant
¼ small fennel bulb
4 kalamata olives
1 small bunch kale
3 large romaine lettuce leaves
1 large handful mixed lettuce leaves
2¾ oz mushrooms
¾ small brown onion
1½ small red onions
1 scallion
4¼ oz pumpkin
1 medium sweet potato
1½ medium tomato
23 cherry tomatoes
¾ medium zucchini

MEAT & ALTERNATIVES

1 lb boneless, skinless chicken breast
¼ lb ground chicken
10 medium raw shrimps
⅓ oz salmon fillet
⅓ oz smoked salmon
4 oz lean beef steak

DAIRY & ALTERNATIVES

⅓ oz low-fat cheddar cheese
1 oz low-fat cottage cheese
4¾ oz low-fat salt-reduced feta
1½ oz mozzarella cheese
1½ oz parmesan cheese
4½ oz low-fat ricotta cheese

HEALTHY FATS

1 (4¾ oz) avocado
½ tsp slivered almonds
2 tsp almond butter
2 tsp chia seeds
1½ oz unsalted pistachio nuts
½ tsp pumpkin seeds
½ tsp sunflower seeds

OTHER

1 small handful fresh regular or Thai basil
1 bay leaf
1 chai teabag
fresh red chilli
1 bunch cilantro
½ tsp cranberry jam
2 tbsp fresh dill, chopped
6¾ garlic cloves
¾ inch fresh ginger
1 lime
¼ tsp matcha powder
microherbs
1 bunch mint
2 nori sheets
1 bunch fresh parsley
½ oz protein powder
raw cacao nibs

Download a copy of this list at kaylaitsines.com/28dayguide/book2/shoppinglist/week1

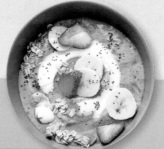

WEEK TWO

	DAY 1	DAY 2	DAY 3	DAY 4	DAY 5	DAY 6	DAY 7
	D	**A**	**B**	**C**	**D**	**A**	**B**
Breakfast	Egg & Bean Smash (page 140)	Spiced Apple & Ricotta Wrap (page 144)	Chia Breakfast Bowl (page 148)	Canteloupe, Walnut and Goat's Cheese Toast Topper (page 152)	Breakfast Hash (page 156)	Acai Pancake Bites (page 160)	Mango Smoothie Bowl (page 164)
Snack A.M.	Frushi (page 140)	Rice Crackers with Pumpkin Hummus (page 144)	Citrus & Chia Seed Salad (page 148)	Banana & Berry Smoothie (page 152)	Crispbreads with Blueberries & Ricotta (page 156)	Pita Triangles with Mexican Salsa (page 160)	Pear & Pistachios (page 164)
Lunch	Tuna Pita Pocket (page 140)	Five Bean Salad (page 144)	Taquitos (page 148)	Chicken & Wild Rice Salad (page 152)	Chicken Quesadilla (page 156)	Edamame Plate (page 160)	Salmon & Salad Roll (page 164)
Snack P.M.	Caprese Salad (page 141)	Mango Swirl (page 145)	Mushroom Pâté with Crispbreads (page 149)	Raisin Bread Toast with Ricotta (page 153)	Bell Pepper & Bocconcini Bruschetta (page 157)	Iced Coffee (page 161)	Rice Crackers with Spinach Dip (page 165)
Dinner	Lamb Tagine (page 141)	Thai Green Curry (page 145)	Tandoori Chicken Pizza (page 149)	Steak with Potato & Fennel Salad (page 153)	Fish with Asparagus & Citrus Soba Salad (page 157)	Coconut-crumbed Chicken & Salad (page 161)	Chicken, Spinach & Ricotta Cannelloni (page 165)

SHOPPING LIST

PANTRY STAPLES

Before you head out to the shops, please make sure that you have a good amount of each of the ingredients on the pantry staples list (see page 101).

GRAINS

2 medium corn tortillas
1 slice raisin bread
60 g wild rice
2 whole wheat pita bread
1 medium whole wheat roll
2 whole wheat wraps
1 slice rye bread
1¾ oz soba noodles

FRUIT

1 medium green apple
2½ medium bananas
5¾ oz blueberries
1 medium pink grapefruit
1 kiwifruit
2 medium mangoes
6 medjool dates
5 medium oranges
3 oz pineapple
½ small pear
4¾ oz canteloupe
13½ oz strawberries

VEGETABLES

1½ large handfuls arugula
6 asparagus spears
4½ large handfuls baby spinach leaves
½ small beetroot
3 oz bok choy
5¼ oz frozen broad beans
1¾ oz broccoli
2 medium carrots
1 celery stalk
10 cherry tomatoes
1 oz frozen corn kernels
1 Lebanese cucumber
1¾ oz frozen edamame
1½ small fennel bulbs
8 green beans
1 oz green cabbage
2 large handfuls lettuce leaves
6 oz mushrooms
1½ small brown onions
2 small red onions
½ medium potato
7½ oz pumpkin
2 medium radishes
1¾ oz red cabbage
1 medium red bell pepper
2 oz snow peas
2 scallions
¾ medium sweet potato
1½ medium tomatoes
8 yellow beans
½ medium zucchini

MEAT & ALTERNATIVES

3½ oz boneless, skinless chicken breast
3½ oz ground chicken
7 oz roast chicken
3½ oz chicken tenders
3½ oz boneless, skinless chicken thigh
4½ oz lean beef steak
3 oz lean lamb leg steaks
3 oz salmon fillet
1½ oz smoked salmon
1½ oz dried yellow split peas
5 medium shrimps

DAIRY & ALTERNATIVES

⅔ oz camembert cheese
⅔ oz low-fat cheddar cheese
⅔ oz salt-reduced low-fat feta
2½ oz low-fat goat's cheese
8 oz low-fat ricotta
⅔ oz parmesan cheese

HEALTHY FATS

1¾ oz avocado
2 tsp flaked almonds
4 tsp chia seeds
⅔ oz pistachio kernels
⅔ oz walnuts

OTHER

2½ tsp acai berry powder
¼ tsp balsamic glaze
coffee beans, to garnish
1 tbsp fresh chives
8 tsp fresh cilantro
1 tbsp fresh dill
5 garlic cloves
1 tsp fresh mint
fresh parsley
1½ fresh red chillis
1 sprig fresh thyme
1 kaffir lime leaf
3–4 lemons
½ tsp rice wine vinegar
2 tsp tandoori paste

Download a copy of this list at kaylaitsines.com/28dayguide/book2/shoppinglist/week2

	DAY 1	DAY 2	DAY 3	DAY 4	DAY 5	DAY 6	DAY 7
	C	**D**	**A**	**B**	**C**	**D**	**A**
Breakfast	Chocolate Overnight Oats (page 168)	"Green Eggs" (page 172)	Grilled Peach Toast Topper (page 176)	Berry Beet Smoothie Bowl (page 180)	Sweet Rice Breakfast Pudding (page 184)	Asparagus Bruschetta (page 188)	Fig & Muesli Breakfast Bowl (page 192)
Snack A.M.	"Mulled" Fruit & Spiced Yoghurt (page 168)	Acai Yoghurt & Muesli (page 172)	Egg & Tomato Rice Cakes (page 176)	Mango, Mint & Macadamia Salad (page 180)	Lemon & Blueberry Parfait (page 184)	Apple "Doughnuts" (page 188)	Tuna & Tomato Rice Cakes (page 192)
Lunch	Sweet Potato & Chickpea Orzo Salad (page 168)	Smoked Salmon Open Sandwich (page 172)	Pickled Vegetable Salad (page 176)	Fattoush Salad (page 180)	Chicken & Salad Roll (page 184)	Freekeh Salad (page 188)	Beef Pita Pocket (page 192)
Snack P.M.	Pita Triangles with Garlic & Cilantro Yoghurt (page 169)	Crispbreads with Cottage Cheese & Tomato Salsa (page 173)	Salted Caramel Yoghurt (page 177)	Salmon & Cucumber on Rice Cakes (page 181)	Crispbreads with Cottage Cheese & Chives (page 185)	Pita Triangles with Beetroot & Yoghurt Dip (page 189)	Ricotta & Cherry Mousse (page 193)
Dinner	Shrimp & Vegetable Asian Omelette (page 169)	Stuffed Sweet Potato (page 173)	Satay Beef Skewers with Rice & Vegetables (page 177)	Moroccan Chickpea Burger (page 181)	Chicken & Succotash (page 185)	Waldorf Salad (page 189)	Chickpea & Spinach Curry (page 193)

SHOPPING LIST

PANTRY STAPLES

Before you head out to the shops, please make sure that you have a good amount of each of the ingredients on the pantry staples list (see page 101).

GRAINS

1½ oz cracked freekeh
2 slices raisin bread
2 medium whole wheat bread rolls
3 whole wheat pita bread

FRUIT

½ medium apple (green or red)
1 medium green apple
2 medium bananas
7 oz blueberries
20 cherries
1 oz dried cranberries
⅔ oz dried currants
2 medium figs
4–5 lemons
lime, juiced, to taste
1 medium mango
5 medjool dates
3 tbsp 100% orange juice
1 orange
1 large peach
1½ oz raspberries
4¼ oz strawberries

VEGETABLES

1 small handful alfalfa sprouts
2 large handfuls arugula
5 asparagus spears
3 large handfuls baby spinach leaves
1 small handful bean sprouts
2 small beetroot
7½ oz bok choy
2½ oz broccoli
2 medium carrots
2 celery stalks
24 cherry tomatoes
1 oz Chinese cabbage (wombok)
3 oz frozen corn kernels
4 Lebanese cucumbers
½ small fennel bulb
1 large handful kale
2 large handfuls lettuce leaves
1 small brown onion
2 small red onions
3 medium radishes
2 medium red bell pepper
3 scallions
1½ oz snow peas
2 medium sweet potatoes
2 medium tomatoes
½ medium zucchini

MEAT & ALTERNATIVES

12⅓ oz boneless, skinless chicken breast
3 oz lean beef steak
3 oz lean beef strips
5 medium raw shrimp
3 oz smoked salmon
6 oz firm tofu

DAIRY & ALTERNATIVES

⅓ oz low-fat cheddar cheese
3 oz low-fat cottage cheese
2 oz low-fat goat's cheese
7 oz low-fat ricotta cheese
3 oz salt-reduced low-fat feta cheese

HEALTHY FATS

1 tsp chia seeds
5 tsp flaked almonds
⅓ oz unsalted macadamia nuts
⅓ oz roasted peanuts
⅓ oz pecans
2 tsp pine nuts
⅓ oz walnut halves

OTHER

2½ tsp acai berry powder
½ tsp arrowroot
4 tbsp fresh basil
cacao nibs
3 fresh red chillis
2 tsp fresh chives
20 tsp (1 large bunch) fresh cilantro
½ tsp fresh dill, chopped
4 garlic cloves
1 tsp grated fresh ginger
1½ tsp preserved lemon rind, finely diced
3 tbsp fresh mint, chopped
1 tbsp oyster sauce
1 bunch fresh parsley
½ cup (125ml) rice wine vinegar
watercress, to garnish (optional)

Download a copy of this list at kaylaitsines.com/28dayguide/book2/shoppinglist/week3

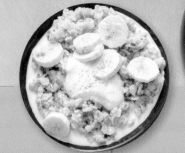

WEEK FOUR

	DAY 1	DAY 2	DAY 3	DAY 4	DAY 5	DAY 6	DAY 7
	B	**C**	**D**	**A**	**B**	**C**	**D**
Breakfast	Chocolate Smoothie Bowl (page 196)	Quinoa Porridge with Coconut Ricotta (page 200)	Spinach & Goat's Cheese Omelette (page 204)	Date & Banana Porridge (page 208)	Coconut Smoothie Bowl (page 212)	Mango & Coconut Bircher (page 216)	Fried Egg Toast Topper (page 220)
Snack A.M.	Strawberries & Coconut (page 196)	Cookie Dough Smoothie (page 200)	Vanilla Yoghurt & Muesli (page 204)	Rice Crackers with Pumpkin Hummus (page 208)	Raspberries with Chocolate Sauce (page 212)	Crackers with Cheese & Fruit Paste (page 216)	Crispbreads with Blueberries & Ricotta (page 220)
Lunch	Turkey & Goat's Cheese Pasta Salad (page 196)	Chicken Fajitas (page 200)	Beetroot Couscous Salad (page 204)	Mason Jar Salad (page 208)	Tuna Sandwich (page 212)	Puttanesca Pasta Salad (page 216)	Warm Chicken Salad (page 220)
Snack P.M.	Pita Triangles with Mexican Salsa (page 197)	Flatbread with Cranberry & Cottage Cheese (page 201)	Bell Pepper & Bocconcini Bruschetta (page 205)	Strawberry Swirl (page 209)	Rice Crackers with Beetroot Hummus (page 213)	Raisin Bread Toast with Ricotta (page 217)	Pita Triangles with Spinach, Cheese & Chive Dip (page 221)
Dinner	Lentil Dhal (page 197)	Salt & Pepper Squid (page 201)	Asian-style Pork with Orange & Avocado Salad (page 205)	Steak Sandwich (page 209)	Chicken, Mushroom & Semi-dried Tomato Risotto (page 213)	Roast Vegetable Salad (page 217)	Thai Shrimp Salad (page 221)

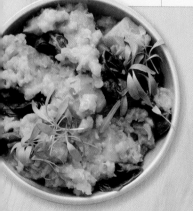

SHOPPING LIST

PANTRY STAPLES

Before you head out to the shops, please make sure that you have a good amount of each of the ingredients on the pantry staples list (see page 101).

GRAINS

1 tbsp brown rice flour
1 slice raisin bread
½ whole wheat lavash
1 whole wheat pita bread
1 whole wheat wrap

FRUIT

1 medium apple
2 medium bananas
5¾ oz blueberries
2 dried figs
2 tbsp goji berries
2–3 lemons
1 lime
2 medium mangoes
6 medjool dates
1 medium orange
1 small pear
5¾ oz raspberries
13¼ oz strawberries

VEGETABLES

1½ large handfuls arugula leaves
4 large handfuls baby spinach leaves
1 small handful bean sprouts
4 small beetroots
1¾ medium red bell peppers
¼ medium yellow bell pepper
1¼ medium carrots
½ celery stalk
15 cherry tomatoes
3½ oz Chinese cabbage (wombok)
1 oz frozen corn kernels
½ small fennel bulb
8 green beans
4 kalamata olives
1 small handful kale
1¾ Lebanese cucumber
1 small handful lettuce leaves
1½ large handfuls mixed lettuce leaves
1 small handful romaine lettuce leaves
2¾ oz mushrooms
1½ small brown onions
1¼ small red onions
4¼ oz pumpkin
3 scallions
1½ oz snow peas
1 medium sweet potato
1½ medium tomatoes
7 semi-dried tomatoes

MEAT & ALTERNATIVES

9 oz boneless, skinless chicken breast
3 oz lean beef minute steak
10 medium shrimps
3 oz pork tenderloin
3 oz roast turkey
8 oz squid tube

DAIRY & ALTERNATIVES

⅔ oz bocconcini
1½ oz camembert cheese
⅔ oz low-fat cheddar cheese
4¼ oz low-fat cottage cheese
4¼ oz low-fat goat's cheese
4¾ oz low-fat ricotta cheese
1 oz low-fat salt-reduced feta cheese
⅔ oz parmesan cheese

HEALTHY FATS

3 oz avocado
1 tsp chia seeds
1 tsp pine nuts
⅔ oz pistachio nuts

OTHER

4 tsp chopped fresh basil
1¼ fresh red chilli
fresh chives
15 tsp (2 small bunches) fresh cilantro
1½ tsp cranberry sauce
1 tsp chopped fresh dill
8¼ garlic cloves
¾ tsp grated fresh ginger
2 tsp hoisin sauce
1 tbsp chopped fresh mint leaves
2 tsp chopped fresh oregano
9 tsp chopped fresh parsley
1 scoop (1 oz) chocolate protein powder
2 tsp raw cacao nibs
½ tsp fresh thyme leaves

Download a copy of this list at kaylaitsines.com/28dayguide/book2/shoppinglist/week4

PART 4

RECIPES

THE MEAL PLAN

I love seeing you make some of my favourite recipes, so make sure you take a photo of your finished dish! Share it with me by posting it to social media, using **#kaylaitsines** so I can see it!

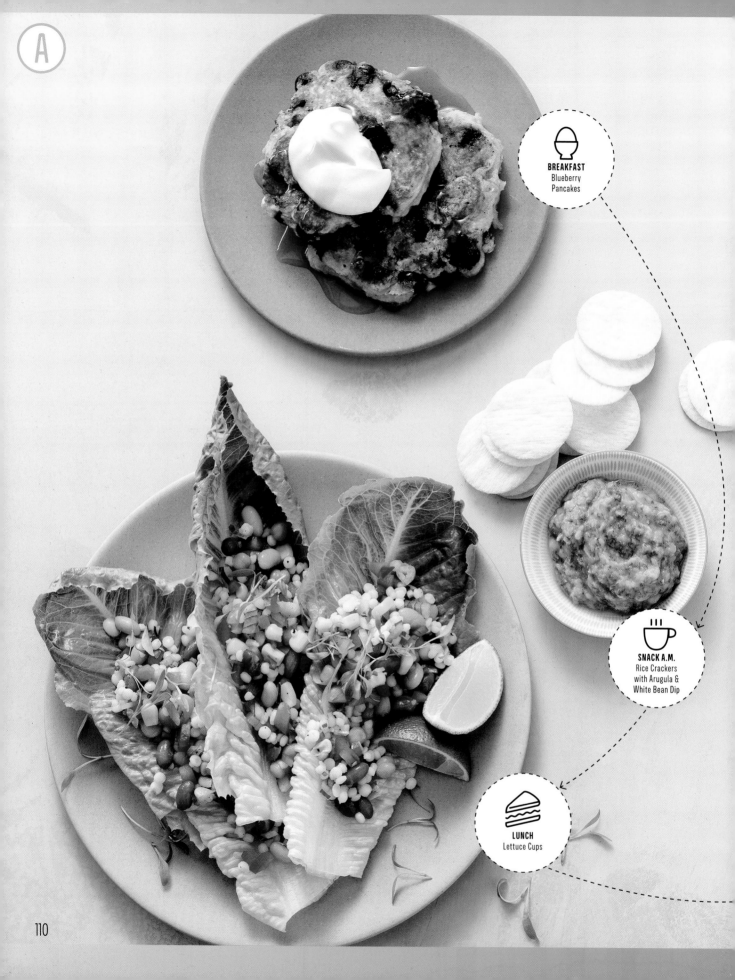

A

BREAKFAST
Blueberry
Pancakes

SNACK A.M.
Rice Crackers
with Arugula &
White Bean Dip

LUNCH
Lettuce Cups

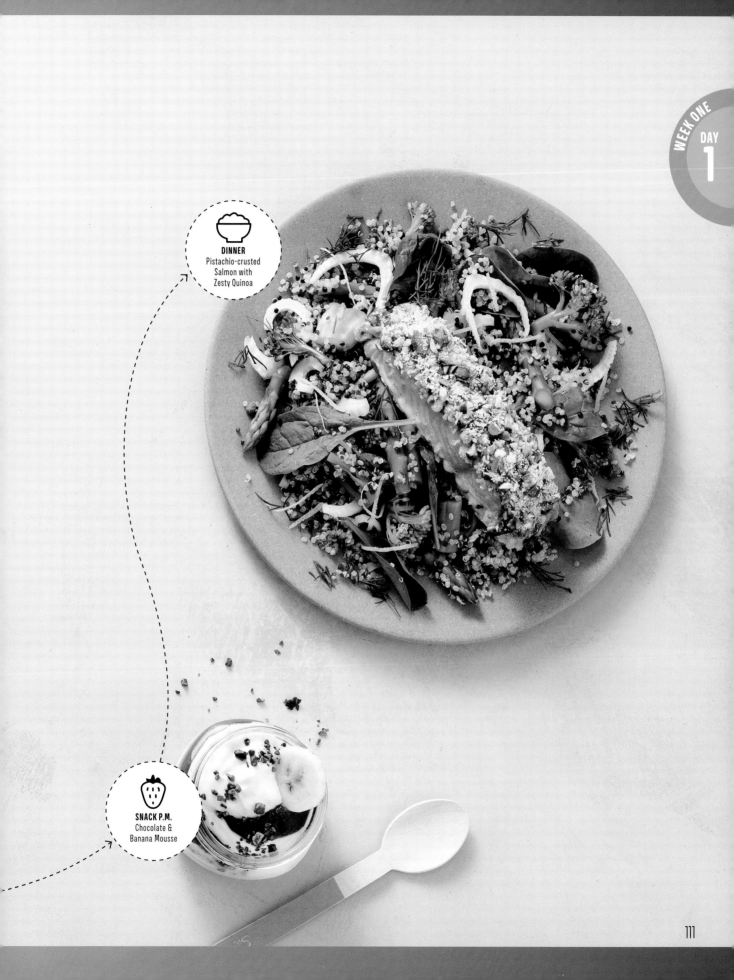

DINNER
Pistachio-crusted
Salmon with
Zesty Quinoa

SNACK P.M.
Chocolate &
Banana Mousse

Blueberry Pancakes

SERVES 1 (MAKES 2 PANCAKES) | **PREP TIME** 5 MINUTES, PLUS 10 MINUTES RESTING TIME | **COOKING TIME** 10 MINUTES | **DIFFICULTY** EASY

2½ oz whole wheat plain flour

1 teaspoon baking powder

½ medium banana,
  peeled and mashed

¼ cup (60 ml) low-fat milk

½ teaspoon pure vanilla extract

3 oz blueberries

oil spray

5¼ oz low-fat plain yoghurt

2 teaspoons pure maple syrup

Place the flour and baking powder in a mixing bowl and mix to combine.

Whisk the banana, milk, and vanilla extract together in a second bowl until well combined. Pour into the dry ingredients and whisk until smooth. Add the blueberries and mix gently. Set aside for 10 minutes to rest.

Heat a non-stick fry pan over medium–high heat and spray lightly with oil spray. Pour a ladleful of the batter into the pan. Cook for 1–2 minutes or until bubbles rise to the surface and the bottom is golden brown. Using a spatula flip the pancake and cook for a further 1–2 minutes or until golden brown and cooked through. Transfer to a plate and cover loosely with foil to keep warm.

Repeat with the remaining batter to make two pancakes in total.

To serve, place the pancakes on a serving plate. Top with the yoghurt and maple syrup.

Rice Crackers with Arugula & White Bean Dip

SERVES 1 | **PREP TIME** 5 MINUTES | **DIFFICULTY** EASY

12 plain rice crackers

ARUGULA & WHITE BEAN DIP

1 large handful arugula leaves,
  roughly chopped

2¾ oz tinned cannellini beans,
  drained and rinsed

¼ garlic clove, crushed

lemon juice, to taste

¼ teaspoon ground cumin

sea salt and ground black
  pepper, to taste

To make the arugula and white bean dip, place the arugula leaves, cannellini beans, garlic, lemon juice, cumin, salt, pepper, and 1 tablespoon of water in a food processor and pulse until smooth and creamy. To save time, you can make the dip the night before and store in an airtight container in the refrigerator.

To serve, place the arugula and white bean dip in a small bowl and serve with the rice crackers.

Lettuce Cups

SERVES 1 | **PREP TIME** 10 MINUTES, PLUS 10 MINUTES COOLING TIME | **COOKING TIME** 15 MINUTES | **DIFFICULTY** EASY

1 oz pearl couscous

5¼ oz tinned four bean mix,
  drained and rinsed

¼ small red onion, diced

¼ medium red bell pepper,
  seeds removed, diced

½ oz corn kernels

1 tablespoon chopped
  fresh cilantro

½ fresh red chilli, finely
  chopped

sea salt and ground black
  pepper, to taste

3 large romaine lettuce leaves,
  left whole, bases trimmed

lime wedges, to serve

micro herbs, to garnish
  (optional)

Fill a saucepan with water and bring to a boil. Stir in the pearl couscous and simmer over medium heat for 10–12 minutes or until al dente. Drain and set aside to cool for 10 minutes.

Place the pearl couscous, four bean mix, onion, bell pepper, corn, cilantro, chilli, salt, and pepper in a mixing bowl and toss gently to combine.

To serve, place the lettuce leaves on a plate and fill with the pearl couscous mixture. Serve with lime wedges on the side, and garnish with micro herbs (if using).

Chocolate & Banana Mousse

SNACK P.M.   **SERVES** 1 | **PREP TIME** 5 MINUTES, PLUS 30 MINUTES SOAKING TIME | **DIFFICULTY** EASY

1½ medjool dates
½ medium banana,
 peeled and sliced
1 teaspoon raw cacao powder
¼ teaspoon pure vanilla extract
10½ oz low-fat plain yoghurt
raw cacao nibs, to garnish

Place the dates in a heatproof bowl, cover with boiling water, and leave to soak for 30 minutes to soften.

Transfer the dates and 2 tablespoons of the soaking water to a high-powered blender, along with half the sliced banana, the cacao powder, and vanilla and blend until smooth.

To serve, layer the date and banana mixture with the yoghurt in a jar or small bowl, top with the remaining slices of banana, and sprinkle over the cacao nibs.

Pistachio-crusted Salmon with Zesty Quinoa

DINNER   **SERVES** 1 | **PREP TIME** 20 MINUTES | **COOKING TIME** 15 MINUTES | **DIFFICULTY** EASY

⅔ oz unsalted pistachio
 kernels, chopped
1 tablespoon panko bread
 crumbs
squeeze of lemon juice,
 to taste
2 teaspoons Dijon mustard
½ teaspoon honey
sea salt and ground black
 pepper, to taste
3 oz salmon fillet, skin
 removed, deboned
oil spray

ZESTY QUINOA

2 oz quinoa
1¾ oz broccolini,
 ends trimmed
5 asparagus spears,
 ends trimmed
¼ small fennel bulb,
 thinly sliced
1 small handful baby
 spinach leaves
2 tablespoons chopped
 fresh dill
2 teaspoons capers, rinsed
pinch of ground cumin
finely grated zest and juice
 of 1 lemon

Preheat the oven to 400°F (350°F convection) and line a baking sheet with baking paper.

Combine the pistachios, bread crumbs, lemon juice, mustard, and honey in a small bowl. Season with salt and pepper, if desired. Spread the mixture evenly over the top of the salmon fillet, pressing lightly to adhere.

Place the salmon fillet on the lined baking sheet and spray lightly with oil spray. Bake in the oven for 10–12 minutes or until cooked to your liking. Transfer to a plate and set aside to rest for 2 minutes.

Meanwhile, to make the zesty quinoa, bring the quinoa and ⅔ cup of water to a boil in a small saucepan over high heat, stirring occasionally. Reduce the heat to low and simmer, covered, for 10–12 minutes or until the liquid has been absorbed and the quinoa is tender.

Meanwhile, add 2 inches of water to a saucepan and insert a steamer basket. Cover with a lid and bring the water to a boil over high heat, then reduce the heat to medium. Add the broccolini and asparagus and steam, covered, for 4–5 minutes or until the vegetables are tender-crisp.

Place the quinoa, broccolini, asparagus, fennel, spinach, dill, capers, cumin, lemon zest, and juice in a mixing bowl and toss gently to combine.

To serve, place the quinoa mixture on a serving plate and top with the pistachio-crusted salmon.

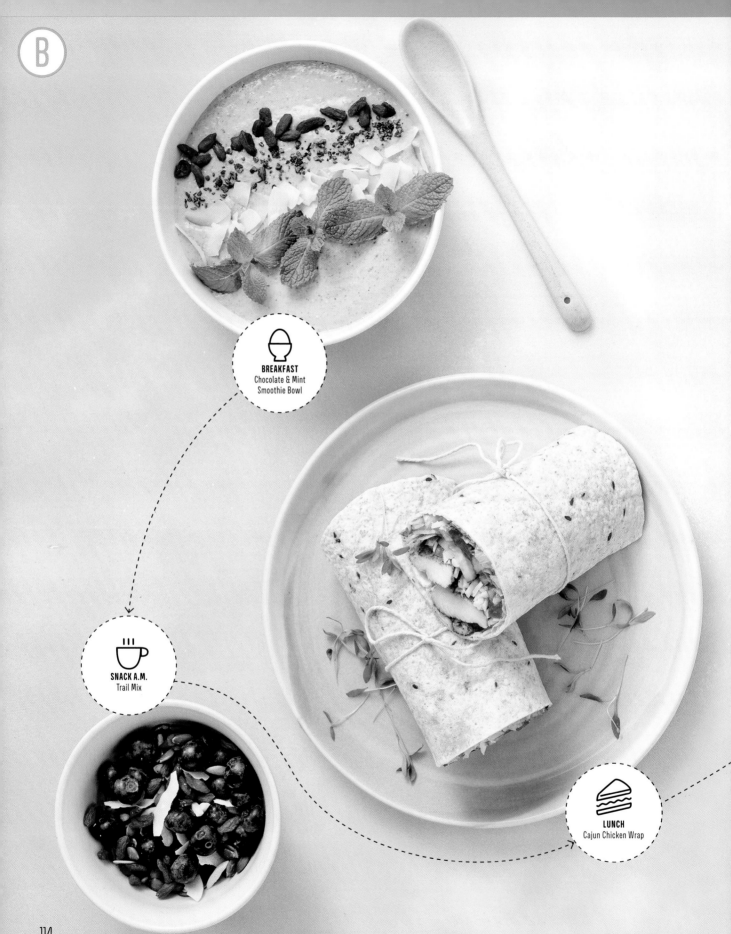

B

BREAKFAST
Chocolate & Mint
Smoothie Bowl

SNACK A.M.
Trail Mix

LUNCH
Cajun Chicken Wrap

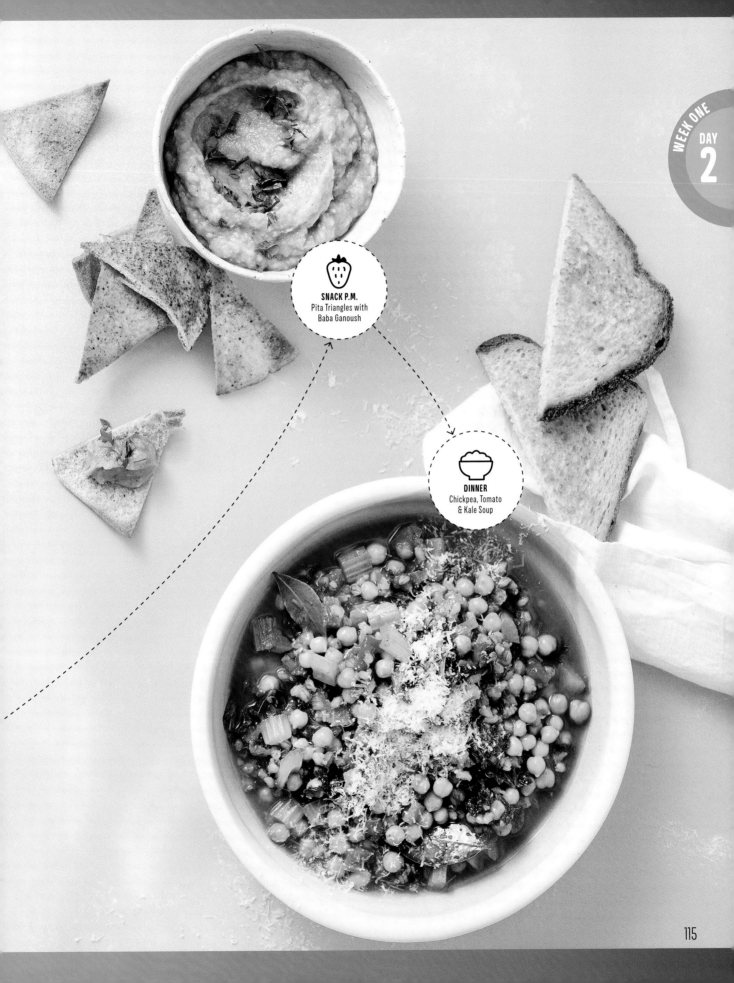

SNACK P.M.
Pita Triangles with
Baba Ganoush

DINNER
Chickpea, Tomato
& Kale Soup

Chocolate & Mint Smoothie Bowl

BREAKFAST **SERVES** 1 | **PREP TIME** 10 MINUTES | **DIFFICULTY** EASY

1 medium banana,
  peeled and sliced
1 oz rolled oats
1 small handful baby
  spinach leaves
½ cup (130 ml) low-fat milk
7 oz low-fat plain yoghurt

1 small handful fresh mint,
  plus extra leaves to garnish
1 teaspoon chia seeds

TOPPINGS
2 teaspoons raw cacao nibs
2 teaspoons coconut flakes
1 tablespoon goji berries

Place the banana, rolled oats, spinach, milk, yoghurt, mint, and chia seeds in a high-powered blender and blend until smooth.

To serve, pour the smoothie mixture into a serving bowl and top with the cacao nibs, coconut flakes, and goji berries. Garnish with the extra mint leaves.

Trail Mix

SNACK A.M. **SERVES** 1 | **PREP TIME** 5 MINUTES | **DIFFICULTY** EASY

½ teaspoon pumpkin seeds
  (pepitas)
½ teaspoon sunflower seeds
½ teaspoon slivered almonds
1 teaspoon coconut flakes
2 teaspoons goji berries
1½ oz blueberries

To serve, place the pumpkin seeds, sunflower seeds, almonds, coconut flakes, goji berries, and blueberries in a small bowl and stir until combined.

Cajun Chicken Wrap

LUNCH **SERVES** 1 | **PREP TIME** 15 MINUTES, PLUS 10 MINUTES CHILLING TIME | **COOKING TIME** 10 MINUTES | **DIFFICULTY** EASY

3½ oz boneless, skinless chicken
  breast, sliced into strips
2 teaspoons Cajun seasoning
oil spray
1¾ oz low-fat plain yoghurt
1 tablespoon chopped
  fresh parsley
1 whole wheat wrap
1 small handful lettuce leaves
¼ small red onion, thinly sliced
⅓ oz low-fat cheddar
  cheese, grated
½ medium tomato, sliced
½ Lebanese cucumber, sliced

Place the chicken strips and Cajun seasoning in a small bowl and mix well to coat. Cover with plastic wrap and marinate in the refrigerator for 10 minutes.

Heat a non-stick fry pan over medium–high heat and spray lightly with oil spray. Add the chicken strips and cook for 3–4 minutes on each side or until cooked through. Transfer to a plate and set aside to rest.

Mix the yoghurt and parsley together in a small bowl.

To serve, place the wrap on a serving plate and spread over the yoghurt. Place the lettuce, onion, cheese, tomato, cucumber, and Cajun spiced chicken down the middle of the wrap. Fold over the end and roll up to enclose the filling.

Pita Triangles with Baba Ganoush

SNACK P.M. **SERVES** 1 | **PREP TIME** 10 MINUTES, PLUS 10 MINUTES COOLING TIME | **COOKING TIME** 35 MINUTES | **DIFFICULTY** EASY

½ medium eggplant

oil spray

½ whole wheat pita bread,
    cut into wedges

2¾ oz tinned cannellini beans,
    drained and rinsed

½ garlic clove, crushed

½ teaspoon tahini

juice of ¼ lemon, plus extra
    if needed

pinch of ground cumin

pinch of sweet paprika,
    plus extra if needed

sea salt, to taste

1 tablespoon chopped
    fresh parsley

Preheat the oven to 400°F (350°F convection) and line two baking sheets with baking paper.

Pierce the eggplant half all over with a fork. Place on one of the lined baking sheets, cut side down, and spray lightly with oil spray. Roast in the oven for 30–35 minutes or until tender.

About 10 minutes before the eggplant is ready, lay the pita wedges in a single layer on the other lined baking sheet and spray lightly with oil spray. Place in the oven and bake for 5 minutes or until they begin to colour. Turn the wedges over and bake for a further 5–8 minutes or until both sides are lightly coloured.

Remove the eggplant and pita triangles from the oven and set aside to cool. Once cool enough to handle, remove the skin from the eggplant.

Place the eggplant, cannellini beans, garlic, tahini, lemon juice, cumin, paprika, salt, and 2 tablespoons of water in a food processor and pulse until smooth and creamy. Transfer to a serving bowl and scatter over the parsley. Season with extra lemon juice, paprika, and salt, if desired.

Serve the pita triangles with the baba ganoush.

Chickpea, Tomato & Kale Soup

DINNER **SERVES** 1 | **PREP TIME** 10 MINUTES, PLUS 1 HOUR SOAKING TIME | **COOKING TIME** 1 HOUR | **DIFFICULTY** EASY

1½ oz pearl barley

oil spray

¼ small brown onion, chopped

½ celery stalk, diced

1 garlic clove, crushed

1 bay leaf

½ teaspoon sweet paprika

pinch of ground coriander

pinch of ground cumin

2 cups (500 ml) salt-reduced
    vegetable stock

5¼ oz tinned crushed tomatoes

5¼ oz tinned chickpeas,
    drained and rinsed

1 small handful kale,
    roughly chopped

sea salt and ground black
    pepper, to taste

1 slice whole wheat bread

⅔ oz parmesan cheese, grated

Rinse the pearl barley under cold running water until the water runs clear. Place in a medium bowl and cover with cold water. Leave to soak for 1 hour, then drain.

Heat a large saucepan over medium heat and spray lightly with oil spray. Add the onion and celery and cook for 5 minutes, stirring occasionally. Add the garlic, bay leaf, paprika, ground coriander, and ground cumin and cook for 1 minute or until fragrant, stirring frequently.

Add the barley and stock and bring to a boil over high heat. Reduce the heat to low and simmer for 30 minutes or until the barley is tender.

Add the tomatoes, chickpeas, and kale and simmer for a further 15–20 minutes, stirring occasionally. Season with salt and pepper, if desired.

Toast the bread to your liking.

To serve, ladle the soup into a serving bowl and sprinkle over the grated cheese. Serve with the toasted bread on the side.

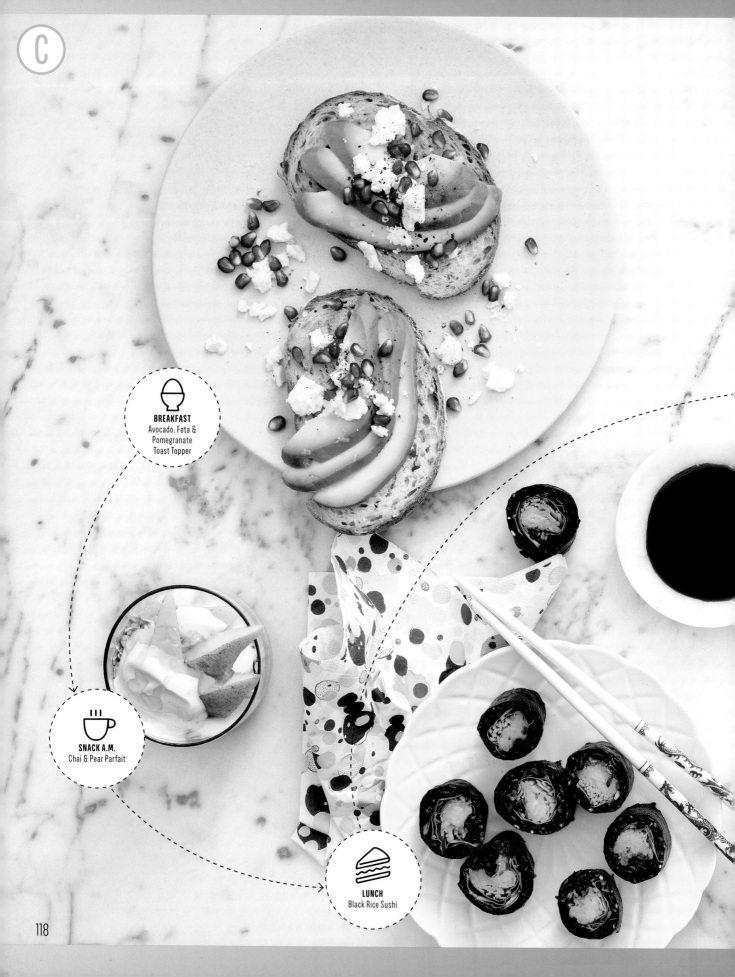

C

BREAKFAST
Avocado, Feta &
Pomegranate
Toast Topper

SNACK A.M.
Chai & Pear Parfait

LUNCH
Black Rice Sushi

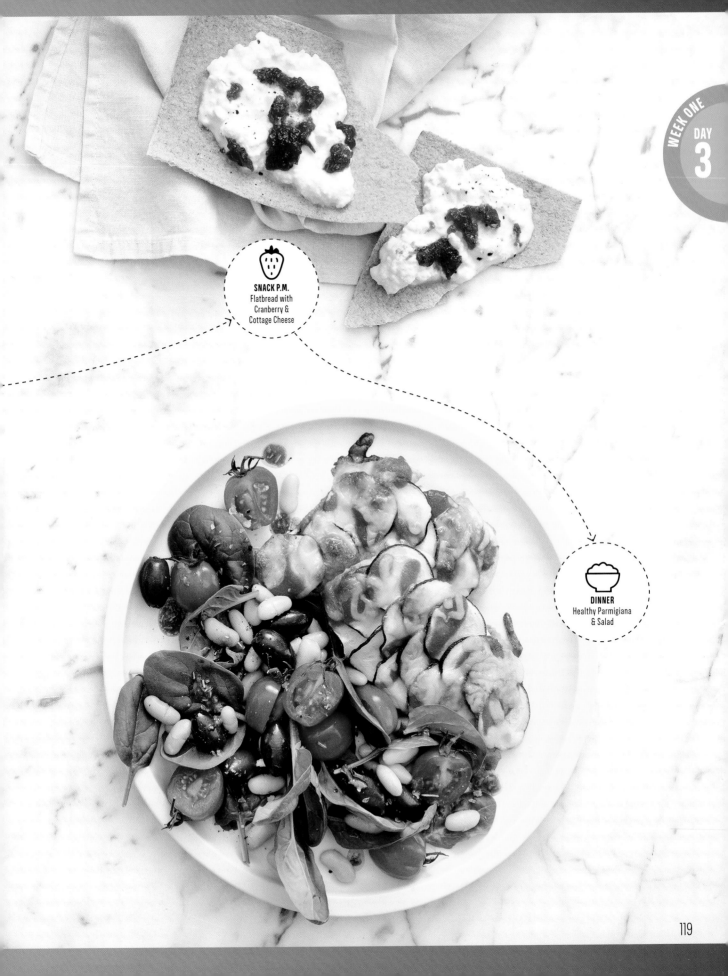

SNACK P.M.
Flatbread with
Cranberry &
Cottage Cheese

DINNER
Healthy Parmigiana
& Salad

Avocado, Feta & Pomegranate Toast Topper

SERVES 1 | **PREP TIME** 5 MINUTES | **COOKING TIME** 2 MINUTES | **DIFFICULTY** EASY

2 slices whole wheat bread
½ pomegranate
1½ oz avocado, sliced
1¾ oz salt-reduced low-fat feta cheese
sea salt and ground black pepper, to taste

Toast the bread to your liking.

Meanwhile, gently tap the pomegranate seeds into a small bowl.

To serve, place the toast on a serving plate and top with the avocado. Sprinkle over the feta and pomegranate seeds and season with salt and pepper, if desired.

Chai & Pear Parfait

SNACK A.M. **SERVES** 1 | **PREP TIME** 10 MINUTES, PLUS 15 MINUTES COOLING AND CHILLING TIME | **DIFFICULTY** EASY

1 chai teabag
7 oz low-fat plain yoghurt
1½ small pears, halved, cored and thinly sliced
1 oz natural muesli
honey, to drizzle

Place the teabag in a mug and add ⅓ cup (80 ml) of boiling water. Allow to infuse for 1 minute or to taste and then remove the teabag. Set aside to cool completely.

Place the yoghurt and chai tea in a small bowl and mix until well combined.

Place the chai yoghurt, pear, and muesli in a glass, then place in the refrigerator to chill for 10 minutes.

To serve, drizzle with honey.

Black Rice Sushi

LUNCH **SERVES** 1 | **PREP TIME** 15 MINUTES, PLUS 20 MINUTES STANDING AND COOLING TIME | **COOKING TIME** 40 MINUTES | **DIFFICULTY** MEDIUM

2 oz black rice
2 nori sheets
3 oz smoked salmon
½ Lebanese cucumber, cut into matchsticks (julienned)
½ medium carrot, cut into matchsticks (julienned)
1 small handful arugula leaves
salt-reduced tamari or soy sauce, for dipping

To cook the rice, bring the rice and 1 cup (250 ml) of water to a boil in a small saucepan over high heat, stirring occasionally. Reduce the heat to low and simmer, covered, for 35–40 minutes or until the liquid has been absorbed and the rice is tender. Remove from the heat and leave to stand, covered, for 10 minutes. Set aside to cool.

Place a sushi mat on a clean board with slats running horizontally. Place one nori sheet on the mat, shiny side down.

Spoon half the cooked rice onto the bottom two-thirds of the nori sheet, leaving a small border around the edge. Top with half the salmon, cucumber, carrot, and arugula.

Hold the filling in place while rolling the mat over to enclose the rice and filling, gently pulling the mat as you go. Continue to roll until the rice and filling are covered with the nori sheet. Shape your hands around the mat to gently tighten the roll.

Repeat with the remaining nori sheet and filling ingredients to make two rolls in total.

Leave the rolls to sit for 2 minutes, then cut into thick rounds with a sharp knife.

To serve, place the sushi on a serving plate and serve with a small dish of tamari or soy sauce for dipping.

Flatbread with Cranberry & Cottage Cheese

SNACK P.M. | **SERVES** 1 | **PREP TIME** 5 MINUTES | **COOKING TIME** 10 MINUTES | **DIFFICULTY** EASY

½ whole wheat lavash

oil spray

1 oz low-fat cottage cheese

½ teaspoon cranberry jam

sea salt and ground black
pepper, to taste

Preheat the oven to 350°F (320°F convection) and line a baking sheet with baking paper.

Place the lavash on the lined baking sheet and spray lightly with oil spray. Bake in the oven for 8–10 minutes or until golden and crispy.

To serve, spread the cottage cheese over the lavash, then spoon over the cranberry jam and season with salt and pepper.

Healthy Parmigiana & Salad

DINNER | **SERVES** 1 | **PREP TIME** 10 MINUTES | **COOKING TIME** 15 MINUTES | **DIFFICULTY** EASY

5¼ oz boneless, skinless
chicken breast

½ medium zucchini,
thinly sliced

2½ oz tomato passata (purée)

⅔ oz mozzarella cheese,
grated

1 large handful baby
spinach leaves

8 cherry tomatoes, halved

1½ oz tinned cannellini beans,
drained and rinsed

4 kalamata olives,
pitted, halved

sea salt and ground black
pepper, to taste

DRESSING

¾ teaspoon olive oil

¼ teaspoon balsamic vinegar

½ garlic clove, crushed

pinch of dried rosemary

Preheat the oven to 400°F (350°F convection) and line a baking sheet with baking paper.

Slice the chicken horizontally through the middle to make two thin fillets.

Place the chicken on the lined baking sheet and spread the sliced zucchini over the top. Spoon over the tomato passata and top with the cheese. Bake in the oven for 15 minutes or until the chicken is cooked through and the cheese has melted.

To make the dressing, whisk the olive oil, balsamic vinegar, garlic, and rosemary together in a small bowl and set aside.

Place the spinach, cherry tomatoes, cannellini beans, and olives in a mixing bowl. Drizzle over the dressing, season with salt and pepper, if desired, and toss gently to combine.

To serve, place the chicken parmigiana on a serving plate with the salad on the side.

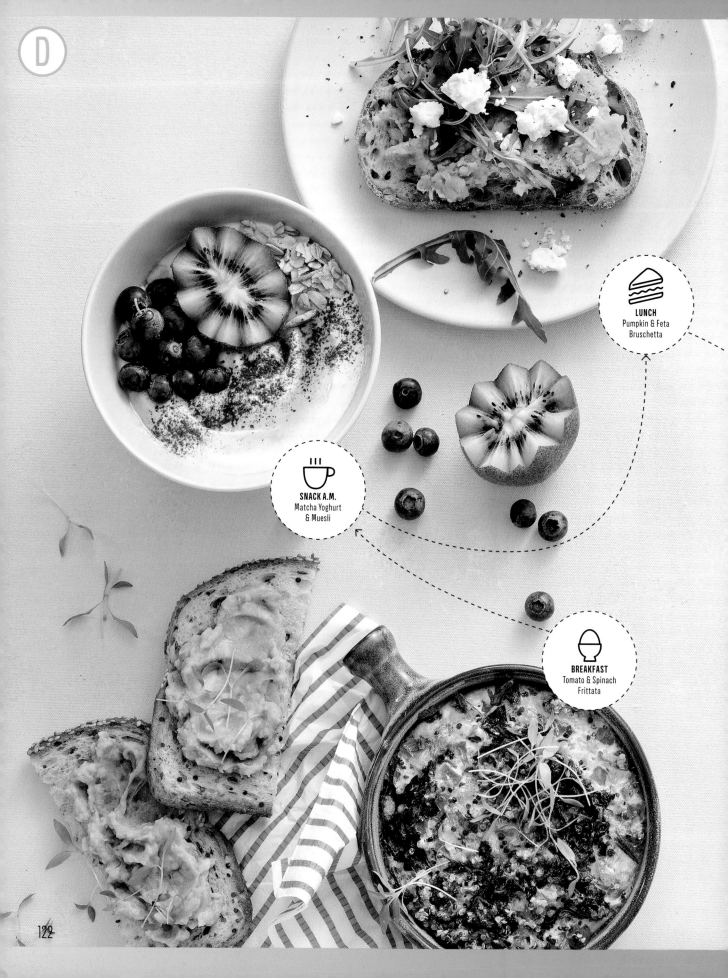

D

LUNCH
Pumpkin & Feta
Bruschetta

SNACK A.M.
Matcha Yoghurt
& Muesli

BREAKFAST
Tomato & Spinach
Frittata

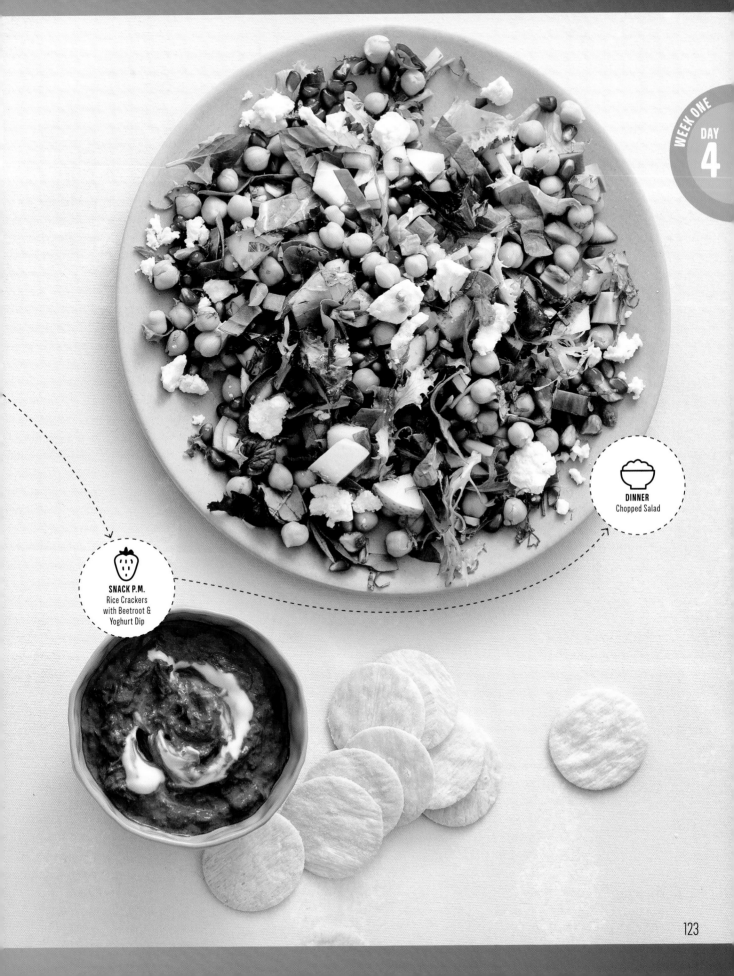

DINNER
Chopped Salad

SNACK P.M.
Rice Crackers
with Beetroot &
Yoghurt Dip

Tomato & Spinach Frittata

BREAKFAST **SERVES** 1 | **PREP TIME** 10 MINUTES, PLUS 10 MINUTES COOLING TIME | **COOKING TIME** 35 MINUTES | **DIFFICULTY** EASY

1 oz quinoa

oil spray

1 small handful baby spinach leaves, shredded

½ medium tomato, diced

1¾ oz low-fat ricotta cheese

2 teaspoons chopped fresh parsley

sea salt and ground black pepper, to taste

2 large eggs

1 slice whole grain bread

1 oz avocado, mashed

micro herbs, to garnish (optional)

Bring the quinoa and ¾ cup (190 ml) of water to a boil in a small saucepan over high heat, stirring occasionally. Reduce the heat to low and simmer, covered, for 10–12 minutes or until the quinoa is tender. Drain off excess liquid and set aside to cool. To save time, the quinoa can be cooked the night before and stored in an airtight container in the refrigerator.

Preheat the oven to 350°F (320°F convection) and grease a 3 inch ramekin with oil spray.

Heat a small non-stick fry pan over medium heat and lightly spray with oil spray. Add the spinach and tomato and cook for 2–3 minutes or until soft, stirring occasionally. Set aside to cool slightly.

Place the quinoa, spinach mixture, cheese, and parsley in a mixing bowl, season with salt and pepper, if desired, and stir until well combined. Transfer to the prepared ramekin. Whisk the eggs and 2 tablespoons of water together in a small bowl. Pour the egg mixture into the ramekin. Bake in the oven for 15–20 minutes or until golden and set.

Meanwhile, toast the bread to your liking and spread with the avocado. Serve the frittata with the toast on the side, garnished with micro herbs (if using).

Matcha Yoghurt & Muesli

SNACK A.M. **SERVES** 1 | **PREP TIME** 5 MINUTES | **DIFFICULTY** EASY

3½ oz low-fat plain yoghurt

¼ teaspoon pure maple syrup

¼ teaspoon matcha powder

1 oz natural muesli or rolled oats

1 kiwifruit, peeled and sliced

3 oz blueberries

Place the yoghurt in a small bowl, drizzle over the maple syrup, then sprinkle with the matcha powder.

To serve, top with the muesli, kiwifruit and blueberries.

Pumpkin & Feta Bruschetta

LUNCH **SERVES** 1 | **PREP TIME** 5 MINUTES, PLUS 5 MINUTES COOLING TIME | **COOKING TIME** 20 MINUTES | **DIFFICULTY** EASY

4¼ oz pumpkin, peeled and cut into 1 inch cubes

oil spray

2¾ oz tinned chickpeas, drained and rinsed

lemon juice, to taste

pinch of ground cumin

sea salt and ground black pepper, to taste

1 slice whole wheat bread

1 oz salt-reduced low-fat feta cheese, crumbled

1 small handful arugula leaves

Preheat the oven to 400°F (350°F convection) and line a baking sheet with baking paper.

Place the pumpkin on the lined baking sheet and spray lightly with oil spray. Bake in the oven for 15–20 minutes or until cooked through, using tongs to turn halfway through. Set aside to cool slightly.

Place the pumpkin and chickpeas in a small bowl and roughly mash with a fork. Season with lemon juice, cumin, salt, and pepper, if desired, and mix until well combined.

Toast the bread to your liking.

To serve, spread the pumpkin mash over the toast. Sprinkle over the feta and top with the arugula.

Rice Crackers with Beetroot & Yoghurt Dip

SERVES 1 | **PREP TIME** 5 MINUTES | **DIFFICULTY** EASY

WEEK ONE DAY 4

12 plain rice crackers

**BEETROOT &
YOGHURT DIP**
½ small beetroot, peeled
  and grated
pinch of ground cumin
pinch of ground coriander
lemon juice, to taste
3½ oz low-fat plain yoghurt
sea salt and ground black
  pepper, to taste

To make the beetroot and yoghurt dip, place the beetroot, cumin, coriander, lemon juice, yoghurt, salt, and pepper in a small bowl and mix until well combined.

Serve the rice crackers with the beetroot yoghurt dip.

Chopped Salad

SERVES 1 | **PREP TIME** 10 MINUTES, PLUS 10 MINUTES COOLING TIME | **COOKING TIME** 15 MINUTES | **DIFFICULTY** EASY

1 oz quinoa
½ pomegranate
1 large handful baby spinach
  leaves, finely chopped
1 small handful mixed lettuce
  leaves, finely chopped
¼ small red onion, chopped
¼ Lebanese cucumber,
  chopped
5¼ oz tinned chickpeas,
  drained and rinsed
½ small pear, chopped
½ oz avocado, diced
1 oz salt-reduced low-fat feta
  cheese, crumbled
⅓ oz unsalted pistachio
  kernels, finely chopped

DRESSING
lemon juice, to taste
2 teaspoons honey
2 teaspoons chopped
  fresh mint
sea salt and ground black
  pepper, to taste

Bring the quinoa and ¾ cup (190 ml) of water to a boil in a small saucepan over high heat, stirring occasionally. Reduce the heat to low and simmer, covered, for 10–12 minutes or until the quinoa is tender. Drain off any excess liquid and set aside to cool. To save time, the quinoa can be cooked the night before and stored in an airtight container in the refrigerator.

To make the dressing, whisk the lemon juice, honey, mint, salt, pepper, and 1 tablespoon of water together in a small bowl and set aside.

Gently tap the pomegranate seeds into a mixing bowl. Add the quinoa, spinach, lettuce, onion, cucumber, chickpeas, pear, avocado, and feta, then drizzle over the dressing and toss gently to combine.

To serve, place the chopped salad in a serving bowl and scatter over the chopped pistachios.

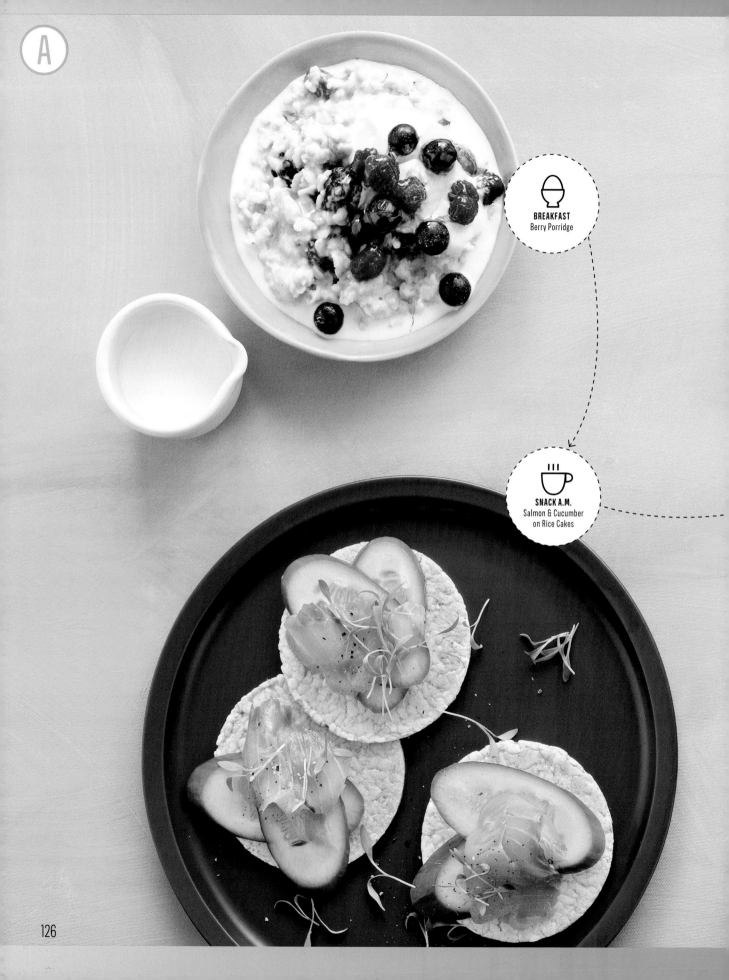

A

BREAKFAST
Berry Porridge

SNACK A.M.
Salmon & Cucumber
on Rice Cakes

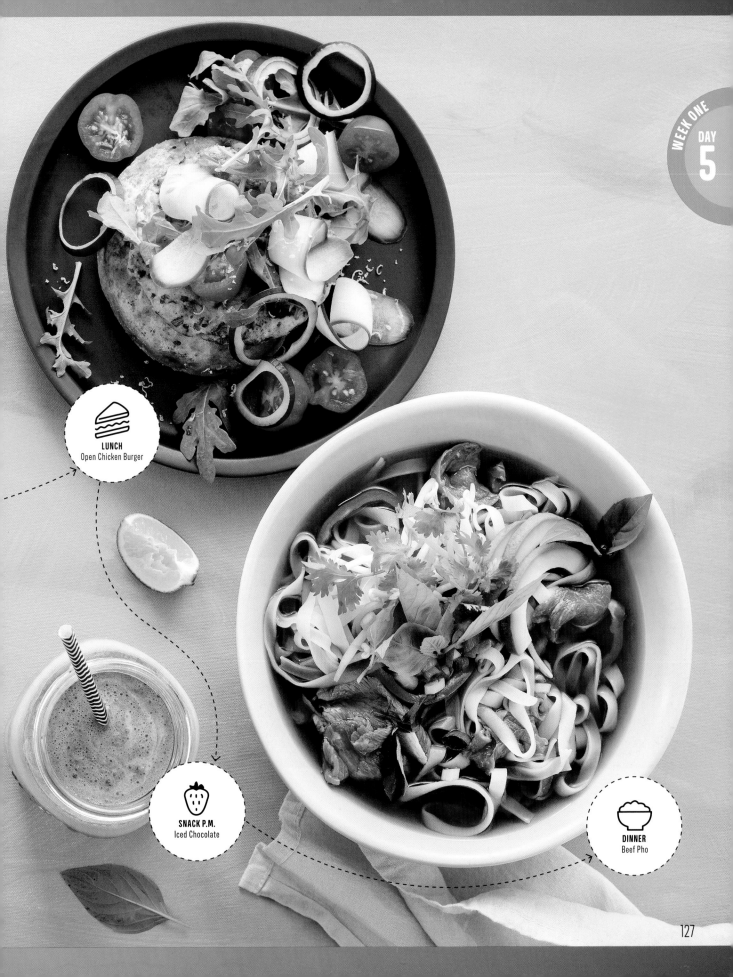

LUNCH
Open Chicken Burger

SNACK P.M.
Iced Chocolate

DINNER
Beef Pho

Berry Porridge

SERVES 1 | **PREP TIME** 5 MINUTES | **COOKING TIME** 10 MINUTES | **DIFFICULTY** EASY

½ cup (125 ml) low-fat milk

2 oz rolled oats

6 oz frozen mixed
  berries, thawed

2 teaspoons honey

3½ oz low-fat plain yoghurt

Combine ¼ cup (50 ml) of the milk and 1 cup (200 ml) of water in a small saucepan and bring to the boil over high heat. Stir in the oats and reduce the heat to medium–low. Simmer for 3 minutes, stirring occasionally.

Add half the berries and 1 teaspoon of the honey and cook for a further 2 minutes or until the porridge has thickened and the berries are warmed through, stirring occasionally.

To serve, pour the berry porridge into a serving bowl. Top with the yoghurt and the remaining milk, honey, and berries.

Salmon & Cucumber on Rice Cakes

SNACK A.M. **SERVES** 1 | **PREP TIME** 5 MINUTES | **DIFFICULTY** EASY

3 rice cakes

1 Lebanese cucumber, sliced

1½ oz smoked salmon

sea salt and ground black
  pepper, to taste

micro herbs, to garnish
  (optional)

To serve, place the rice cakes on a serving plate and top with the cucumber and salmon. Season with salt and pepper and scatter with micro herbs (if using).

Open Chicken Burger

LUNCH **SERVES** 1 | **PREP TIME** 10 MINUTES, PLUS 30 MINUTES CHILLING TIME | **COOKING TIME** 10 MINUTES | **DIFFICULTY** EASY

3½ oz ground chicken

2 teaspoons chopped
  fresh cilantro

2 teaspoons chopped
  fresh mint

¼ teaspoon ground cumin

¼ teaspoon sweet paprika

½ garlic clove, crushed

2 teaspoons panko bread
  crumbs

sea salt and ground black
  pepper, to taste

oil spray

¾ Lebanese cucumber

1 small handful arugula leaves

5 cherry tomatoes, halved

¼ small red onion, sliced

finely grated zest and juice
  of 1 lemon

½ medium whole wheat roll

Place the ground chicken, cilantro, mint, cumin, paprika, garlic, bread crumbs, salt, and pepper in a mixing bowl and mix to combine.

Using slightly damp hands, shape the chicken mixture into a patty. Place on a plate, cover with plastic wrap, and refrigerate for 30 minutes.

Heat a non-stick fry pan over medium heat and spray lightly with oil spray. Cook the patty for 4–5 minutes on each side or until cooked through and golden. To save time, the patty can be prepared and cooked the night before and once cooled, stored in an airtight container in the refrigerator.

Meanwhile, use a vegetable peeler to carefully slice the cucumber lengthwise into long, thin ribbons.

Place the arugula, cucumber, tomatoes, onion, and lemon zest in a mixing bowl. Drizzle over the lemon juice and toss gently to combine.

To serve, lightly toast the bread roll half in a toaster or under a hot oven grill. Top the toasted bread with the patty and the arugula salad.

Iced Chocolate

SNACK P.M. | **SERVES** 1 | **PREP TIME** 5 MINUTES, PLUS 30 MINUTES SOAKING TIME | **DIFFICULTY** EASY

WEEK ONE DAY 5

3 medjool dates

2 tablespoons raw
  cacao powder

1 cup (250 ml) low-fat milk

3½ oz low-fat plain yoghurt

¼ teaspoon pure vanilla extract

1 small handful ice cubes

Place the dates in a heatproof bowl, cover with boiling water, and leave to soak for 30 minutes to soften. Drain.

Whisk the cacao powder with a dash of boiling water to combine.

Place the dates, milk, yoghurt, cacao mixture, vanilla extract, and ice in a high-powered blender and blend until smooth.

To serve, pour into a glass or jar.

Beef Pho

DINNER | **SERVES** 1 | **PREP TIME** 10 MINUTES, PLUS 10 MINUTES SOAKING TIME | **COOKING TIME** 20 MINUTES | **DIFFICULTY** EASY

2 cups (500 ml) salt-reduced
  beef stock

¾-inch piece fresh ginger,
  peeled and sliced

¼ small brown onion, chopped

½ cinnamon stick

1 star anise

1 garlic clove, sliced

1 teaspoon fish sauce

1 teaspoon honey

3½ oz rice stick noodles

3 oz lean beef steak,
  very thinly sliced

1 large handful bean sprouts

1 scallion, sliced

¼ medium red bell pepper,
  seeds removed, thinly sliced

1¾ oz avocado, sliced

1 small handful fresh cilantro

1 small handful fresh Thai basil
  or regular basil

lime wedges, to serve

Place the stock, ginger, brown onion, cinnamon stick, star anise, garlic, fish sauce, and honey in a medium saucepan. Bring to a boil, then reduce the heat to low. Cover and simmer for 20 minutes. Strain the soup and discard the solid ingredients. Return the soup to the heat, cover, and keep hot over medium–low heat.

Place the noodles in a heatproof bowl and cover with boiling water. Leave for 10 minutes, then loosen the noodles with a fork. Drain and refresh under cool running water. Drain well.

To serve, place the noodles in a serving bowl and top with the thinly sliced beef. Pour over the hot soup and top with the bean sprouts, scallion, bell pepper, and avocado. Garnish with the cilantro and basil leaves and serve with lime wedges on the side.

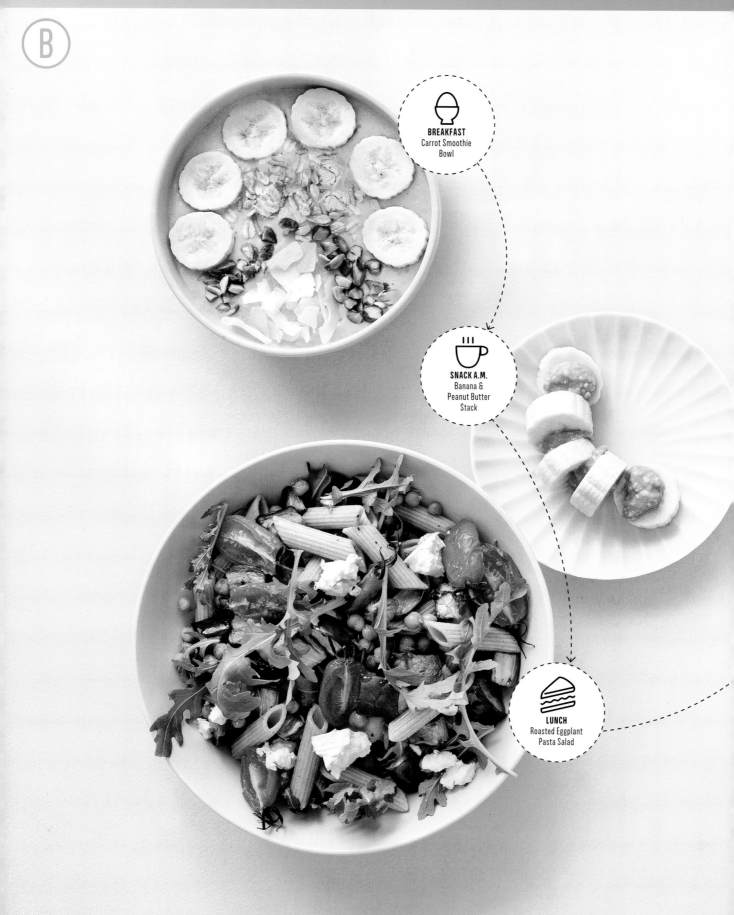

BREAKFAST
Carrot Smoothie
Bowl

SNACK A.M.
Banana &
Peanut Butter
Stack

LUNCH
Roasted Eggplant
Pasta Salad

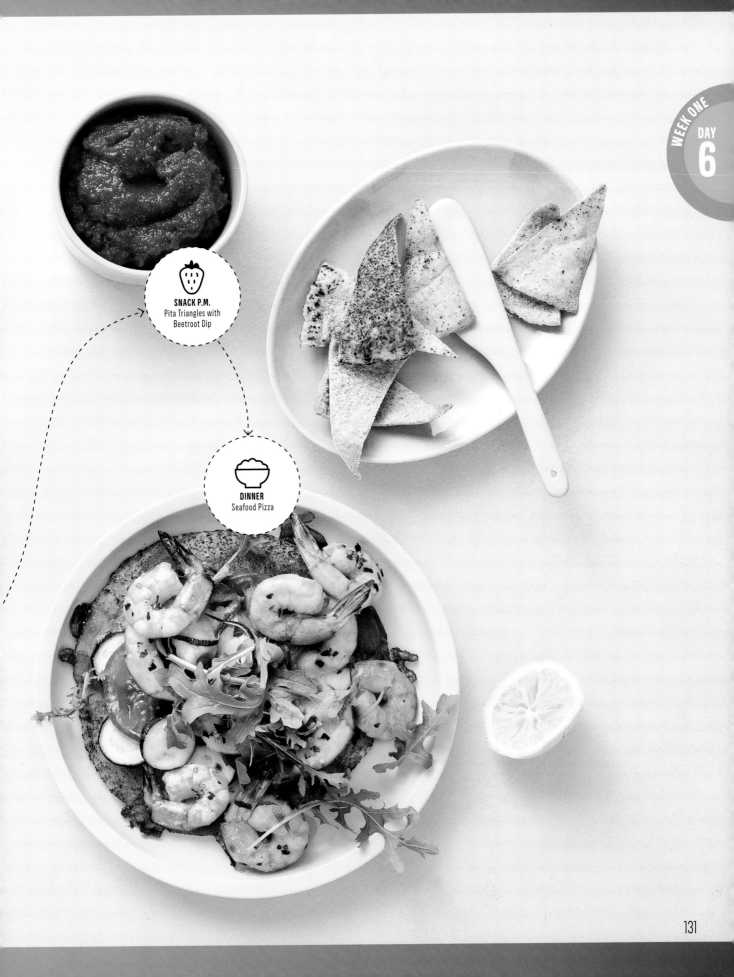

SNACK P.M.
Pita Triangles with
Beetroot Dip

DINNER
Seafood Pizza

Carrot Smoothie Bowl

BREAKFAST **SERVES** 1 | **PREP TIME** 10 MINUTES | **DIFFICULTY** EASY

½ medium carrot,
  roughly chopped

½ medium orange, peeled
  and chopped

¾ cup (190 ml) low-fat milk

5¼ oz low-fat plain yoghurt

½ teaspoon pure
  vanilla extract

1 medium banana, peeled
  and sliced

TOPPINGS

1 oz natural muesli

2 teaspoons coconut flakes

⅓ oz unsalted pistachio
  kernels, roughly chopped

Steam the carrot for 2–3 minutes until soft.

Place the carrot, orange, milk, yoghurt, vanilla, and half the banana in a high-powered blender and blend until smooth.

To serve, pour the smoothie mixture into a serving bowl and top with the muesli, coconut flakes, pistachios, and remaining banana.

Banana & Peanut Butter Stack

SNACK A.M. **SERVES** 1 | **PREP TIME** 5 MINUTES | **DIFFICULTY** EASY

2 teaspoons 100% natural
  peanut butter

½ medium banana, peeled and
  cut into ½-inch thick slices

Spread a small amount of peanut butter in between each of the banana slices to make a "stack."

Repeat until all of the peanut butter and banana are used.

Roasted Eggplant Pasta Salad

LUNCH **SERVES** 1 | **PREP TIME** 10 MINUTES | **COOKING TIME** 20 MINUTES | **DIFFICULTY** EASY

¼ medium eggplant, cut into
  ¾ inch cubes

oil spray

5 cherry tomatoes, halved

5¼ oz tinned chickpeas,
  drained and rinsed

3 oz whole wheat pasta

1 small handful arugula leaves

sea salt and ground black
  pepper, to taste

1 oz salt-reduced low-fat
  feta cheese, crumbled

DRESSING

½ garlic clove, crushed

1 tablespoon chopped
  fresh parsley

lemon juice, to taste

Preheat the oven to 350°F (325°F convection) and line a baking sheet with baking paper.

Place the eggplant on the lined baking sheet and spray lightly with oil spray. Roast the eggplant for 20 minutes or until golden, adding the tomatoes and chickpeas for the last 10 minutes of the cooking time. Using tongs, turn the eggplant once during the cooking time.

Meanwhile, fill a large saucepan with water, add a pinch of salt, and bring to a boil. Add the pasta and cook until al dente (see the pasta packet for the recommended cooking time). Drain and refresh under cool running water. Set aside to cool. To save time, the pasta can be cooked the night before and stored in an airtight container in the refrigerator.

To make the dressing, whisk the garlic, parsley, lemon juice, and 1 tablespoon of water together in a small bowl and set aside.

Place the pasta, eggplant, tomatoes, chickpeas, and arugula in a mixing bowl. Drizzle over the dressing, season with salt and pepper, if desired, and toss gently to combine.

To serve, place the salad in a serving bowl and sprinkle over the feta.

Pita Triangles with Beetroot Dip

½ whole wheat pita bread,
  cut into wedges
oil spray

BEETROOT DIP

1 small beetroot, peeled
  and chopped
2¾ oz tinned cannellini beans,
  drained and rinsed
¼ garlic clove, crushed
pinch of ground coriander
pinch of ground cumin
pinch of sweet paprika
lemon juice, to taste
sea salt and ground black
  pepper, to taste

Preheat the oven to 400°F (350°F convection) and line a baking sheet with baking paper.

Lay the pita wedges in a single layer on the lined baking sheet and spray lightly with oil spray. Bake in the oven for 5 minutes or until they begin to colour. Turn the wedges over and bake for a further 5–8 minutes or until both sides are lightly coloured. Set aside to cool.

To make the beetroot dip, place the beetroot, cannellini beans, garlic, coriander, cumin, paprika, and 2 teaspoons of water in a food processor and process until smooth. Season with lemon juice, salt, and pepper, if desired.

To serve, place the beetroot dip in a small bowl and serve with the pita triangles.

Seafood Pizza

¼ teaspoon dried chilli flakes
1 garlic clove, crushed
1 teaspoon honey
lemon juice, to taste
6–8 medium raw shrimps,
  peeled and deveined,
  tails intact
1 whole wheat pita bread
2¾ oz tomato passata (purée)
¼ small red onion, thinly sliced
¼ medium zucchini,
  thinly sliced
½ medium tomato, sliced
sea salt and ground black
  pepper, to taste
⅔ oz mozzarella cheese,
  grated
1 small handful arugula leaves
lemon wedges, to serve

Preheat the oven to 350°F (325°F convection) and line a baking sheet with baking paper.

Whisk the chilli, garlic, honey and lemon juice together in a small bowl. Add the shrimps and toss gently to combine. Ensure that all the shrimps are coated with the sauce.

Lay the pita bread on a clean work surface and spread over the passata. Scatter over the red onion, zucchini, tomato, and shrimps. Season with salt and pepper, if desired, and sprinkle over the cheese.

Place the pizza on the lined baking sheet and bake for 8–10 minutes or until the shrimps are cooked through and the cheese has melted.

To serve, top the pizza with the arugula and serve the lemon wedges on the side.

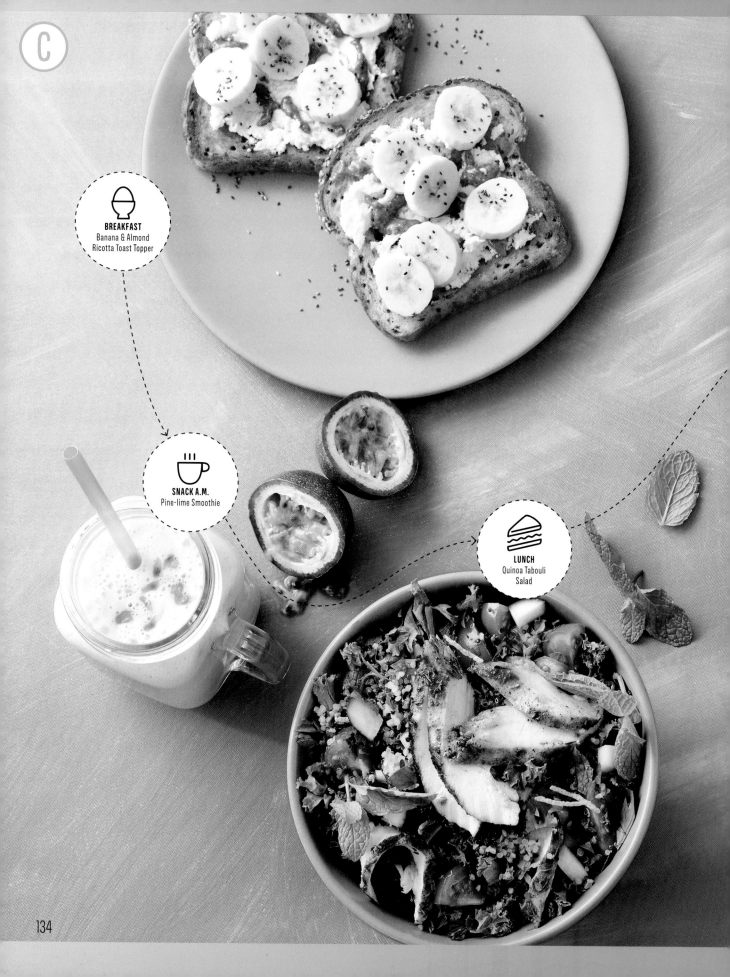

C

BREAKFAST
Banana & Almond
Ricotta Toast Topper

SNACK A.M.
Pine-lime Smoothie

LUNCH
Quinoa Tabouli
Salad

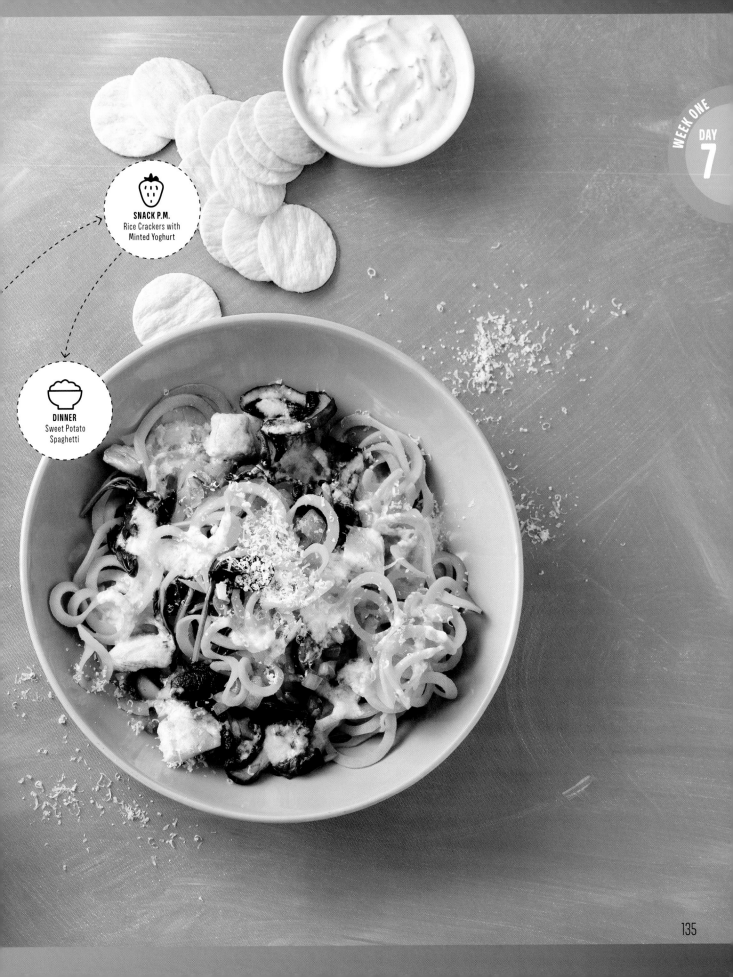

SNACK P.M.
Rice Crackers with
Minted Yoghurt

DINNER
Sweet Potato
Spaghetti

135

Banana & Almond Ricotta Toast Topper

SERVES 1 | **PREP TIME** 5 MINUTES | **COOKING TIME** 2 MINUTES | **DIFFICULTY** EASY

2 slices whole wheat bread
2 teaspoons almond butter
2¾ oz low-fat ricotta cheese
½ medium banana,
  peeled and sliced
1 teaspoon chia seeds

Toast the bread to your liking.

To serve, spread the almond butter and the ricotta over the toast and top with the banana. Sprinkle over the chia seeds.

Pine-lime Smoothie

SERVES 1 | **PREP TIME** 5 MINUTES | **DIFFICULTY** EASY

6 oz peeled pineapple,
  chopped
lime juice, to taste
1 oz rolled oats
¾ cup (190 ml) low-fat milk

1¾ oz low-fat plain yoghurt
½ scoop (½ oz) protein
  powder (optional)
3 passionfruit, halved

Place the pineapple, lime juice, oats, milk, yoghurt, and protein powder (if using) in a high-powered blender and blend until smooth.

To serve, pour into a glass or jar and stir through the passionfruit pulp.

Quinoa Tabouli Salad

SERVES 1 | **PREP TIME** 15 MINUTES, PLUS 25 MINUTES COOLING AND CHILLING TIME | **COOKING TIME** 25 MINUTES | **DIFFICULTY** EASY

2 oz quinoa
½ teaspoon smoked paprika
¼ teaspoon dried thyme
¼ teaspoon ground cumin
3½ oz boneless, skinless
  chicken breast
½ Lebanese cucumber,
  finely chopped
5 cherry tomatoes, quartered
¼ small red onion, finely
  chopped
1 small handful kale,
  finely shredded
1 small handful fresh
  parsley, chopped
1 small handful fresh mint,
  chopped, plus extra leaves
  to garnish
lemon juice, to taste
sea salt and ground black
  pepper, to taste
oil spray
finely grated lemon zest,
  to taste

Bring the quinoa and 1 cup (250 ml) of water to a boil in a small saucepan over high heat, stirring occasionally. Reduce the heat to low and simmer, covered, for 10–12 minutes or until the liquid has been absorbed and the quinoa is tender. Set aside to cool. To save time, the quinoa can be cooked the night before and stored in an airtight container in the refrigerator.

Meanwhile, place the paprika, thyme, and cumin in a medium bowl and mix to combine. Rub the spice mix over the chicken, cover with plastic wrap, and refrigerate for 10 minutes.

Place the quinoa, cucumber, tomatoes, onion, kale, parsley, mint, and lemon juice in a mixing bowl. Season with salt and pepper, if desired, and toss gently to combine.

Heat a chargrill pan over medium heat and spray lightly with oil spray. Add the chicken and cook for 5–6 minutes on each side or until cooked through. Transfer to a plate, cover with foil, and set aside to rest for 5 minutes. Cut into thick slices.

To serve, place the quinoa tabouli in a serving bowl and top with the sliced chicken. Garnish with extra mint leaves and lemon zest.

Rice Crackers with Minted Yoghurt

SNACK P.M. | **SERVES** 1 | **PREP TIME** 5 MINUTES | **DIFFICULTY** EASY

12 plain rice crackers

MINTED YOGHURT
1¾ oz low-fat plain yoghurt
2 tablespoons chopped
  fresh mint
¼ garlic clove, crushed
lemon juice, to taste
sea salt and ground black
  pepper, to taste

To make the minted yoghurt, whisk the yoghurt, mint, garlic, lemon juice, salt, and pepper together in a small bowl. To save time, the minted yoghurt can be made the night before and stored in an airtight container in the refrigerator.

Serve the rice crackers with the minted yoghurt.

Sweet Potato Spaghetti

DINNER | **SERVES** 1 | **PREP TIME** 10 MINUTES | **COOKING TIME** 25 MINUTES | **DIFFICULTY** EASY

¾ teaspoon olive oil
3½ oz boneless, skinless
  chicken breast, cut into
  ¾ inch cubes
1 medium sweet
  potato, spiralised
oil spray
¼ small brown onion, diced
1 garlic clove, crushed
2¾ oz mushrooms, sliced
1 small handful baby
  spinach leaves
1 large egg, lightly whisked
⅔ oz parmesan cheese, grated
sea salt and ground black
  pepper, to taste

Heat the oil in a non-stick fry pan over medium–high heat. Add the chicken and cook for 7–10 minutes or until lightly browned and cooked through. Set aside on a plate and cover with foil to keep warm.

Meanwhile, fill a medium saucepan with water, add a pinch of salt, and bring to a boil. Add the sweet potato and cook for 2–3 minutes or until just starting to soften but not completely tender, gently stirring occasionally. Reserve 2 tablespoons of the cooking water, then drain. Return the sweet potato spaghetti to the saucepan, off the heat.

Wipe the non-stick fry pan clean. Heat the pan over medium heat and spray lightly with oil spray. Add the onion and cook for 5 minutes or until soft and translucent, stirring occasionally. Add the garlic and mushrooms and cook for 6–7 minutes or until the mushrooms are tender and juicy, stirring frequently. Add the spinach and cook for 1–2 minutes or until the spinach wilts.

Place the egg, half the cheese, reserved water, salt, and pepper in a small bowl and mix well to combine. Pour over the warm spaghetti and, using tongs, gently toss until evenly coated.

Add the vegetables and chicken to the sweet potato spaghetti and gently toss to combine. Season with salt and pepper, if desired.

To serve, place the sweet potato spaghetti in a serving bowl and top with the remaining cheese.

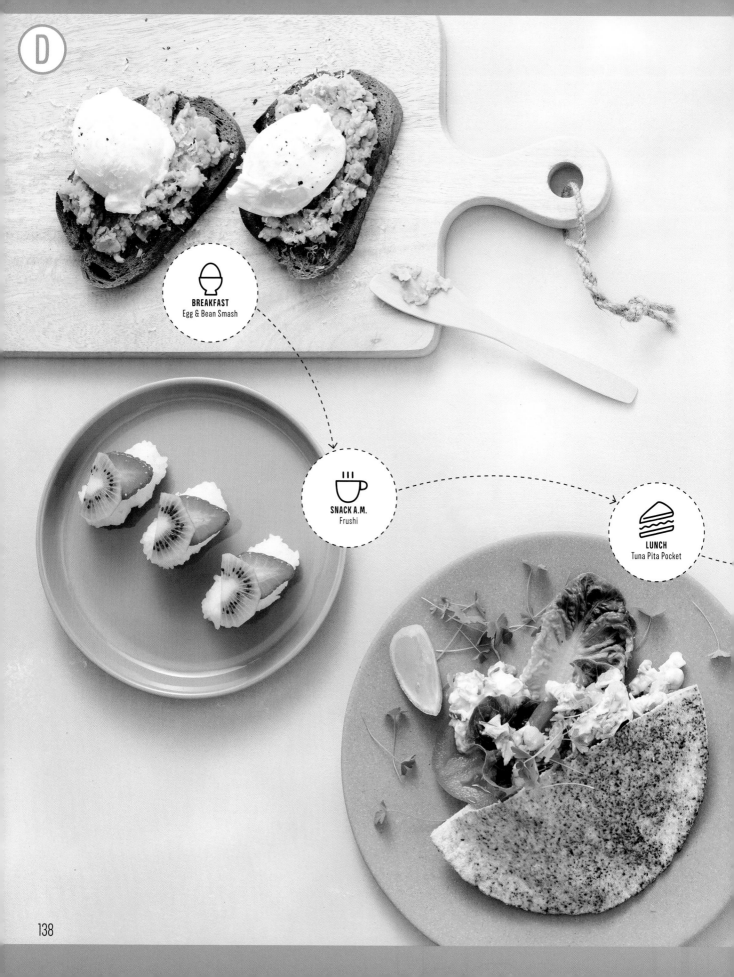

D

BREAKFAST
Egg & Bean Smash

SNACK A.M.
Frushi

LUNCH
Tuna Pita Pocket

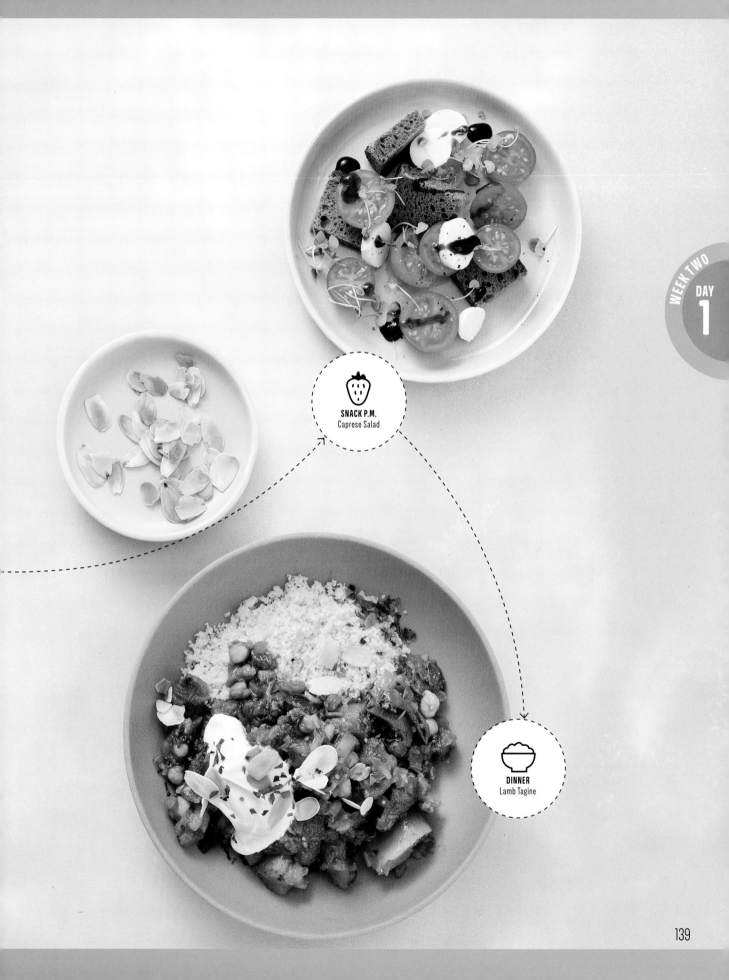

SNACK P.M.
Caprese Salad

DINNER
Lamb Tagine

Egg & Bean Smash

SERVES 1 | **PREP TIME** 10 MINUTES | **COOKING TIME** 10 MINUTES | **DIFFICULTY** EASY

3½ oz frozen broad beans, thawed

1 oz avocado (about ⅛ avocado)

lemon juice, to taste

2 teaspoons chopped fresh mint

⅔ oz parmesan cheese, grated

sea salt and ground black pepper, to taste

1 teaspoon white vinegar

2 large eggs

2 slices whole wheat bread

Fill a medium saucepan with water, add a pinch of salt, and bring to a boil. Add the broad beans and cook for 3–4 minutes. Drain and set aside until cool enough to handle. Gently squeeze each bean out of the shell, so that you are left with the brighter green bean.

Place the beans, avocado, lemon juice, mint, and parmesan in a small bowl. Season with salt and pepper, if desired, and roughly mash using a fork until a chunky paste has formed.

To poach the eggs, fill a saucepan with water to 3 inches deep. Add the vinegar and bring to a boil over medium heat, then reduce the heat to medium–low. Break the eggs into the water and cook for 2–3 minutes for a semi-soft yolk or 3–4 minutes for a firm yolk. Remove the eggs from the water using a slotted spoon and allow to drain on paper towels.

Meanwhile, toast the bread to your liking.

To serve, spread the bean smash over the toast, then top with the eggs.

Frushi

SERVES 1 | **PREP TIME** 10 MINUTES, PLUS 45 MINUTES COOLING AND CHILLING TIME | **COOKING TIME** 40 MINUTES | **DIFFICULTY** EASY

1 oz arborio rice

½ cup (125 ml) low-fat milk

1 tablespoon pure maple syrup

pinch of ground cinnamon

1 kiwifruit, peeled and sliced

4½ oz strawberries, hulled and sliced

Line a baking sheet with baking paper.

Put the rice in a medium saucepan, cover with cold water, and bring to a boil. Reduce the heat to medium–low and cook, uncovered, for 10 minutes. Drain the rice and then return to the saucepan.

Add the milk, ¼ cup (60 ml) of water, maple syrup, and cinnamon and bring to a boil. Reduce the heat to low and simmer, uncovered, for 25–30 minutes or until the rice is tender and the liquid is absorbed, stirring frequently. Remove from the heat and transfer to a medium bowl to cool to room temperature. You can refrigerate the rice if you want to speed up the cooling process.

Scoop out 1 heaped tablespoon of the cooled rice mixture and shape into an oval using wet hands. Place on the lined baking sheet and continue until all of the rice mixture has been shaped. Top the rice ovals with the sliced fruit. Cover with plastic wrap and refrigerate for 15–30 minutes.

To serve, place the frushi on a serving plate.

Tuna Pita Pocket

SERVES 1 | **PREP TIME** 10 MINUTES | **DIFFICULTY** EASY

3½ oz low-fat plain yoghurt

lemon juice, to taste

1 tablespoon chopped fresh parsley

1¾ oz tinned tuna in springwater, drained

⅔ oz tinned chickpeas, drained and rinsed

¼ small red onion, chopped

½ celery stalk, chopped

sea salt and ground black pepper, to taste

½ whole wheat pita bread

1 small handful lettuce leaves

½ medium tomato, sliced

Whisk the yoghurt, lemon juice, and parsley together in a small bowl.

Place the tuna, chickpeas, onion, and celery in a mixing bowl. Add the yoghurt dressing, season with salt and pepper, if desired, and toss gently to combine.

To serve, fill the pita with the lettuce, tomato, and the tuna mixture.

Caprese Salad

SNACK P.M. **SERVES** 1 | **PREP TIME** 5 MINUTES | **COOKING TIME** 2 MINUTES | **DIFFICULTY** EASY

1 slice whole wheat bread

5 cherry tomatoes, halved

⅔ oz baby bocconcini, sliced

finely chopped fresh basil or micro herbs, to taste

sea salt and ground black pepper, to taste

balsamic glaze, to serve

Toast the bread to your liking. Cut into small squares.

To serve, place the toasted croutons, tomatoes, and bocconcini on a small plate. Garnish with basil or micro herbs, season with salt and pepper, and drizzle over the balsamic glaze.

WEEK TWO
DAY
1

Lamb Tagine

DINNER **SERVES** 1 | **PREP TIME** 15 MINUTES | **COOKING TIME** 45 MINUTES | **DIFFICULTY** EASY

oil spray

3 oz lean lamb leg steaks, cut into ¾ inch cubes

¼ small brown onion, diced

½ garlic clove, crushed

½ teaspoon sweet paprika

½ teaspoon ground coriander

½ teaspoon ground ginger

¼ teaspoon chilli powder

¾ cup (190 ml) salt-reduced beef stock

2¾ oz tinned crushed tomatoes

3 oz pumpkin, peeled and cut into ¾ inch cubes

1½ oz tinned chickpeas, drained and rinsed

3 medjool dates, pitted and sliced

finely grated zest and juice of 1 medium orange

sea salt and ground black pepper, to taste

¼ teaspoon olive oil

¼ teaspoon ground turmeric

1½ oz couscous

1 tablespoon chopped fresh cilantro

3½ oz low-fat plain yoghurt

2 teaspoons flaked almonds, toasted

Lightly spray a large saucepan with oil and heat over medium heat. Add half the lamb and cook for 2–3 minutes or until browned on all sides, stirring frequently. Transfer to a plate and set aside. Repeat with the remaining lamb.

Reheat the saucepan over medium heat. Add the onion and garlic and cook for 3–4 minutes or until the onion is soft, stirring frequently. Add the paprika, ground coriander, ginger, and chilli powder and cook for 1 minute or until fragrant, stirring constantly.

Return the lamb to the pan and add the stock, tomatoes, pumpkin, chickpeas, dates, orange zest, and juice. Season with salt and pepper, if desired, and stir to combine. Reduce the heat to low and simmer, covered, for 30–35 minutes or until the lamb is cooked through and the pumpkin is tender, stirring occasionally. If the sauce is too thick towards the end of cooking time, stir in a small amount of water.

Meanwhile, in a small saucepan, bring the oil, turmeric and ½ cup (125 ml) of water to a boil. Add the couscous and remove the pan from the heat. Leave to stand, covered, for 2–3 minutes before fluffing with a fork to help separate the grains. Set aside.

Stir half the cilantro through the tagine.

To serve, place the couscous in a serving bowl and top with the tagine and yoghurt. Sprinkle over the almonds and remaining cilantro.

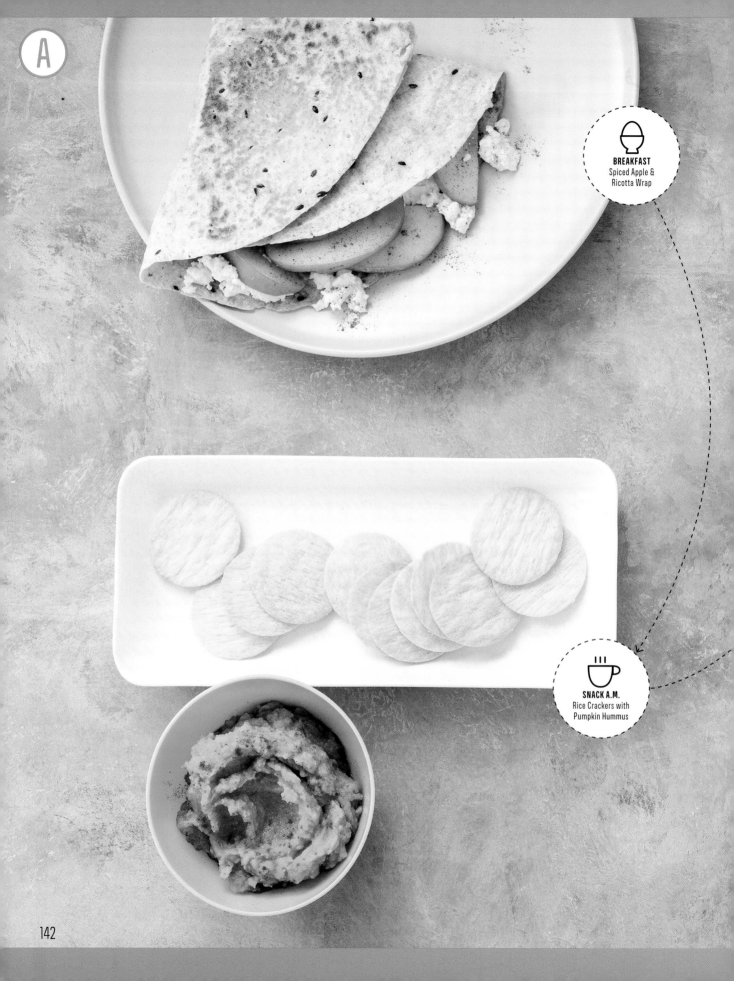

A

BREAKFAST
Spiced Apple &
Ricotta Wrap

SNACK A.M.
Rice Crackers with
Pumpkin Hummus

142

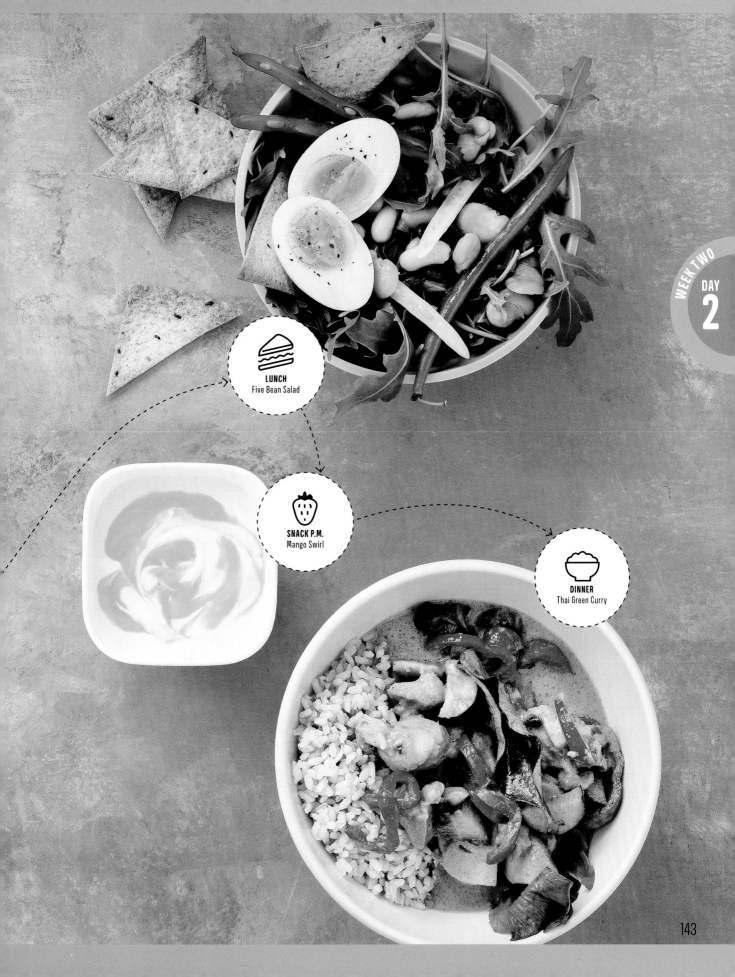

LUNCH
Five Bean Salad

SNACK P.M.
Mango Swirl

DINNER
Thai Green Curry

Spiced Apple & Ricotta Wrap

SERVES 1 | **PREP TIME** 5 MINUTES, PLUS 10 MINUTES COOLING TIME | **COOKING TIME** 10 MINUTES | **DIFFICULTY** EASY

1 medium green apple,
  cored and sliced

lemon juice, to taste

½ teaspoon ground cinnamon

3½ oz low-fat ricotta cheese

1 whole wheat wrap

Heat a small saucepan over medium heat. Add the apple, lemon juice, cinnamon, and 1 tablespoon of water and cook, covered, for 4 minutes or until the apple is soft, stirring occasionally. Set aside to cool. To save time, the apple can be cooked the night before and stored in an airtight container in the refrigerator.

Preheat a sandwich press. Spread the ricotta over one-third of the wrap. Top with the spiced apple, then roll or fold up to enclose the filling. Place the wrap in the sandwich press and toast for 3–4 minutes or until the wrap is golden and the mixture is heated through, then serve.

Rice Crackers with Pumpkin Hummus

SERVES 1 | **PREP TIME** 5 MINUTES, PLUS 10 MINUTES COOLING TIME | **COOKING TIME** 15 MINUTES | **DIFFICULTY** EASY

12 plain rice crackers

PUMPKIN HUMMUS

4¼ oz pumpkin, peeled and cut
  into ¾ in cubes

2¾ oz tinned chickpeas,
  drained and rinsed

¼ garlic clove, crushed

lemon juice, to taste

sea salt, to taste

pinch of smoked paprika

To make the pumpkin hummus, add 2 inches of water to a saucepan and insert a steamer basket. Cover with a lid and bring the water to a boil over high heat, then reduce the heat to medium. Add the pumpkin and steam, covered, for 12–15 minutes or until soft. Alternatively, microwave on high for 8–10 minutes. Set aside to cool.

Place the pumpkin, chickpeas, garlic, lemon juice, and salt in a food processor and pulse until smooth and creamy. To save time, the pumpkin hummus can be made the night before and stored in an airtight container in the refrigerator.

Sprinkle the paprika over the hummus and serve with the rice crackers.

Five Bean Salad

SERVES 1 | **PREP TIME** 10 MINUTES | **COOKING TIME** 20 MINUTES | **DIFFICULTY** EASY

½ whole wheat wrap

oil spray

1¾ oz frozen broad beans,
  thawed

8 green beans and 8 yellow
  beans, trimmed and sliced

1½ oz tinned red kidney beans,
  drained and rinsed

1½ oz tinned cannellini beans,
  drained and rinsed

½ scallion, sliced

1 small handful arugula leaves

lemon juice, to taste

sea salt and ground black
  pepper, to taste

1 large hard-boiled egg
  (see page 176), halved

Preheat the oven to 350°F (325°F convection) and line a baking sheet with baking paper. Cut the wrap into wedges, place on the lined baking sheet and spray lightly with oil spray. Bake in the oven for 4 minutes or until they begin to colour. Turn the wedges over and bake for a further 4–6 minutes or until both sides are lightly coloured, then set aside to cool.

Meanwhile, fill a medium saucepan with water, add a pinch of salt and bring to a boil. Add the broad beans and cook for 3–4 minutes. Drain and set aside until cool enough to handle. Gently squeeze each bean out of the shell, so that you are left with the brighter green bean.

Add 2 inches of water to a saucepan and insert a steamer basket. Cover with a lid and bring the water to a boil over high heat, then reduce the heat to medium. Add the green and yellow beans and steam, covered, for 3–4 minutes or until just tender. Place in a bowl of iced water to stop them from cooking and set aside for 1–2 minutes. Drain and set aside.

Place the beans, scallion, and arugula leaves in a mixing bowl. Drizzle with lemon juice and toss to combine. Season with salt and pepper, if desired. To serve, place the five bean salad in a serving bowl and top with the egg. Serve with the baked wedges on the side.

Mango Swirl

SERVES 1 | **PREP TIME** 5 MINUTES | **DIFFICULTY** EASY

1 medium mango, peeled
  and sliced
10¾ oz low-fat plain yoghurt

Place the mango and 2 tablespoons of the yoghurt in a high-powered blender and blend until smooth.

To serve, place the remaining yoghurt in a serving bowl. Add the mango yoghurt and swirl through with a spoon.

Thai Green Curry

DINNER **SERVES** 1 | **PREP TIME** 15 MINUTES, PLUS 5 MINUTES STANDING TIME | **COOKING TIME** 30 MINUTES | **DIFFICULTY** EASY

2 oz brown rice
oil spray
½ scallion, sliced
½ garlic clove, crushed
1 tablespoon green curry paste
3½ oz boneless, skinless
  chicken thigh, cut into
  1 inch cubes
½ cup (120 ml) light coconut milk
1 kaffir lime leaf
½ teaspoon fish sauce
½ medium zucchini, halved
  and sliced
3 oz bok choy, roughly chopped
¼ medium red bell pepper,
  seeds removed, sliced
1 small handful fresh basil
finely grated lime zest, to taste
  (optional)

Bring the rice and 1 cup (250 ml) of water to a boil in a small saucepan over high heat, stirring occasionally. Reduce the heat to low and simmer, covered, for 20–25 minutes or until the liquid has been absorbed and the rice is tender. Remove from the heat and leave to stand, covered, for 5 minutes.

Meanwhile, lightly spray a large saucepan with oil and heat over medium heat. Add the scallion, garlic, and curry paste and cook for 1–2 minutes or until fragrant, stirring frequently. Add the chicken and stir to coat in the paste mixture.

Add the coconut milk and lime leaf and bring to a boil. Reduce the heat to medium–low and simmer for 18–20 minutes, stirring occasionally, or until the chicken is cooked through.

Add the fish sauce, zucchini, bok choy, and bell pepper and cook for 3–5 minutes or until the vegetables are just tender.

Just before serving, remove the curry from the heat and stir through the basil leaves.

To serve, place the rice in a serving bowl and top with the green curry. Sprinkle over the lime zest (if using).

WEEK TWO
DAY
2

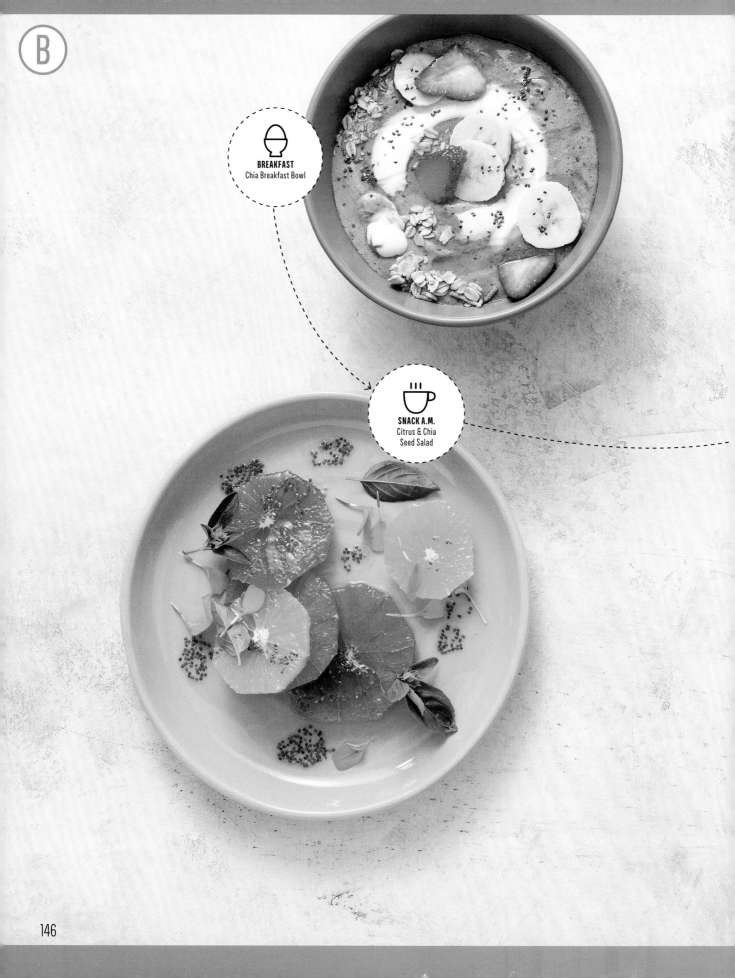

B

BREAKFAST
Chia Breakfast Bowl

SNACK A.M.
Citrus & Chia
Seed Salad

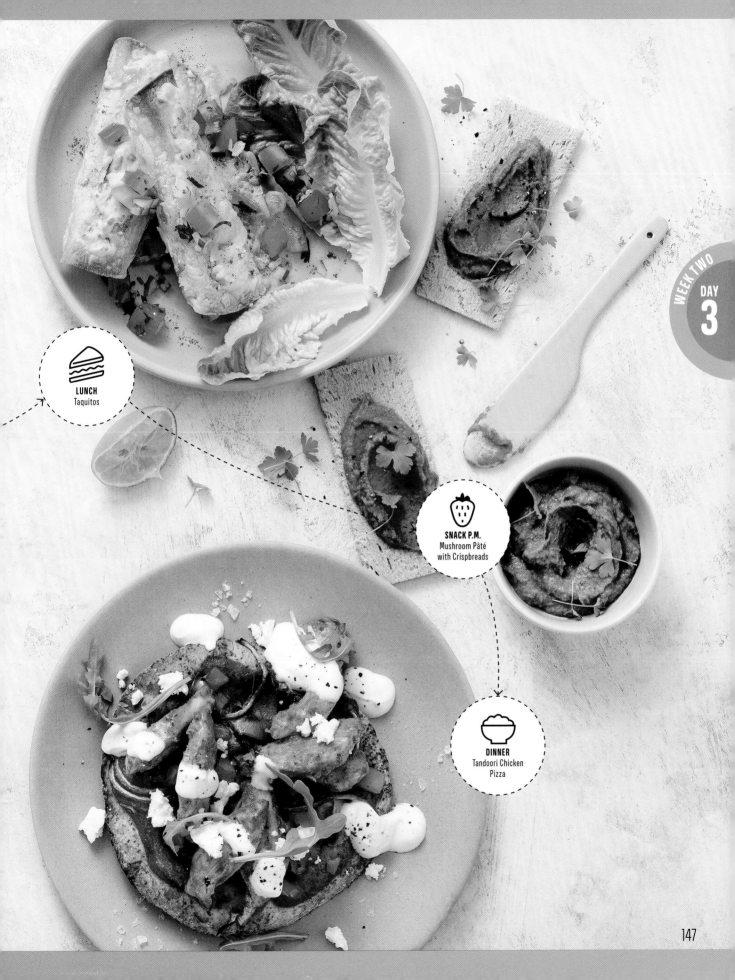

LUNCH
Taquitos

SNACK P.M.
Mushroom Pâté
with Crispbreads

DINNER
Tandoori Chicken
Pizza

147

Chia Breakfast Bowl

SERVES 1 | **PREP TIME** 15 MINUTES, PLUS 3 HOURS SETTING TIME | **DIFFICULTY** EASY

½ small beetroot, chopped
1 cup (250 ml) low-fat milk
4½ oz strawberries, hulled
2 teaspoons chia seeds
2 teaspoons honey
1 medium banana, peeled
3½ oz low-fat plain yoghurt
1 oz natural muesli

Place the beetroot, milk, and half the strawberries in a high-powered blender and blend until smooth. Pour into a bowl, add the chia seeds (reserving a pinch for later) and half the honey and mix until well combined. Pour into a 2 cup (500 ml) capacity jar and cover with plastic wrap. Place in the refrigerator to set for 2–3 hours or overnight.

Mash half the banana in a small bowl, add the yoghurt, and mix well to combine. Swirl the banana yoghurt through the beetroot chia mixture.

Slice the remaining strawberries and banana. To serve, top the breakfast bowl with the muesli, remaining sliced fruit, chia seeds, and honey.

Citrus & Chia Seed Salad

SERVES 1 | **PREP TIME** 5 MINUTES | **DIFFICULTY** EASY

2 teaspoons chia seeds
2 teaspoons honey
2 teaspoons lime juice
¼ medium pink grapefruit
¼ medium orange
basil leaves, to garnish

Whisk the chia seeds, honey, and lime juice together in a small bowl. Peel and slice the grapefruit and orange.

To serve, place the grapefruit and orange on a serving plate and drizzle over the dressing. Garnish with basil.

Taquitos

SERVES 1 | **PREP TIME** 15 MINUTES, PLUS 10 MINUTES COOLING TIME | **COOKING TIME** 30 MINUTES | **DIFFICULTY** EASY

oil spray
¼ small brown onion, diced
¼ garlic clove, crushed
¼ teaspoon smoked paprika
¼ teaspoon ground cumin
lime juice, to taste
3 oz roast chicken, shredded
sea salt and ground black
   pepper, to taste
⅔ oz low-fat cheddar cheese
2 medium corn tortillas
1 small handful lettuce leaves

SALSA

½ medium tomato, diced
¼ small red onion, diced
pinch of dried chilli flakes
2 teaspoons chopped
   fresh cilantro
lime juice, sea salt, and ground
   black pepper, to taste

Preheat the oven to 400°F (350°F convection) and line a baking sheet with baking paper.

Lightly spray a medium saucepan with oil and heat over medium heat. Add the brown onion and cook for 3–4 minutes or until soft, stirring frequently. Add the garlic and cook for 1 minute or until fragrant, stirring frequently. Reduce the heat to low, add the paprika, cumin, and lime juice and stir until well combined. Add the chicken, salt, and pepper, if desired, and toss gently to combine.

Transfer to a bowl and set aside to cool for 5–10 minutes. Grate the cheese and stir through.

Warm the corn tortillas, one at a time, in a dry fry pan over medium heat for 15 seconds on each side. Place one tortilla on a clean work surface. Place half of the chicken mixture on the lower third of the tortilla and tightly roll up to enclose the filling. Place, seam side down, on the lined baking sheet. Repeat with the remaining ingredients to create two tortillas in total.

Bake in the oven for 15–20 minutes or until golden brown and crispy.

Meanwhile, to make the salsa, place the tomato, red onion, chilli flakes, cilantro, lime juice, salt, and pepper, if desired, in a small bowl and toss gently to combine.

To serve, place the taquitos on a serving plate. Top with the salsa and serve with the lettuce leaves on the side.

Mushroom Pâté with Crispbreads

SERVES 1 | **PREP TIME** 5 MINUTES, PLUS 30 MINUTES CHILLING TIME | **COOKING TIME** 15 MINUTES | **DIFFICULTY** EASY

2 rye crispbreads
parsley leaves, to garnish

MUSHROOM PÂTÉ
oil spray
¼ small brown onion, chopped
½ garlic clove, crushed
2¾ oz mushrooms, thinly sliced
1 sprig fresh thyme, chopped
2¾ oz tinned cannellini beans,
   drained and rinsed
orange juice, to taste
¼ teaspoon balsamic glaze
sea salt and ground black
   pepper, to taste

To make the mushroom pâté, lightly spray a medium saucepan with oil and place over a medium heat. Add the onion and cook for 3–4 minutes or until soft, stirring frequently. Add the garlic, mushrooms, and thyme and cook for 6–7 minutes or until the mushrooms are tender and juicy, stirring occasionally. Add the beans, orange juice, and balsamic glaze and cook for a further minute. Season with salt and pepper, if desired.

Using a stick blender or food processor, blend the mushroom mixture until smooth. Place in a small bowl, cover with plastic wrap and refrigerate for 30 minutes or overnight. This can be made the night before and stored in an airtight container in the refrigerator.

To serve, place the crispbreads on a serving plate and spread over the mushroom pâté. Top with the parsley leaves.

WEEK TWO
DAY
3

Tandoori Chicken Pizza

DINNER **SERVES** 1 | **PREP TIME** 10 MINUTES, PLUS 30 MINUTES MARINATING TIME | **COOKING TIME** 15 MINUTES | **DIFFICULTY** EASY

2 teaspoons tandoori paste
lemon juice, to taste
1¾ oz low-fat plain yoghurt
3½ oz boneless, skinless
   chicken breast, thinly sliced
1 whole wheat pita bread
1½ oz tomato passata (purée)
¼ small red onion, thinly sliced
1¾ oz mushrooms, thinly sliced
¼ medium red bell pepper,
   seeds removed, thinly sliced
⅔ oz salt-reduced low-fat feta
   cheese, crumbled
sea salt and ground black
   pepper, to taste
1 small handful arugula leaves

Whisk the tandoori paste, lemon juice, and half the yoghurt together in a medium bowl. Add the chicken and mix well to coat. Cover with plastic wrap and marinate in the refrigerator for 30 minutes or overnight.

Preheat the oven to 350°F (325°F convection) and line a baking sheet with baking paper.

Place the chicken on the lined baking sheet and bake in the oven for 5 minutes. Transfer the chicken to a plate and set aside to rest. Re-line the baking sheet with baking paper.

Lay the pita bread on the lined baking sheet and spread over the passata. Scatter over the onion, mushrooms, and bell pepper. Top with the tandoori chicken and sprinkle over the feta. Season with salt and pepper, if desired.

Bake in the oven for 8–10 minutes or until the toppings are hot, the cheese has melted, and the edges are golden brown.

To serve, dollop the remaining yoghurt over the pizza and top with the arugula and more ground black pepper, if desired.

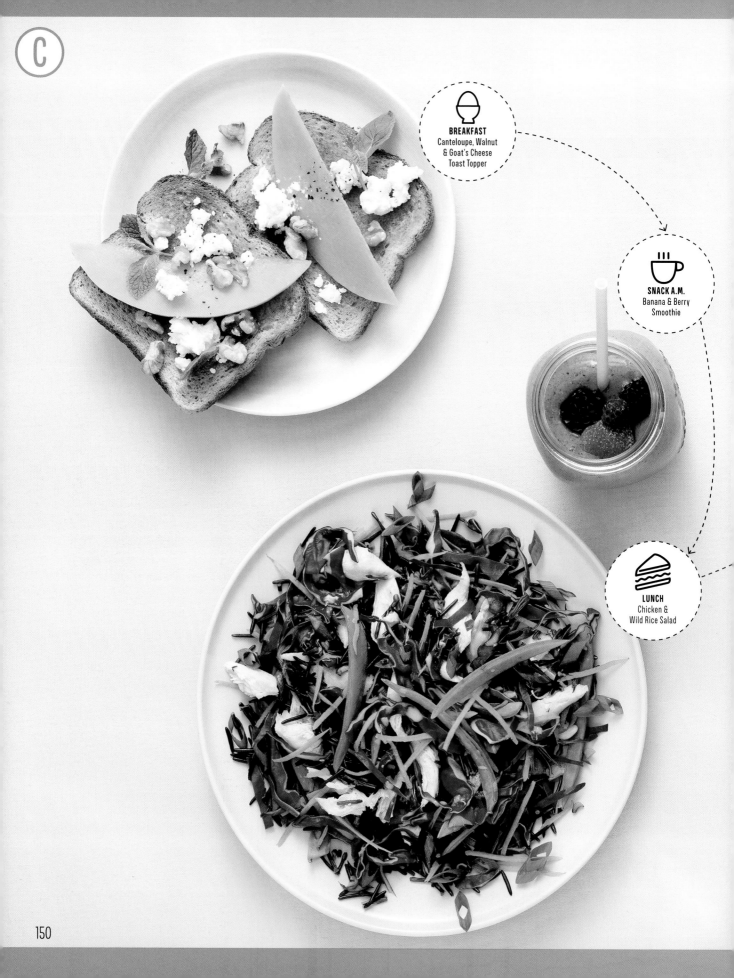

C

BREAKFAST
Canteloupe, Walnut
& Goat's Cheese
Toast Topper

SNACK A.M.
Banana & Berry
Smoothie

LUNCH
Chicken &
Wild Rice Salad

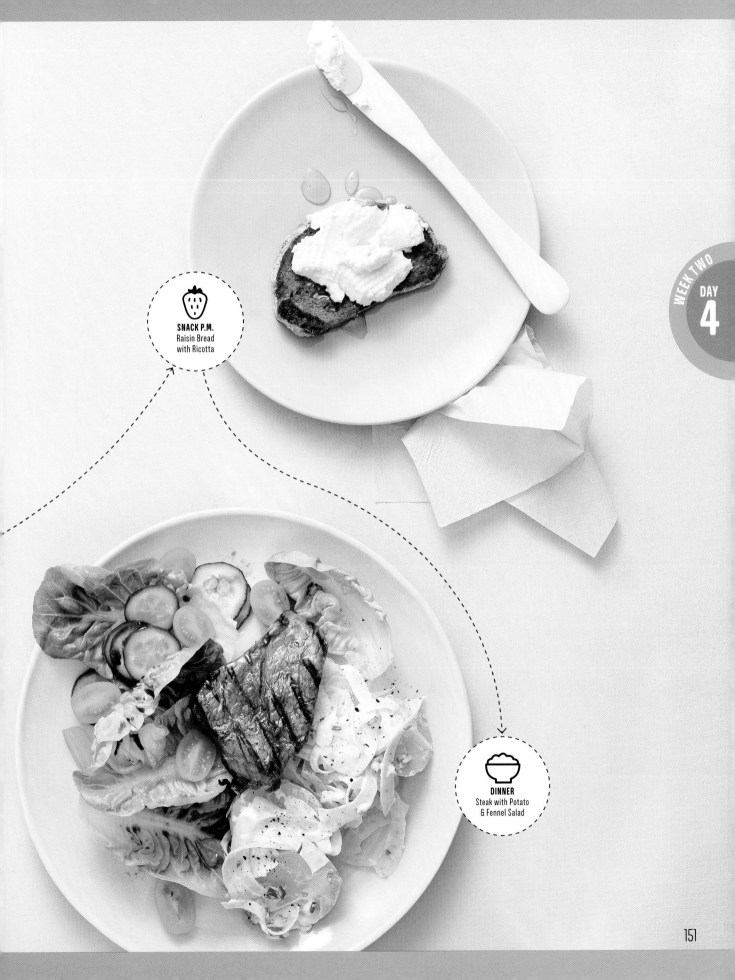

SNACK P.M.
Raisin Bread
with Ricotta

DINNER
Steak with Potato
& Fennel Salad

Canteloupe, Walnut & Goat's Cheese Toast Topper

SERVES 1 | **PREP TIME** 5 MINUTES | **COOKING TIME** 2 MINUTES | **DIFFICULTY** EASY

2 slices whole wheat bread
4½ oz canteloupe, sliced
1½ oz low-fat goat's cheese, crumbled
¾ oz walnuts, roughly chopped
ground black pepper, to taste
1 teaspoon chopped fresh mint (optional)

Toast the bread to your liking.

To serve, place the toast on a serving plate and top with the canteloupe, goat's cheese, and walnuts. Season with pepper and garnish with mint (if using).

Banana & Berry Smoothie

SERVES 1 | **PREP TIME** 5 MINUTES | **DIFFICULTY** EASY

1 medium banana, peeled and chopped
3 oz frozen mixed berries
1 oz rolled oats
¾ cup (190 ml) low-fat milk
1¾ oz low-fat plain yoghurt
½ teaspoon acai berry powder (optional)

Place the banana, three-quarters of the berries, oats, milk, yoghurt, and acai powder (if using) in a high-powered blender and blend until smooth.

To serve, pour into a glass or jar and top with the remaining berries.

Chicken & Wild Rice Salad

SERVES 1 | **PREP TIME** 15 MINUTES, PLUS 5 MINUTES STANDING TIME | **COOKING TIME** 40 MINUTES | **DIFFICULTY** EASY

2 oz wild rice
2¾ oz roast chicken, shredded
1 oz red cabbage, finely shredded
½ medium carrot, grated
1½ oz snow peas, trimmed and thinly sliced
½ scallion, sliced

DRESSING

¼ garlic clove, crushed
lemon juice, to taste
¼ teaspoon Dijon mustard
sea salt and ground black pepper, to taste

Bring the rice and 1 cup (250 ml) of water to a boil in a small saucepan over high heat, stirring occasionally. Reduce the heat to medium–low and simmer, covered, for 35–40 minutes or until the liquid has been absorbed and the rice is tender. Remove from the heat and leave to stand, covered, for 5 minutes. Set aside to cool. To save time, the rice can be cooked the night before and stored in an airtight container in the refrigerator.

To make the dressing, whisk the garlic, lemon juice, mustard, salt, pepper, and 2 teaspoons of water together in a small bowl.

Place the rice, chicken, cabbage, carrot, snow peas, and scallion in a mixing bowl. Drizzle over the dressing and toss gently to combine, then serve.

Raisin Bread Toast with Ricotta

SNACK P.M. **SERVES** 1 | **PREP TIME** 5 MINUTES | **COOKING TIME** 2 MINUTES | **DIFFICULTY** EASY

1 slice raisin bread
1 oz low-fat ricotta cheese
¼ teaspoon honey

Toast the bread to your liking.

Meanwhile, place the ricotta and honey in a small bowl and mix until well combined.

To serve, spread the ricotta over the toast.

Steak with Potato & Fennel Salad

DINNER **SERVES** 1 | **PREP TIME** 15 MINUTES, PLUS 10 MINUTES COOLING TIME | **COOKING TIME** 25 MINUTES | **DIFFICULTY** EASY

½ medium potato
3½ oz low-fat plain yoghurt
lemon juice, to taste
½ fresh red chilli, seeds removed, finely chopped
1 small fennel bulb, thinly sliced
1 tablespoon finely chopped fresh chives
sea salt and ground black pepper, to taste
4¾ oz lean beef steak
oil spray
¾ teaspoon olive oil
¼ teaspoon balsamic vinegar
1 small handful lettuce leaves
½ Lebanese cucumber, sliced
5 cherry tomatoes, halved

Fill a large saucepan with water, add a pinch of salt, and bring to a boil. Cook the potato for 12–15 minutes or until just tender. Drain, then leave to cool for 10 minutes. When cool enough to handle, slice into rounds.

Whisk the yoghurt, lemon juice, chilli, and 2 teaspoons of water together in a medium bowl. Add the potato, fennel, and chives. Season with salt and pepper, if desired, and toss gently to combine.

Heat a barbecue grill-plate or chargrill pan over medium–high heat.

Place the steak on a plate and lightly spray both sides with oil spray. Season with salt and pepper, if desired.

Meanwhile, whisk the oil and balsamic vinegar together in a small bowl.

Place the lettuce, cucumber, and tomatoes in a mixing bowl, drizzle over the balsamic dressing, and toss gently to combine.

Grill the steak for 4–5 minutes or until slightly charred. Turn the steak over and cook for a further 5 minutes for medium or continue until cooked to your liking. Loosely cover with foil and set aside to rest for 2 minutes.

To serve, place the steak on a serving plate with the potato salad and lettuce salad on the side.

WEEK TWO
DAY
4

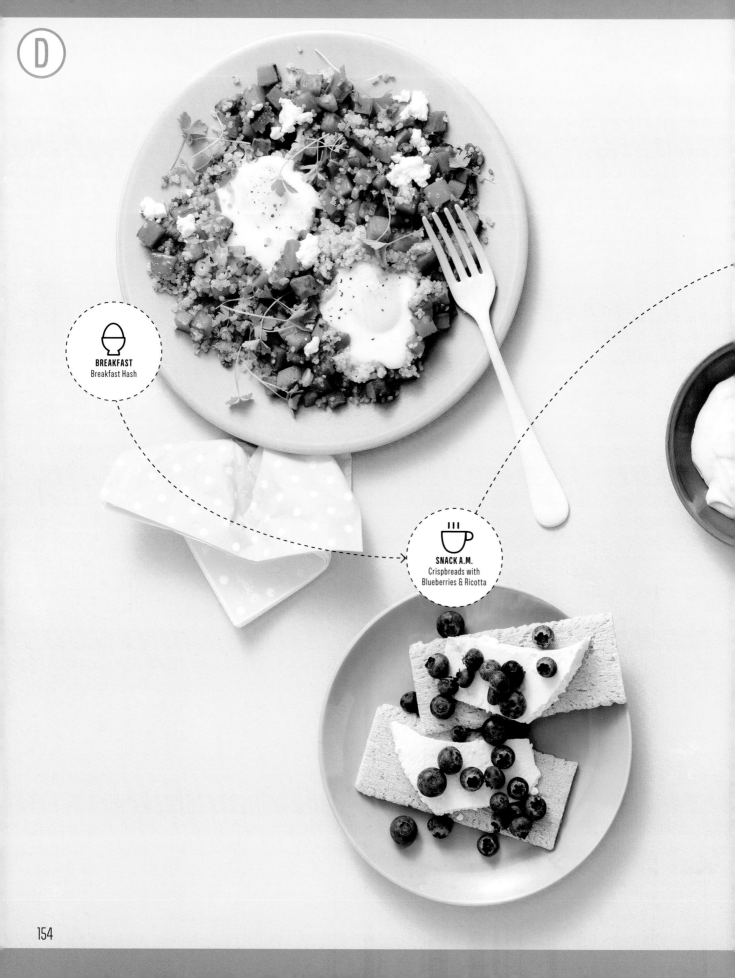

D

BREAKFAST
Breakfast Hash

SNACK A.M.
Crispbreads with
Blueberries & Ricotta

154

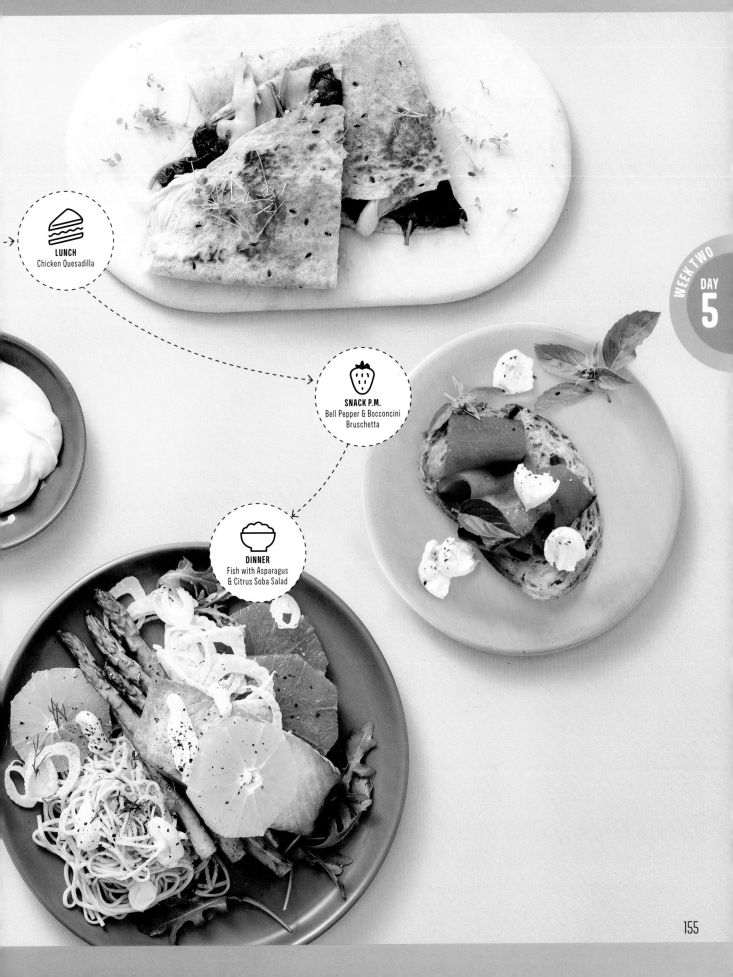

LUNCH
Chicken Quesadilla

SNACK P.M.
Bell Pepper & Bocconcini
Bruschetta

DINNER
Fish with Asparagus
& Citrus Soba Salad

WEEK TWO

DAY
5

155

Breakfast Hash

SERVES 1 | **PREP TIME** 10 MINUTES | **COOKING TIME** 20 MINUTES | **DIFFICULTY** EASY

2 oz quinoa

1½ teaspoons olive oil

¾ medium sweet potato, peeled and cut into ½ inch cubes

½ garlic clove, crushed

½ scallion, sliced

sea salt and ground black pepper, to taste

2 large eggs

1 oz low-fat goat's cheese, crumbled

micro herbs, to garnish (optional)

Bring the quinoa and 1 cup (250 ml) of water to a boil in a small saucepan over high heat, stirring occasionally. Reduce the heat to low and simmer, covered, for 10–12 minutes or until the liquid has been absorbed and the quinoa is tender. To save time, the quinoa can be cooked the night before and stored in an airtight container in the refrigerator.

Meanwhile, heat the oil in a non-stick fry pan over medium heat. Add the sweet potato and cook for 8–10 minutes or until the sweet potato starts to colour, stirring occasionally. Stir in the garlic and scallion and cook, covered, for 2–3 minutes or until the sweet potato is tender, stirring occasionally. Stir in the quinoa and season with salt and pepper, if desired.

Reduce the heat to medium–low and carefully crack the eggs over the sweet potato mixture. Cover and cook for another 2–3 minutes or until the eggs are cooked to your liking.

To serve, transfer to a serving plate, sprinkle over the goat's cheese, and scatter with micro herbs (if using).

Crispbreads with Blueberries & Ricotta

SERVES 1 | **PREP TIME** 5 MINUTES | **DIFFICULTY** EASY

1¾ oz low-fat ricotta cheese

2 rye crispbreads

5¾ oz blueberries

To serve, spread the ricotta over the crispbreads and top with the blueberries.

Chicken Quesadilla

SERVES 1 | **PREP TIME** 5 MINUTES, PLUS 10 MINUTES COOLING TIME | **COOKING TIME** 20 MINUTES | **DIFFICULTY** EASY

oil spray

¼ small brown onion, chopped

¼ garlic clove, crushed

1¾ oz mushrooms, sliced

1½ oz roast chicken, shredded

1 large handful baby spinach leaves

½ whole wheat wrap

⅔ oz camembert cheese, sliced

micro herbs, to garnish (optional)

Lightly spray a non-stick fry pan with oil and heat over medium heat. Add the onion and cook for 3–4 minutes or until soft, stirring frequently. Add the crushed garlic and mushrooms and cook for 6–7 minutes or until the mushrooms are tender and juicy, stirring occasionally. Add the chicken and spinach and cook for 1 minute or until the spinach wilts. Remove from the heat and drain off any liquid. Transfer the chicken and mushroom mixture to a heatproof bowl and set aside to cool slightly.

Preheat a sandwich press.

Lay the wrap down on the sandwich press and top half of the wrap with the chicken and mushroom mixture and camembert slices. Fold in half to enclose the filling and gently press the sandwich press lid down.

Toast for 3–5 minutes until the wrap is crisp and golden brown. Serve with micro herbs (if using).

Bell Pepper & Bocconcini Bruschetta

SERVES 1 | **PREP TIME** 5 MINUTES, PLUS 5 MINUTES RESTING TIME | **COOKING TIME** 10 MINUTES | **DIFFICULTY** EASY

¼ medium red bell pepper, seeds removed

⅔ oz baby bocconcini, sliced

1 small handful fresh basil

lemon juice, to taste

sea salt and ground black pepper, to taste

1 slice rye bread

oil spray

½ garlic clove

Heat a small non-stick fry pan over high heat. Place the bell pepper, skin side down, in the hot pan. Cook for 5–7 minutes or until the skin starts to blister and turn brown. Transfer to a bowl, cover with plastic wrap, and leave to sweat for 5 minutes. Peel off the skin and cut into ¾ inch pieces.

Place the bell pepper, bocconcini, basil, lemon juice, and salt and pepper, if desired, in a small bowl and toss gently to combine.

Toast the bread to your liking. Lightly spray the toast with oil spray and rub with the cut side of the garlic clove.

To serve, place the toast on a serving plate and top with the bell pepper and bocconcini mixture. Season with additional ground black pepper, if desired.

WEEK TWO
DAY
5

Fish with Asparagus & Citrus Soba Salad

DINNER **SERVES** 1 | **PREP TIME** 15 MINUTES | **COOKING TIME** 20 MINUTES | **DIFFICULTY** EASY

1¾ oz soba noodles

6 asparagus spears, trimmed

oil spray

3 oz salmon fillet, skin removed, deboned

½ medium pink grapefruit, peeled and sliced

½ medium orange, peeled and sliced

1 small handful arugula leaves

½ small fennel bulb, thinly sliced

1 tablespoon chopped fresh dill

sea salt and ground black pepper, to taste

AVOCADO DRESSING

1 oz avocado, mashed

3½ oz low-fat plain yoghurt

½ garlic clove, crushed

lime juice, to taste

sea salt and ground black pepper, to taste

Fill a large saucepan with water, add a pinch of salt, and bring to a boil. Add the noodles and cook for 7–8 minutes. Drain and place in a bowl of cold water. Using your hands, grab handfuls of the noodles and vigorously rub. This will help to wash off the excess starch and separate the noodles. Refresh under cold water and drain well.

To make the avocado dressing, place the avocado, yoghurt, garlic, lime juice, and 1 tablespoon of water in a high-powered blender and blend until smooth. If the dressing is a little thick for your liking, gradually add extra water until the desired consistency is reached. Season with salt and pepper, if desired.

Heat a non-stick fry pan over medium–high heat. Add the asparagus spears and cook for 3–5 minutes or until they change colour and are at the desired tenderness. Set aside on a heatproof plate.

Lightly spray the non-stick fry pan with oil and heat over medium heat. Add the salmon and cook for 5–6 minutes or until cooked to your liking, turning occasionally. Transfer to a plate and set aside to rest for 2 minutes.

To serve, place the noodles, asparagus, citrus slices, salmon, arugula, fennel, and dill on a plate and spoon over the dressing. Season to taste.

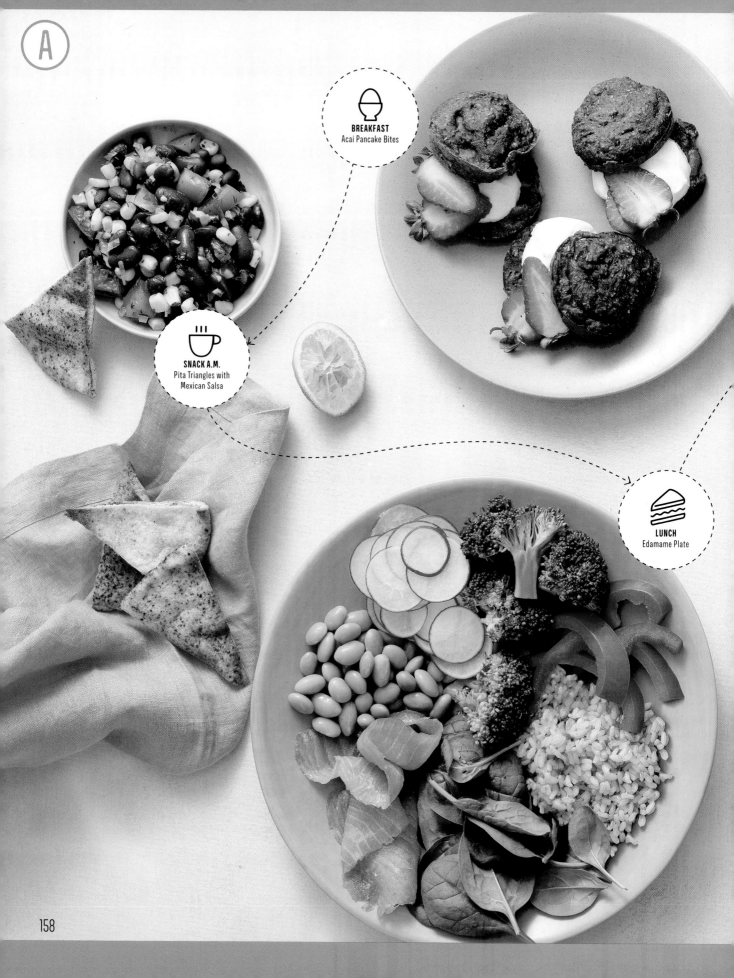

BREAKFAST
Acai Pancake Bites

SNACK A.M.
Pita Triangles with
Mexican Salsa

LUNCH
Edamame Plate

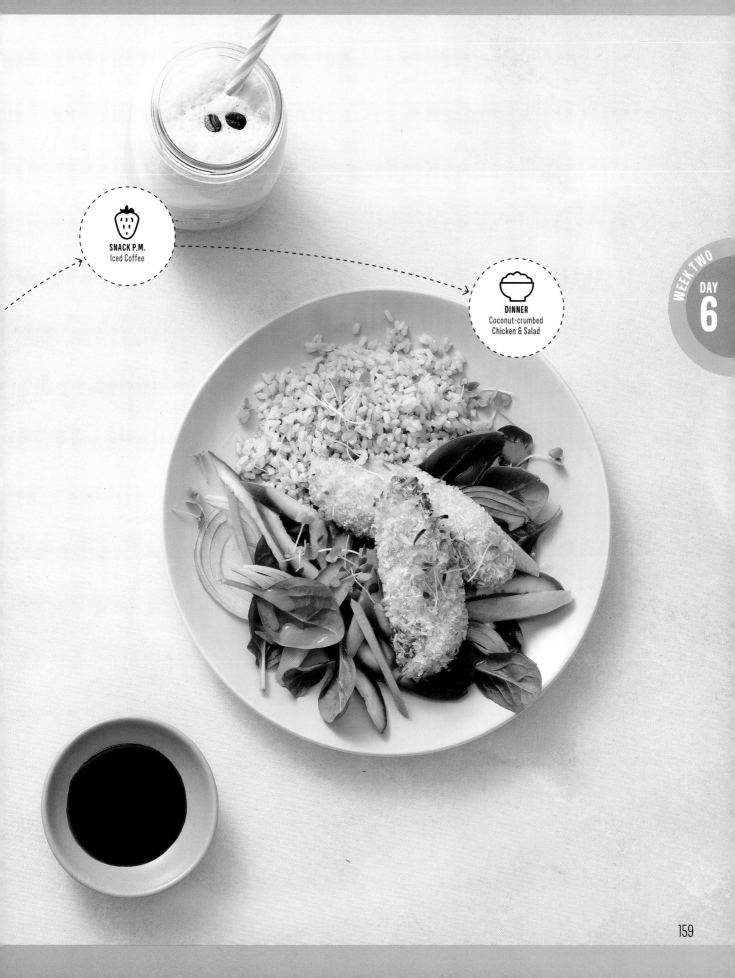

SNACK P.M.
Iced Coffee

DINNER
Coconut-crumbed
Chicken & Salad

Acai Pancake Bites

BREAKFAST | **SERVES** 1 | **PREP TIME** 5 MINUTES, PLUS 10 MINUTES RESTING TIME | **COOKING TIME** 15 MINUTES | **DIFFICULTY** EASY

oil spray
2½ oz whole wheat plain flour
1 teaspoon baking powder
2 teaspoons acai berry powder
½ medium banana, peeled
¼ cup (60 ml) low-fat milk
½ teaspoon pure
  vanilla extract
4¾ oz strawberries, sliced
5¼ oz low-fat plain yoghurt

Preheat the oven to 350°F (325°F convection) and lightly spray 3 cups of a 6-cup muffin tin with oil spray.

Place the flour, baking powder, and acai powder, in a mixing bowl and mix until well combined. Mash the banana in a second bowl, then whisk it together with the milk and vanilla extract until well combined. Pour into the dry ingredients and whisk until smooth. Stir through half the strawberries and set aside for 10 minutes to rest.

Evenly fill 3 of the muffin cups with the acai pancake mixture. Bake in the oven for 15 minutes or until firm to the touch. Leave in the muffin tin to cool for 5 minutes, then remove from the tin and place on a wire rack to cool completely.

Slice the pancake bites in half horizontally, then fill with the yoghurt and remaining sliced strawberries and serve.

Pita Triangles with Mexican Salsa

SNACK A.M. | **SERVES** 1 | **PREP TIME** 10 MINUTES, PLUS 10 MINUTES COOLING TIME | **COOKING TIME** 15 MINUTES | **DIFFICULTY** EASY

½ whole wheat pita bread
oil spray

MEXICAN SALSA

1½ oz tinned black beans,
  drained and rinsed
1½ oz tinned red kidney beans,
  drained and rinsed
½ medium tomato, diced
1 oz frozen corn kernels,
  thawed

2 teaspoons chopped
  fresh cilantro
2 teaspoons finely
  diced red onion
½ teaspoon chopped
  fresh red chilli, seeds
  removed (optional)
lime juice, to taste
sea salt and ground
  black pepper, to taste

Preheat the oven to 400°F (350°F convection) and line a baking sheet with baking paper. Cut the pita into wedges, place them in a single layer on the lined baking sheet and spray lightly with oil spray. Bake in the oven for 5 minutes or until they begin to colour. Turn the wedges over and bake for a further 5–8 minutes or until both sides are lightly coloured. Set aside to cool.

To make the Mexican salsa, place the black beans, kidney beans, tomato, corn, cilantro, onion and chilli (if using) in a small serving bowl. Season with lime juice, salt and pepper, if desired, and stir until well combined. Serve the pita triangles with the Mexican salsa.

Edamame Plate

LUNCH | **SERVES** 1 | **PREP TIME** 10 MINUTES, PLUS 5 MINUTES STANDING TIME | **COOKING TIME** 30 MINUTES | **DIFFICULTY** EASY

1 oz brown rice
1¾ oz broccoli, cut into florets
1¾ oz frozen edamame, thawed
2 teaspoons salt-reduced
  tamari or soy sauce
½ teaspoon rice wine vinegar
2 teaspoons honey
2 medium radishes
¼ medium red bell pepper,
  seeds removed
1½ oz smoked salmon
1 small handful baby
  spinach leaves

Bring the rice and 1 cup (250 ml) of water to a boil in a small saucepan over high heat, stirring occasionally. Reduce the heat to low and simmer, covered, for 20–25 minutes or until the liquid has been absorbed and the rice is tender. Remove from the heat and leave to stand, covered, for 5 minutes. To save time, the rice can be cooked the night before and stored in an airtight container in the refrigerator.

Add 2 inches of water to a saucepan and insert a steamer basket. Cover with a lid and bring the water to the boil over high heat, then reduce the heat to medium. Steam the broccoli for 2–3 minutes, add the edamame, and continue to steam for a further minute until tender-crisp. Refresh under cold running water and drain.

Whisk the tamari or soy sauce, vinegar, honey, and 2 teaspoons of water together in a small bowl. Thinly slice the radishes and bell pepper.

To serve, arrange all the ingredients on a plate and serve with the dressing on the side.

Iced Coffee

SNACK P.M. **SERVES** 1 | **PREP TIME** 5 MINUTES, PLUS 30 MINUTES SOAKING TIME | **DIFFICULTY** EASY

3 medjool dates

1 shot of coffee

1 cup (250 ml) low-fat milk

3½ oz low-fat plain yoghurt

pinch of ground cinnamon,
  plus extra to garnish (optional)

1 small handful ice cubes

coffee beans, to garnish
  (optional)

Place the dates in a heatproof bowl, cover with boiling water, and leave to soak for 30 minutes to soften. Drain.

Place the dates, coffee, milk, yoghurt, cinnamon, and ice in a high-powered blender and blend until smooth.

To serve, pour into a glass or jar. Garnish with coffee beans and a dusting of cinnamon (if using).

WEEK TWO
DAY
6

Coconut-crumbed Chicken & Salad

DINNER **SERVES** 1 | **PREP TIME** 15 MINUTES, PLUS 5 MINUTES STANDING TIME | **COOKING TIME** 25 MINUTES | **DIFFICULTY** EASY

2 oz brown rice

2 tablespoons whole wheat
  plain flour

1 large egg

1½ oz shredded coconut

1 tablespoon panko bread
  crumbs

sea salt and ground black
  pepper, to taste

3½ oz chicken tenders

oil spray

½ Lebanese cucumber, halved
  and thinly sliced

½ medium carrot, halved and
  thinly sliced

¼ small red onion, thinly sliced

1 large handful baby
  spinach leaves

micro herbs, to garnish
  (optional)

DRESSING

½ teaspoon Dijon mustard

2 teaspoons white vinegar

2 teaspoons honey

Preheat the oven to 375°F (350°F convection) and line a baking sheet with baking paper.

Bring the rice and 1 cup (250 ml) of water to a boil in a small saucepan over high heat, stirring occasionally. Reduce the heat to low and simmer, covered, for 20–25 minutes or until the liquid has been absorbed and the rice is tender. Remove from the heat and leave to stand, covered, for 5 minutes.

Meanwhile, place the flour on a flat plate. Crack the egg into a small bowl and whisk until well combined. In a separate bowl, combine the coconut, bread crumbs, salt, and pepper.

Lightly coat the chicken tenders in the flour. Shake off any excess and then dip into the beaten egg. Coat the chicken in the coconut crumb mixture, pressing firmly to ensure that it is evenly coated.

Place the crumbed chicken on the lined baking sheet and spray lightly with oil spray. Bake in the oven for 20–25 minutes or until the chicken is cooked through, turning once during the cooking time.

To make the dressing, whisk the mustard, vinegar, honey, and 1 tablespoon of water together in a small bowl and set aside.

To serve, place the rice, cucumber, carrot, onion, and spinach on a serving plate and top with the coconut-crumbed chicken. Spoon over the dressing and top with micro herbs (if using).

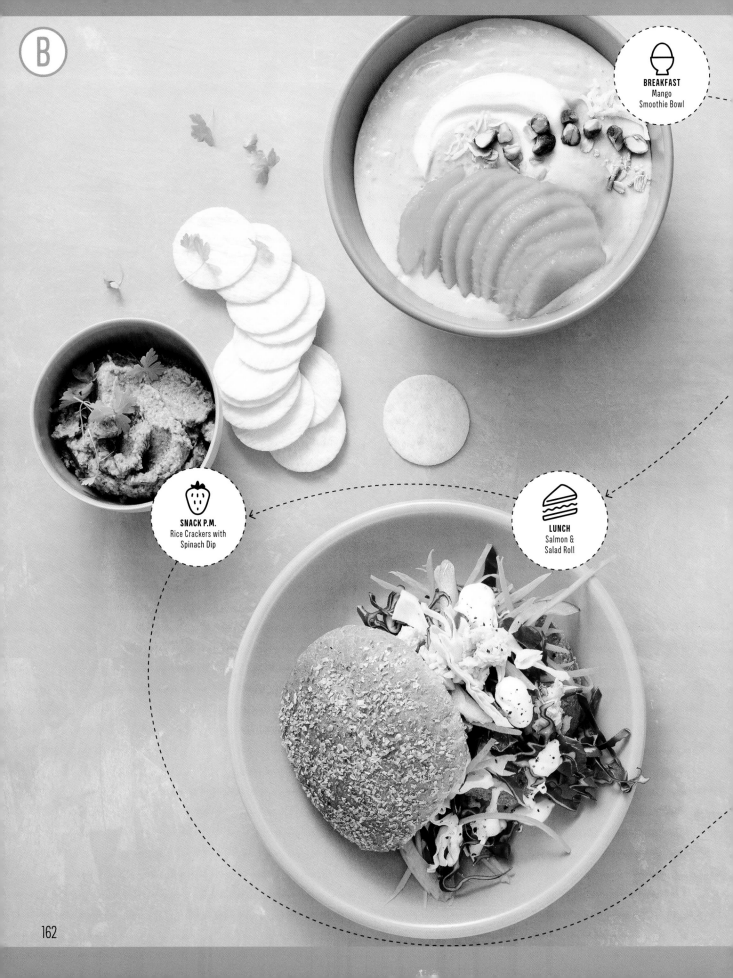

BREAKFAST
Mango
Smoothie Bowl

LUNCH
Salmon &
Salad Roll

SNACK P.M.
Rice Crackers with
Spinach Dip

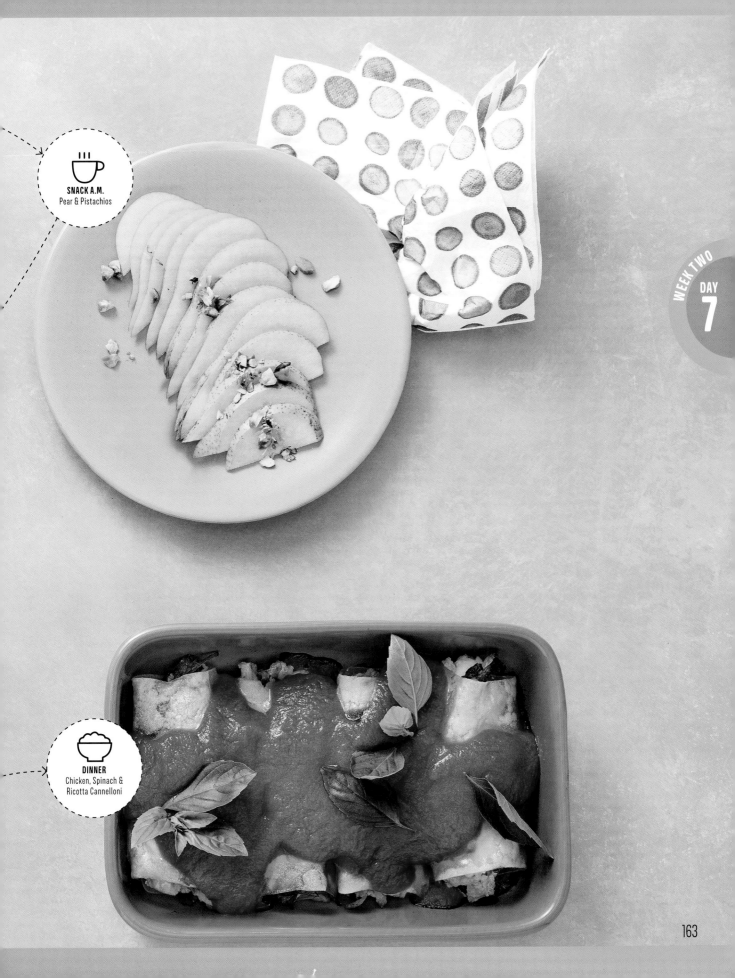

SNACK A.M.
Pear & Pistachios

DINNER
Chicken, Spinach &
Ricotta Cannelloni

Mango Smoothie Bowl

BREAKFAST **SERVES** 1 | **PREP TIME** 15 MINUTES | **DIFFICULTY** EASY

1 medium mango, peeled

3 oz pineapple, peeled and chopped

1½ oz tinned chickpeas, drained and rinsed

1 tablespoon light coconut milk

¾ cup (190 ml) low-fat milk

5¼ oz low-fat plain yoghurt

TOPPINGS

1 oz natural muesli

2 teaspoons shredded coconut

⅓ oz unsalted pistachio kernels, roughly chopped

Place half the mango, the pineapple, chickpeas, coconut milk, milk, and yoghurt in a high-powered blender and blend until smooth. Slice the remaining mango.

To serve, pour the smoothie mixture into a serving bowl and top with the muesli, coconut, pistachios, and mango slices.

Pear & Pistachios

SNACK A.M. **SERVES** 1 | **PREP TIME** 5 MINUTES | **DIFFICULTY** EASY

½ small pear, thinly sliced

⅓ oz unsalted pistachio kernels, chopped

To serve, place the pear on a small serving plate and top with the pistachios.

Salmon & Salad Roll

LUNCH **SERVES** 1 | **PREP TIME** 10 MINUTES | **DIFFICULTY** EASY

2½ oz tinned salmon, drained

1¾ oz red cabbage, finely shredded

1 oz green cabbage, finely shredded

¼ small red onion, thinly sliced

¼ medium carrot, grated

½ celery stalk, thinly sliced

2 teaspoons chopped fresh parsley

1 medium whole wheat roll, halved

DIJON YOGHURT DRESSING

3½ oz low-fat plain yoghurt

½ teaspoon white vinegar

½ teaspoon Dijon mustard

To make the Dijon yoghurt dressing, whisk the yoghurt, vinegar, and mustard together in a small bowl.

Place the salmon, red and green cabbage, onion, carrot, celery, and parsley in a mixing bowl. Drizzle over the dressing and toss gently to combine.

To serve, spoon the salmon and salad mixture onto one half of the roll. Top with the other half of the roll.

Rice Crackers with Spinach Dip

SNACK P.M. **SERVES** 1 | **PREP TIME** 10 MINUTES | **COOKING TIME** 30 MINUTES | **DIFFICULTY** EASY

12 plain rice crackers

SPINACH DIP

4½ oz dried yellow split peas

1 teaspoon white vinegar

oil spray

¼ small brown onion, finely chopped

½ garlic clove, crushed

1 large handful baby spinach leaves

1 tablespoon chopped fresh parsley, plus extra parsley leaves to garnish

lemon juice, to taste

sea salt and ground black pepper, to taste

To make the spinach dip, place the split peas, vinegar, and 1½ cups (300 ml) of cold water in a medium saucepan and bring to a boil. Reduce the heat to medium–low and simmer for 25–30 minutes or until soft. Drain and rinse under cold running water.

Meanwhile, lightly spray a non-stick fry pan with oil and heat over medium heat. Add the onion and cook for 5 minutes or until soft and translucent, stirring occasionally. Add the garlic and spinach and cook for 1 minute or until the spinach has wilted, stirring occasionally. Remove from the heat and set aside to cool slightly.

Place the peas, spinach mixture, parsley, and 2 teaspoons of water in a food processor and process until smooth. Season with lemon juice, salt, and pepper, if desired.

Place the spinach dip in a small bowl, garnish with the extra parsley, and serve with the rice crackers.

WEEK TWO
DAY
7

Chicken, Spinach & Ricotta Cannelloni

DINNER **SERVES** 1 | **PREP TIME** 15 MINUTES | **COOKING TIME** 45 MINUTES | **DIFFICULTY** EASY

oil spray

4 whole wheat lasagne sheets

¼ small brown onion, chopped

½ garlic clove, crushed

3½ oz ground chicken

1 large handful baby spinach leaves, chopped

1¾ oz low-fat ricotta cheese

pinch of ground nutmeg

sliced fresh basil, to taste, plus extra leaves to garnish

sea salt and ground black pepper, to taste

2¾ oz tomato passata (purée)

Preheat the oven to 350°F (325°F convection). Spray a medium-sized, shallow baking dish with oil spray.

Fill a large saucepan with water, add a pinch of salt, and bring to a boil. Add the lasagne sheets and cook until al dente (see the pasta packet for the recommended cooking time). Drain well and set aside, ensuring the sheets are flat.

Meanwhile, lightly spray a non-stick fry pan with oil and heat over medium heat. Add the onion and cook for 3–4 minutes or until soft, stirring occasionally. Add the garlic and ground chicken and cook for 8–10 minutes or until cooked through, stirring frequently with a wooden spoon to break up the chicken. Drain off any excess liquid.

Stir in the spinach, ricotta, nutmeg, and basil and cook for 2–3 minutes or until the spinach has wilted, stirring occasionally. Season with salt and pepper, if desired.

Spread one-quarter of the tomato passata over the base of the baking dish.

Place one-quarter of the spinach and ricotta mixture along the length of one lasagne sheet and roll to enclose the filling. Place the cannelloni, seam side down, in the baking dish. Repeat with the remaining mixture and lasagne sheets, making four cannelloni in total.

Spoon the remaining tomato passata evenly over the cannelloni and bake in the oven for 20–25 minutes or until heated through. Serve garnished with extra basil leaves.

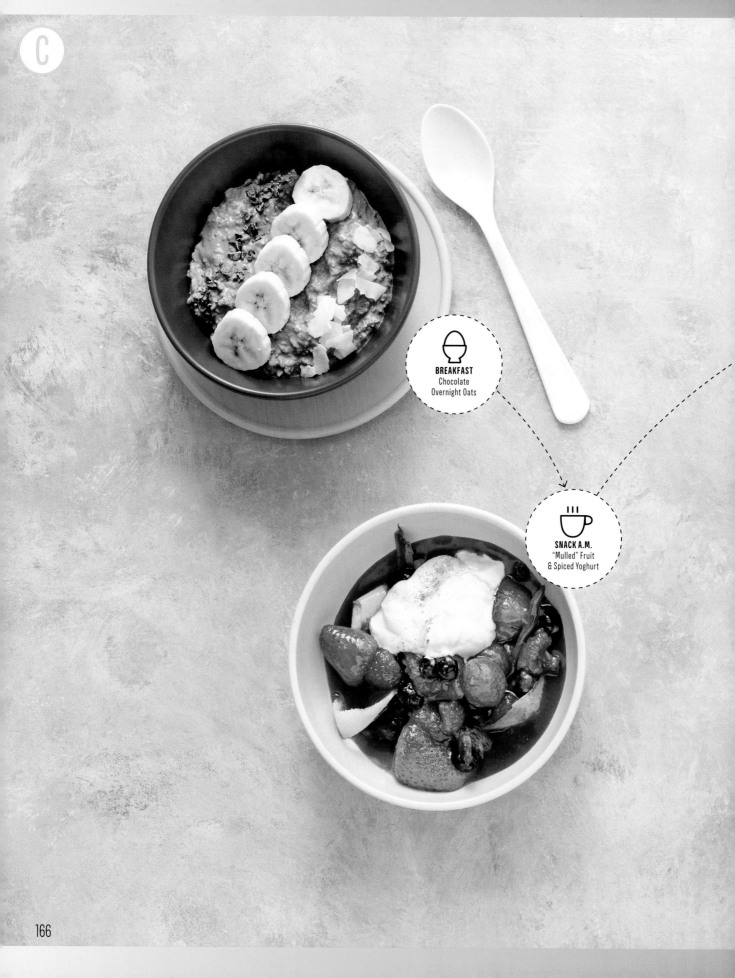

BREAKFAST
Chocolate
Overnight Oats

SNACK A.M.
"Mulled" Fruit
& Spiced Yoghurt

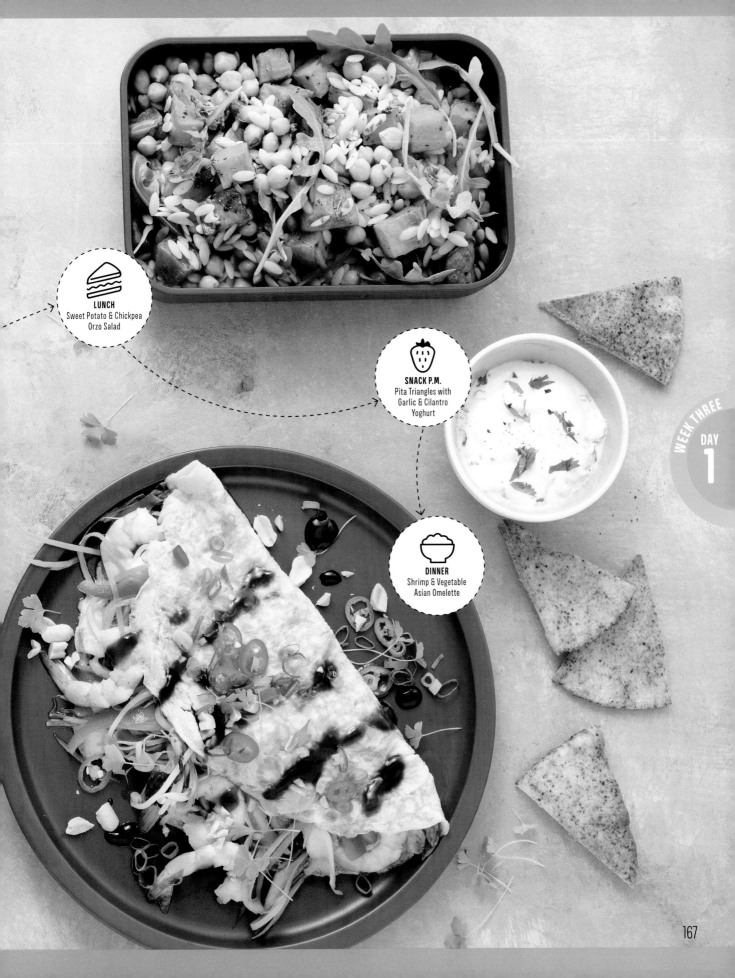

LUNCH
Sweet Potato & Chickpea
Orzo Salad

SNACK P.M.
Pita Triangles with
Garlic & Cilantro
Yoghurt

DINNER
Shrimp & Vegetable
Asian Omelette

WEEK THREE

DAY
1

Chocolate Overnight Oats

SERVES 1 | **PREP TIME** 5 MINUTES, PLUS OVERNIGHT CHILLING TIME | **DIFFICULTY** EASY

2 oz rolled oats
½ cup (125 ml) low-fat milk
1½ tablespoons light
  coconut milk
1¾ oz low-fat plain yoghurt

1 tablespoon raw
  cacao powder
½ medium banana, peeled
  and sliced
1 tablespoon coconut flakes
raw cacao nibs, to garnish

Place the oats, milk, coconut milk, yoghurt, and cacao powder in a bowl and mix until well combined. Cover with plastic wrap and place in the refrigerator to chill overnight.

To serve, stir the oats, then top with the sliced banana, coconut flakes, and cacao nibs.

"Mulled" Fruit & Spiced Yoghurt

SERVES 1 | **PREP TIME** 10 MINUTES + 15 MINUTES CHILLING TIME | **COOKING TIME** 10 MINUTES | **DIFFICULTY** EASY

7 oz low-fat plain yoghurt
pinch of ground cinnamon,
  plus an extra small pinch
  for dusting (optional)
pinch of ground nutmeg
pinch of ground cloves
¼ teaspoon pure
  vanilla extract
1 teaspoon honey
1 oz natural muesli

"MULLED" FRUIT
¼ cup (60 ml) 100%
  cranberry juice

1½ tablespoons 100%
  orange juice
peeled zest of ½ an orange
2 teaspoons honey
½ cinnamon stick
½ star anise
2 cloves
2 oz strawberries, hulled
1½ oz blueberries
1½ oz raspberries
½ teaspoon arrowroot

To make the "mulled" fruit, place the cranberry juice, orange juice, orange zest, honey, cinnamon stick, star anise, and cloves in a medium saucepan. Bring to a gentle boil over medium–high heat, then reduce the heat to medium–low and simmer for 4–5 minutes or until reduced and syrupy. Add the berries and simmer for 1 minute.

Meanwhile, dissolve the arrowroot in 1 tablespoon of water. Add to the pan and simmer for 2 minutes until thickened, stirring gently. Remove from the heat and transfer to a bowl. Cover with plastic wrap and chill in the refrigerator for 15 minutes. Remove the whole spices before serving.

Whisk the yoghurt, cinnamon, nutmeg, cloves, vanilla, and honey together in a small bowl. To serve, place the "mulled" fruit in a serving bowl and top with the spiced yoghurt, muesli, and an extra pinch of cinnamon (if using).

Sweet Potato & Chickpea Orzo Salad

SERVES 1 | **PREP TIME** 10 MINUTES + COOLING TIME | **COOKING TIME** 20 MINUTES | **DIFFICULTY** EASY

½ medium sweet potato,
  peeled
oil spray
sea salt and ground black
  pepper, to taste
3 oz orzo
lemon juice, to taste
1 tablespoon chopped
  fresh parsley
1 small handful arugula leaves
5¼ oz tinned chickpeas,
  drained and rinsed

Preheat the oven to 400°F (350°F convection) and line a baking sheet with baking paper. Cut the sweet potato into ¾ inch cubes, then place in a single layer on the lined tray and spray lightly with oil. Season with salt and pepper, if desired. Bake in the oven for 15–20 minutes or until tender and lightly browned, turning with tongs halfway through.

Meanwhile, fill a large saucepan with water, add a pinch of salt and bring to the boil. Add the orzo and cook until al dente (see the packet for the recommended cooking time). Drain and refresh under cool running water. Set aside to cool.

Whisk the lemon juice, parsley and 1 tablespoon of water together in a small bowl. Place the orzo, sweet potato, arugula, and chickpeas in a mixing bowl. Drizzle over the dressing, season with salt and pepper, if desired, and toss gently to combine.

To serve, place the sweet potato and chickpea salad in a serving bowl.

Pita Triangles with Garlic & Cilantro Yoghurt

SNACK P.M. **SERVES** 1 | **PREP TIME** 5 MINUTES | **COOKING TIME** 15 MINUTES | **DIFFICULTY** EASY

½ whole wheat pita bread,
  cut into wedges
oil spray

**GARLIC & CILANTRO
YOGHURT**

1¾ oz low-fat plain yoghurt
2 teaspoons chopped fresh
  cilantro
¼ garlic clove, crushed
lemon juice, to taste
sea salt and ground black
  pepper, to taste

Preheat the oven to 400°F (350°F convection) and line a baking sheet with baking paper.

Lay the pita wedges in a single layer on the lined baking sheet and spray lightly with oil spray. Bake in the oven for 5 minutes or until they begin to colour. Turn the wedges over and bake for a further 5–8 minutes or until both sides are lightly coloured. Set aside to cool.

To make the garlic and cilantro yoghurt, whisk the yoghurt, cilantro, garlic, lemon juice, salt, and pepper together in a small bowl.

Serve the pita triangles with the garlic and cilantro yoghurt.

Shrimp & Vegetable Asian Omelette

DINNER **SERVES** 1 | **PREP TIME** 20 MINUTES | **COOKING TIME** 15 MINUTES | **DIFFICULTY** MEDIUM

WEEK THREE
DAY
1

oil spray
5 medium raw shrimp, peeled
  and deveined, tails intact
¼ small red onion, thinly sliced
¾ medium carrot, thinly sliced
¾ medium red bell pepper,
  seeds removed, thinly sliced
3 oz bok choy, chopped
1 small handful bean sprouts
2 large eggs
¼ cup (60 ml) low-fat milk
½ teaspoon fish sauce
sea salt and ground black
  pepper, to taste
⅓ oz low-fat cheddar
  cheese, grated
1 tablespoon oyster sauce
1 scallion, thinly sliced
½ fresh red chilli, seeds
  removed and thinly sliced
1 tablespoon chopped
  fresh cilantro
⅓ oz roasted peanuts,
  roughly chopped

Lightly spray a non-stick fry pan with oil and heat over medium–high heat. Cook the shrimp for 2–3 minutes or until they are pink. Transfer to a plate and set aside to rest.

Reheat the non-stick fry pan over medium heat. Add the onion, carrot, bell pepper, and bok choy and cook for 3–4 minutes or until tender-crisp. Add the bean sprouts and cook for a further minute. Transfer to a bowl and set aside.

Whisk the eggs, milk, and fish sauce together in a small bowl. Season with salt and pepper, if desired.

Lightly spray the non-stick fry pan with oil and heat over medium heat. Pour in the egg mixture and swirl to cover the base of the pan. Cook for 1–2 minutes or until the egg starts to set and the underside is golden in colour. Reduce the heat to medium–low and sprinkle the cheese, shrimp, and vegetable mixture over the omelette. Cook for 1 minute or until the egg is golden and set. Fold in half to cover the filling and, using a spatula, transfer to a serving plate.

Whisk the oyster sauce and 1 tablespoon of warm water together in a small bowl.

To serve, top the shrimp and vegetable omelette with the scallion, chilli, and cilantro. Drizzle over the oyster sauce and garnish with the peanuts.

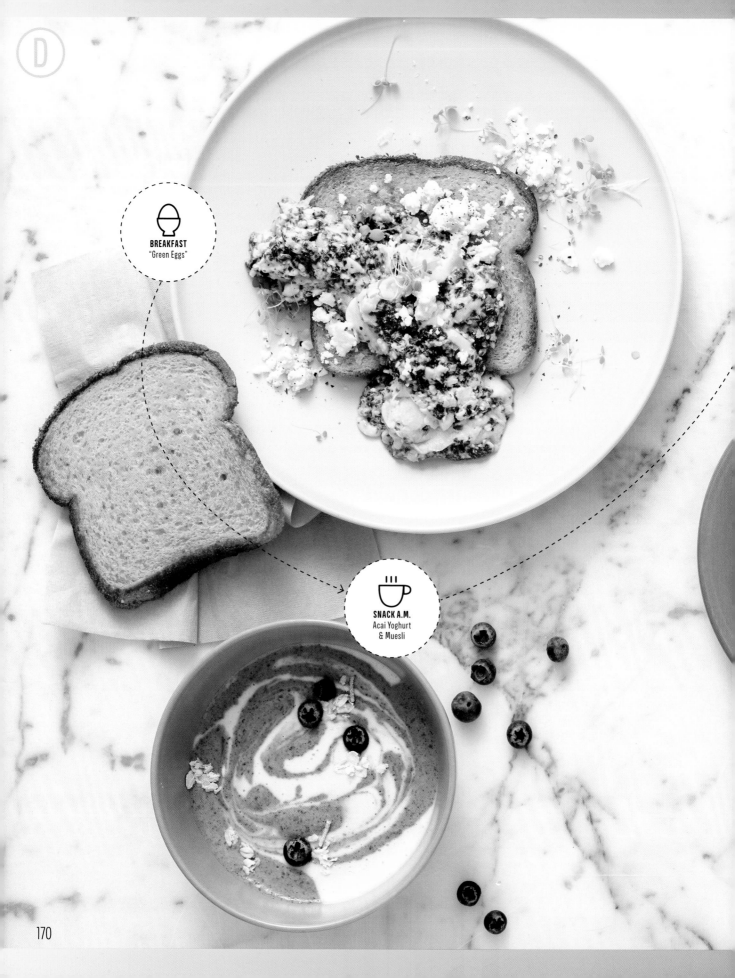

D

BREAKFAST
"Green Eggs"

SNACK A.M.
Acai Yoghurt
& Muesli

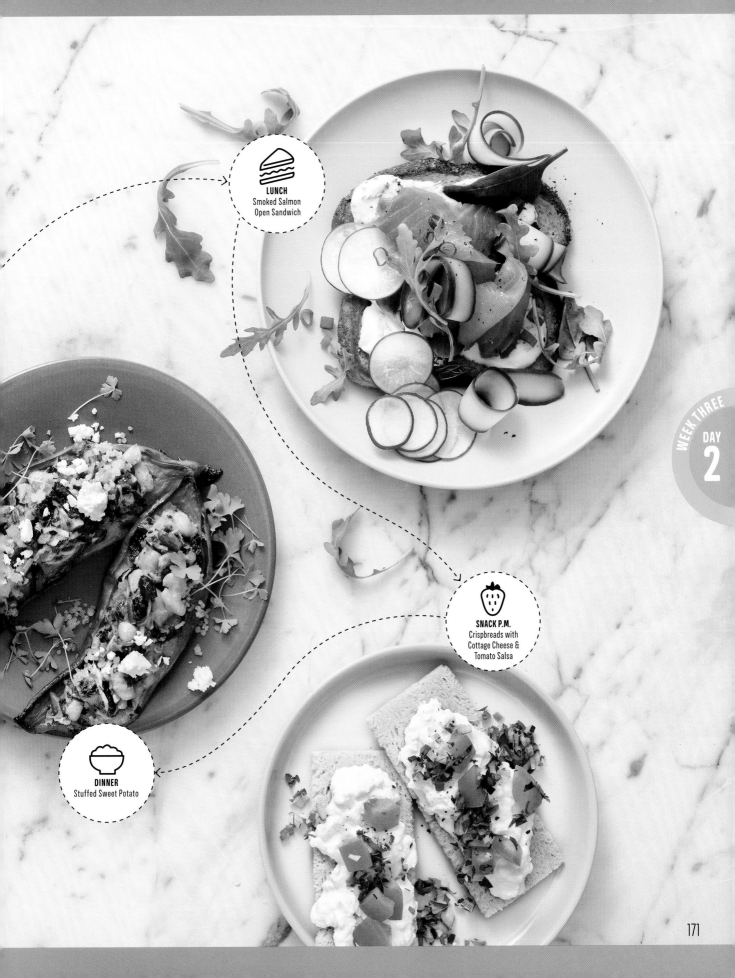

LUNCH
Smoked Salmon
Open Sandwich

SNACK P.M.
Crispbreads with
Cottage Cheese &
Tomato Salsa

DINNER
Stuffed Sweet Potato

WEEK THREE

DAY
2

"Green Eggs"

SERVES 1 | **PREP TIME** 10 MINUTES | **COOKING TIME** 10 MINUTES | **DIFFICULTY** MEDIUM

2 large eggs
¼ cup (60 ml) low-fat milk
sea salt and ground black
  pepper, to taste
2 slices whole wheat bread
⅔ oz salt-reduced low-fat
  feta cheese, crumbled

KALE PESTO

1 small handful kale,
  roughly chopped
1 scallion, sliced
2 teaspoons pine nuts
½ garlic clove, crushed
lemon juice, to taste
sea salt and ground black
  pepper, to taste

To make the pesto, place the kale, scallion, pine nuts, garlic, and lemon juice in a food processor and pulse until finely chopped. Add ¼ cup (60 ml) of water and process until smooth. If the mixture is too thick, add 1 tablespoon of water at a time until the desired consistency is reached. Season with salt and pepper, if desired.

Whisk the eggs, milk, salt, and pepper together in a bowl. Heat a non-stick fry pan over medium heat. When the pan is hot, pour in the egg mixture, followed by the pesto. As the mixture begins to set, gently push it across the pan with a wooden spoon to form large folds. Ensure that you push the mixture from different directions and include the egg from around the edge of the pan. Do not stir constantly. Continue to cook until no visible liquid egg remains, then immediately remove from the heat.

Toast the bread to your liking.

To serve, place the toast on a serving plate and top with the "green eggs" and the feta.

Acai Yoghurt & Muesli

SERVES 1 | **PREP TIME** 5 MINUTES | **DIFFICULTY** EASY

½ medium banana, peeled
2 teaspoons acai
  berry powder
½ teaspoon honey
3½ oz low-fat plain yoghurt
3 oz blueberries
1 oz natural muesli

Place the banana, acai berry powder, honey, half the yoghurt, and three-quarters of the blueberries in a high-powered blender and blend until smooth.

To serve, pour the acai yoghurt into a serving bowl. Swirl through the remaining yoghurt, then top with the muesli and remaining blueberries.

Smoked Salmon Open Sandwich

SERVES 1 | **PREP TIME** 10 MINUTES | **COOKING TIME** 2 MINUTES | **DIFFICULTY** EASY

1 slice whole wheat bread
½ Lebanese cucumber
1½ oz smoked salmon
1 small handful arugula leaves
1 small handful baby
  spinach leaves
1 medium radish, thinly sliced
½ scallion, sliced

DILL YOGHURT

3½ oz low-fat plain yoghurt
½ teaspoon chopped fresh dill
¼ garlic clove, crushed
finely grated zest and juice
  of ¼ lemon
sea salt and ground black
  pepper, to taste

To make the dill yoghurt, place the yoghurt, dill, garlic, lemon zest, and juice in a small bowl. Season with salt and pepper, if desired, and mix until well combined.

Toast the bread to your liking. Meanwhile, use a vegetable peeler to carefully slice the cucumber lengthwise into long, thin ribbons.

To serve, place the toast on a serving plate and spread over the dill yoghurt. Top with the salmon, arugula, spinach, cucumber, radish, and scallion.

Crispbreads with Cottage Cheese & Tomato Salsa

SERVES 1 | **PREP TIME** 10 MINUTES | **DIFFICULTY** EASY

2 oz low-fat cottage cheese

2 rye crispbreads

TOMATO SALSA

½ medium tomato, diced

2 teaspoons finely diced red onion

2 teaspoons chopped fresh cilantro

lime juice, to taste

¼ teaspoon finely chopped fresh red chilli (optional)

sea salt and ground black pepper, to taste

To make the tomato salsa, place the tomato, onion, cilantro, lime juice, and chilli (if using) in a small bowl. Season with salt and pepper, if desired, and mix until well combined.

To serve, spread the cottage cheese over the crispbreads and top with the tomato salsa.

Stuffed Sweet Potato

SERVES 1 | **PREP TIME** 15 MINUTES, PLUS 10 MINUTES COOLING TIME | **COOKING TIME** 50 MINUTES | **DIFFICULTY** EASY

1 small sweet potato, halved lengthwise

oil spray

1 oz quinoa

1¼ cups (300 ml) salt-reduced vegetable stock

¼ small brown onion, chopped

½ garlic clove, crushed

1 small handful kale, finely shredded

½ medium zucchini, grated

2¾ oz tinned cannellini beans, drained and rinsed

1 oz salt-reduced low-fat feta cheese, crumbled

1 oz dried cranberries

⅓ oz pecans, roughly chopped

sea salt and ground black pepper, to taste

1 large egg, lightly whisked

fresh parsley leaves, to garnish

Preheat the oven to 400°F (350°F convection) and line a baking sheet with baking paper.

Lightly spray the sweet potato halves with oil, ensuring they are lightly coated all over. Place the sweet potato halves on the lined baking sheet, cut side up, and bake in the oven for 30–35 minutes or until tender. Set aside to cool slightly.

Meanwhile, bring the quinoa and stock to a boil in a small saucepan over high heat, stirring occasionally. Reduce the heat to low and simmer, covered, for 10–12 minutes or until the quinoa is tender. Drain off any excess liquid.

Lightly spray a non-stick fry pan with oil and heat over medium heat. Add the onion and cook for 3–4 minutes or until it starts to soften, stirring occasionally. Add the garlic and cook for 1 minute or until fragrant. Add the kale and zucchini and cook for 3–5 minutes or until soft, stirring occasionally. Remove from the heat.

Stir the quinoa, cannellini beans, feta, cranberries, and pecans through the kale mixture and season with salt and pepper, if desired. Set aside.

Leaving the sweet potato shells intact, scoop out the flesh and place in a mixing bowl, then roughly mash with a fork. Add the egg and mix until well combined. Add the sweet potato mash to the kale and cannellini bean mixture and mix until well combined.

Spoon the sweet potato and kale mixture into the sweet potato shells and return to the lined baking sheet. Lightly spray the top with oil and bake in the oven for 15 minutes or until heated through and light golden in colour.

To serve, place the stuffed sweet potato halves on a serving plate and sprinkle over the parsley leaves.

WEEK THREE DAY 2

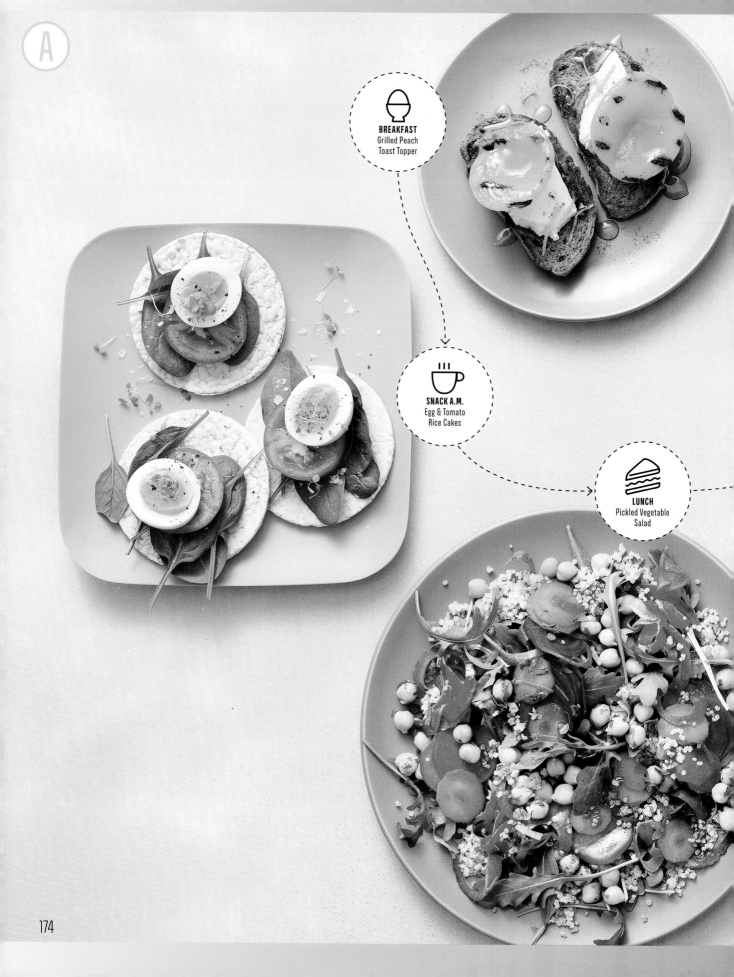

BREAKFAST
Grilled Peach
Toast Topper

SNACK A.M.
Egg & Tomato
Rice Cakes

LUNCH
Pickled Vegetable
Salad

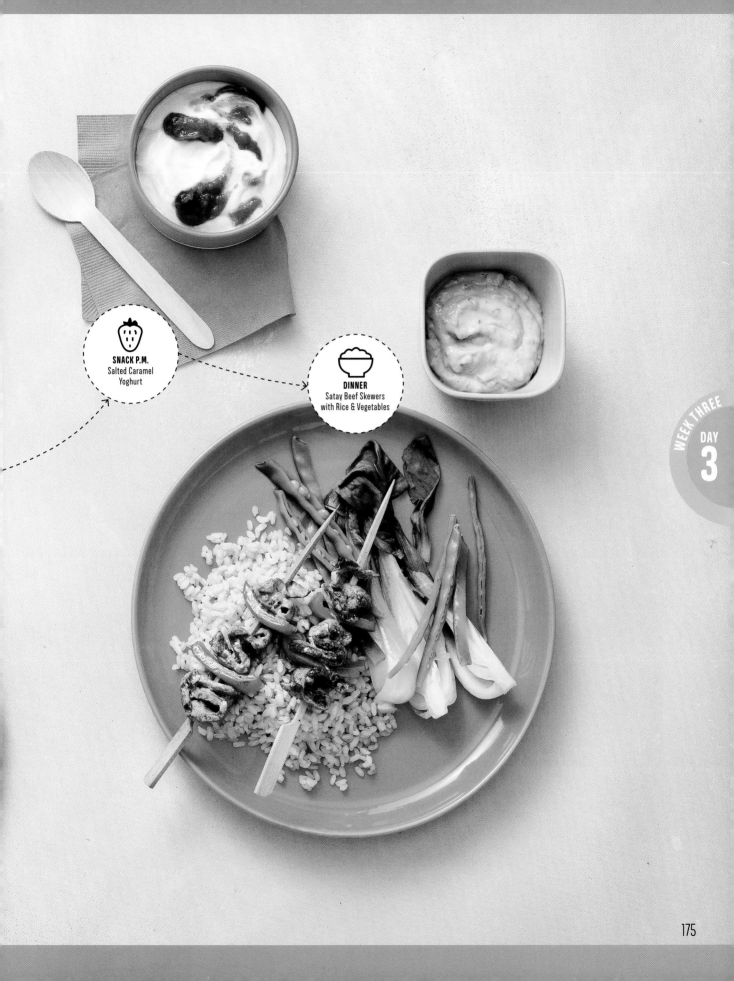

SNACK P.M.
Salted Caramel
Yoghurt

DINNER
Satay Beef Skewers
with Rice & Vegetables

Grilled Peach Toast Topper

SERVES 1 | **PREP TIME** 5 MINUTES | **COOKING TIME** 10 MINUTES | **DIFFICULTY** EASY

1 large peach
oil spray
2 slices raisin bread
3½ oz low-fat ricotta cheese
½ teaspoon honey
finely grated zest and juice
  of ¼ medium orange
pinch of ground cinnamon

Cut the peach in half and remove the stone. Lightly spray a barbecue grill-plate or chargrill pan with oil and heat over medium heat. Grill the peach halves for about 2–4 minutes on each side or until soft and nicely charred.

Meanwhile, toast the raisin bread to your liking.

To serve, place the toast on a serving plate and top with the ricotta. Place the grilled peach halves on top and drizzle with the honey and orange juice. Garnish with the orange zest and a dash of cinnamon.

Egg & Tomato Rice Cakes

SERVES 1 | **PREP TIME** 5 MINUTES | **COOKING TIME** 10 MINUTES | **DIFFICULTY** EASY

1 large egg
3 rice cakes
1 small handful baby
  spinach leaves
½ medium tomato, sliced
sea salt and ground black
  pepper, to taste
micro herbs, to garnish
  (optional)

To hard-boil the egg, place it in a small saucepan and fill with cold water until it is covered by ¾ inch. Bring the water to a boil over high heat. Reduce the heat to low and simmer, covered, for 7–8 minutes. Remove the egg from the pan with a slotted spoon and place in a bowl of iced water. Leave for 1 minute. Tap the egg gently on the bench to crack the shell, then peel and slice into rounds.

To serve, place the rice cakes on a serving plate and top with the spinach, tomato, and egg. Season with salt and pepper, if desired, and garnish with micro herbs (if using).

Pickled Vegetable Salad

SERVES 1 | **PREP TIME** 10 MINUTES, PLUS 20 MINUTES COOLING AND STANDING TIME | **COOKING TIME** 15 MINUTES | **DIFFICULTY** EASY

1 oz quinoa
½ small beetroot, peeled
½ small fennel bulb
½ medium carrot
1 medium radish
½ cup (125 ml) rice
  wine vinegar
2 teaspoons honey
finely grated zest of ½ lemon
finely grated zest of ½
  medium orange
sea salt, to taste
5¼ oz tinned chickpeas,
  drained and rinsed
1 small handful arugula leaves
2 teaspoons chopped
  fresh parsley

Bring the quinoa and about 1 cup (200 ml) of water to a boil in a small saucepan over high heat, stirring occasionally. Reduce the heat to low and simmer, covered, for 10–12 minutes or until the quinoa is tender. Drain off any excess liquid. Set aside to cool. To save time, the quinoa can be cooked the night before and stored in an airtight container in the refrigerator.

Using a mandoline, shave the beetroot, fennel, carrot, and radish and place in a bowl.

Place the vinegar, ½ cup (125 ml) of water, honey, lemon zest, orange zest, and salt in a small saucepan and bring to a boil. Reduce the heat to medium–low and simmer for 2 minutes. Pour the pickling liquid over the shaved vegetables and leave to stand for 10 minutes or until the vegetables are just tender. Drain.

Place the quinoa, pickled vegetables, chickpeas, and arugula in a mixing bowl and toss gently to combine.

To serve, place the salad on a serving plate and scatter over the parsley.

Salted Caramel Yoghurt

SERVES 1 | **PREP TIME** 10 MINUTES, PLUS 30 MINUTES SOAKING TIME | **DIFFICULTY** EASY

3 medjool dates, pitted
¼ teaspoon sea salt
10¾ oz low-fat plain yoghurt

Place the dates in a heatproof bowl, cover with boiling water, and leave to soak for 30 minutes to soften. Drain.

Place the dates, salt, and 2 tablespoons of water in a high-powered blender and blend until smooth.

To serve, place the yoghurt and half of the salted caramel in a small bowl and mix until well combined. Top with the remaining caramel.

Satay Beef Skewers with Rice & Vegetables

SERVES 1 | **PREP TIME** 10 MINUTES | **COOKING TIME** 40 MINUTES | **DIFFICULTY** EASY

2 oz brown rice
3 oz lean beef strips
¼ medium red bell pepper, seeds removed, chopped
oil spray
4¼ oz bok choy, trimmed and halved
1½ oz snow peas, trimmed

SATAY SAUCE
oil spray
2 teaspoons finely diced brown onion
½ garlic clove, crushed
¼ teaspoon finely grated fresh ginger
pinch of dried chilli flakes
2 teaspoons 100% natural peanut butter
½ teaspoon salt-reduced tamari or soy sauce
lime juice, to taste
¼ cup (60 ml) light coconut milk

Bring the rice and 1 cup (250 ml) of water to the boil in a small saucepan over high heat, stirring occasionally. Reduce the heat to low and simmer, covered, for 20–25 minutes or until the liquid has been absorbed and the rice is tender. Remove from the heat and leave to stand, covered, for 5 minutes.

Meanwhile, soak two wooden skewers in cold water for 30 minutes. This will help stop the skewers from burning during cooking.

To make the satay sauce, lightly spray a small saucepan with oil and heat over medium heat. Add the onion and cook for 3 minutes, stirring occasionally. Add the garlic, ginger, and chilli flakes and cook for 1 minute, stirring frequently. Add the peanut butter, tamari or soy sauce, lime juice, and coconut milk and stir until smooth. Add 2 tablespoons of water and bring to a boil. Reduce the heat to medium–low and simmer for 8–10 minutes or until thickened to your liking, stirring occasionally. Remove from the heat and set aside.

Preheat a barbecue grill-plate or chargrill pan over medium–high heat.

Thread the beef and bell pepper onto the skewers, alternating as you go. Spray lightly with oil and grill for 6–8 minutes or until cooked to your liking, turning frequently.

Add 2 inches of water to a saucepan and insert a steamer basket. Cover with a lid and bring the water to the boil over high heat, then reduce the heat to medium. Add the bok choy and steam, covered, for 3 minutes. Add the snow peas and steam for a further 2–3 minutes or until the vegetables are tender-crisp.

To serve, place the rice and steamed vegetables on a serving plate and top with the beef skewers. Serve the satay sauce on the side.

WEEK THREE
DAY
3

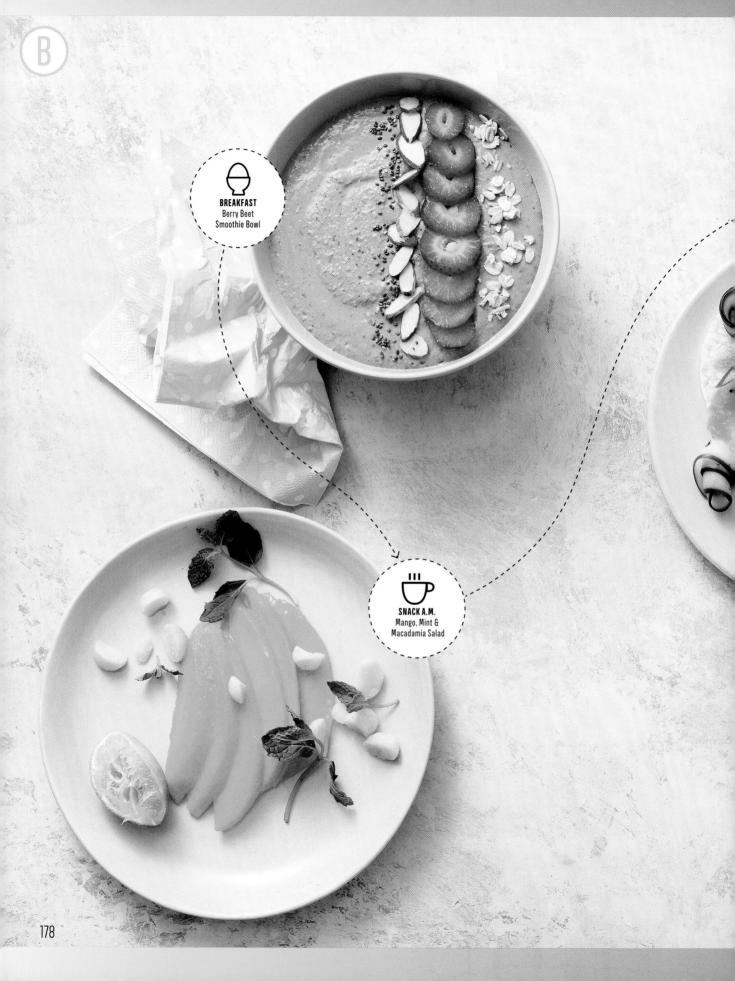

BREAKFAST
Berry Beet
Smoothie Bowl

SNACK A.M.
Mango, Mint &
Macadamia Salad

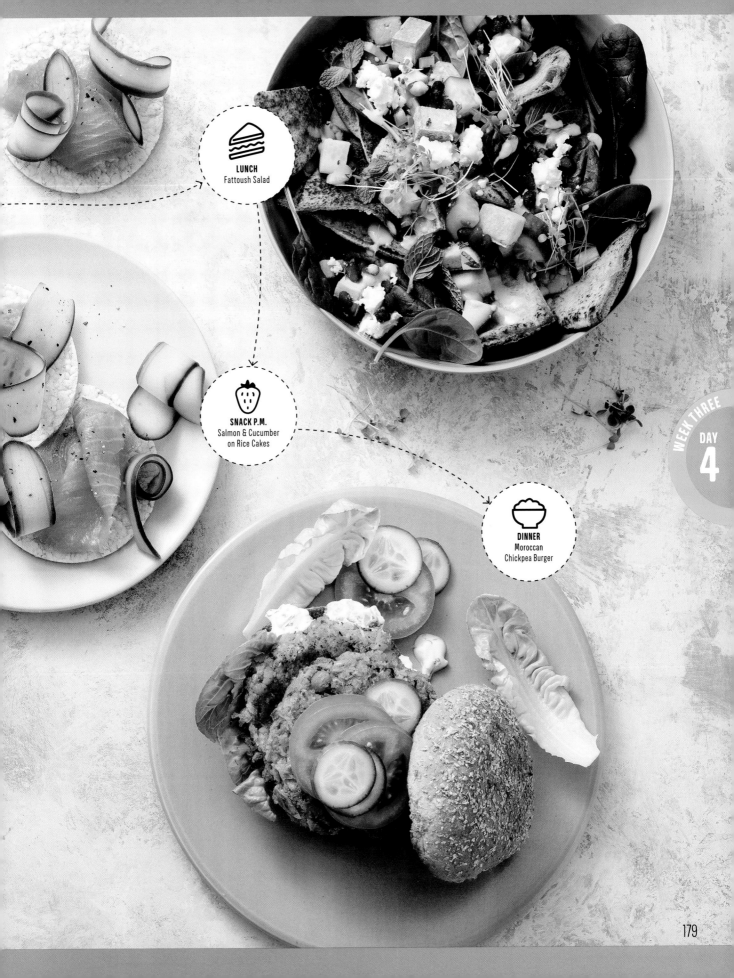

LUNCH
Fattoush Salad

SNACK P.M.
Salmon & Cucumber
on Rice Cakes

DINNER
Moroccan
Chickpea Burger

Berry Beet Smoothie Bowl

SERVES 1 | **PREP TIME** 10 MINUTES, PLUS 30 MINUTES SOAKING TIME | **DIFFICULTY** EASY

1½ medjool dates, pitted
½ small beetroot, peeled
   and chopped
4¾ oz frozen mixed berries,
   thawed
¼ teaspoon pure
   vanilla extract
5¼ oz low-fat plain yoghurt
¾ cup (190 ml) low-fat milk

TOPPINGS
1 oz natural muesli
2 oz strawberries, hulled
   and sliced
1 teaspoon chia seeds
1 teaspoon raw
   flaked almonds

Place the dates in a heatproof bowl, cover with boiling water, and leave to soak for 30 minutes to soften. Drain.

Place the dates, beetroot, mixed berries, vanilla, yoghurt, and milk in a high-powered blender and blend until smooth.

To serve, pour the smoothie mixture into a serving bowl and top with the muesli, strawberries, chia seeds, and flaked almonds.

Mango, Mint & Macadamia Salad

SERVES 1 | **PREP TIME** 5 MINUTES | **DIFFICULTY** EASY

½ medium mango, peeled
   and sliced
⅓ oz unsalted macadamia
   nuts, roughly chopped
1 small handul fresh mint
juice of ¼ lime

Place the mango slices, macadamias, and mint on a serving plate. Drizzle over the lime juice and serve.

Fattoush Salad

SERVES 1 | **PREP TIME** 10 MINUTES | **COOKING TIME** 15 MINUTES | **DIFFICULTY** EASY

1 whole wheat pita bread,
   cut into wedges
oil spray
1 celery stalk, chopped
½ Lebanese cucumber, diced
1 small handful baby
   spinach leaves
6 oz firm tofu, cut into
   ¾ inch cubes or 3½ oz tinned
   tuna in springwater, drained
1 oz salt-reduced low-fat
   feta cheese, crumbled
1 small handul fresh mint

sea salt and ground black
   pepper, to taste
watercress, to garnish

DRESSING
1 teaspoon white vinegar
1 teaspoon Dijon mustard
sea salt, to taste

Preheat the oven to 400°F (350°F convection) and line a baking sheet with baking paper.

Lay the pita wedges in a single layer on the lined baking sheet and spray lightly with oil spray. Bake in the oven for 5 minutes or until they begin to colour. Turn the wedges over and bake for a further 5–8 minutes or until both sides are lightly coloured, then set aside to cool.

Meanwhile, to make the dressing, whisk the vinegar, mustard, salt, and 2 teaspoons of water together in a small bowl and set aside.

Place the celery, cucumber, spinach, tofu or tuna, feta, pita crisps, and half the mint in a mixing bowl. Drizzle over the dressing, season with salt and pepper, if desired, and toss gently to combine.

To serve, place the salad in a serving bowl. Sprinkle over the watercress and remaining mint.

Salmon & Cucumber on Rice Cakes

SNACK P.M. **SERVES** 1 | **PREP TIME** 5 MINUTES | **DIFFICULTY** EASY

1 Lebanese cucumber
3 rice cakes
1½ oz smoked salmon
sea salt and ground black
  pepper, to taste

Using a vegetable peeler, carefully slice the cucumber lengthways into long, thin ribbons.

To serve, place the rice cakes on a serving plate and top with the salmon and cucumber. Season with salt and pepper, if desired.

Moroccan Chickpea Burger

DINNER **SERVES** 1 | **PREP TIME** 15 MINUTES, PLUS 30 MINUTES CHILLING TIME | **COOKING TIME** 15 MINUTES | **DIFFICULTY** EASY

oil spray
1 medium whole wheat roll
1 small handful lettuce leaves
½ Lebanese cucumber, sliced
½ medium tomato, sliced

CHICKPEA PATTIES
5¼ oz tinned chickpeas,
  drained and rinsed
¼ medium carrot, grated
¼ small brown onion, chopped
½ garlic clove, crushed
¼ teaspoon ground cumin
¼ teaspoon ground coriander
¼ teaspoon cayenne pepper
pinch of ground cinnamon
¼ teaspoon ground turmeric
1 teaspoon finely diced
  preserved lemon rind
2 teaspoons chopped
  fresh cilantro
2 teaspoons quinoa flour
sea salt and ground black
  pepper, to taste

**LEMON & CILANTRO
YOGHURT**
3½ oz low-fat plain yoghurt
½ teaspoon finely diced
  preserved lemon rind
¼ teaspoon honey
2 teaspoons chopped fresh
  cilantro
sea salt and ground black
  pepper, to taste

To make the chickpea patties, place the chickpeas in a mixing bowl and coarsely mash with a potato masher. Don't mash the chickpeas completely as the mixture should be chunky. Add the carrot, onion, garlic, cumin, ground coriander, cayenne pepper, cinnamon, turmeric, preserved lemon, fresh cilantro, flour, salt, and pepper and mix until well combined.

Shape the chickpea mixture into two even patties. Place on a plate, cover with plastic wrap, and refrigerate for 30 minutes.

To make the lemon and cilantro yoghurt, whisk the yoghurt, preserved lemon, honey, and cilantro together in a small bowl. Season with salt and pepper, if desired. Cover and refrigerate until needed.

Lightly spray a non-stick fry pan with oil and heat over medium heat. Add the chickpea patties and cook for 4–5 minutes on each side or until cooked through.

To serve, cut the bread roll in half and toast lightly in a toaster or under a hot oven grill. On one half of the roll, layer the lemon and cilantro yoghurt, lettuce, chickpea patties, cucumber, and tomato. Top with the other half of the roll.

WEEK THREE
DAY
4

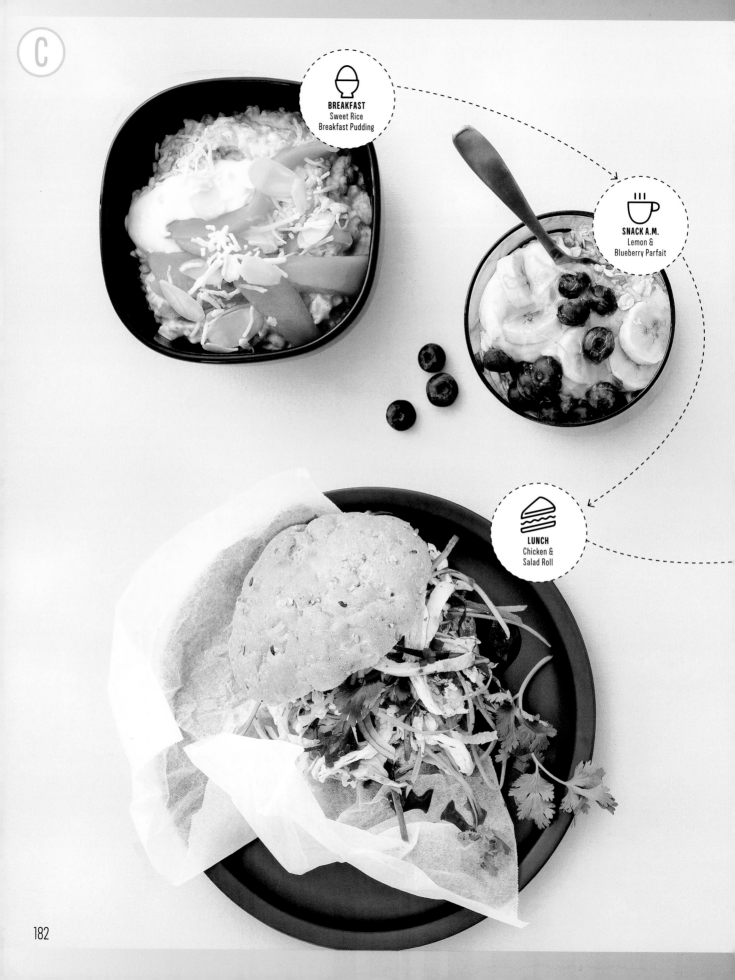

BREAKFAST
Sweet Rice
Breakfast Pudding

SNACK A.M.
Lemon &
Blueberry Parfait

LUNCH
Chicken &
Salad Roll

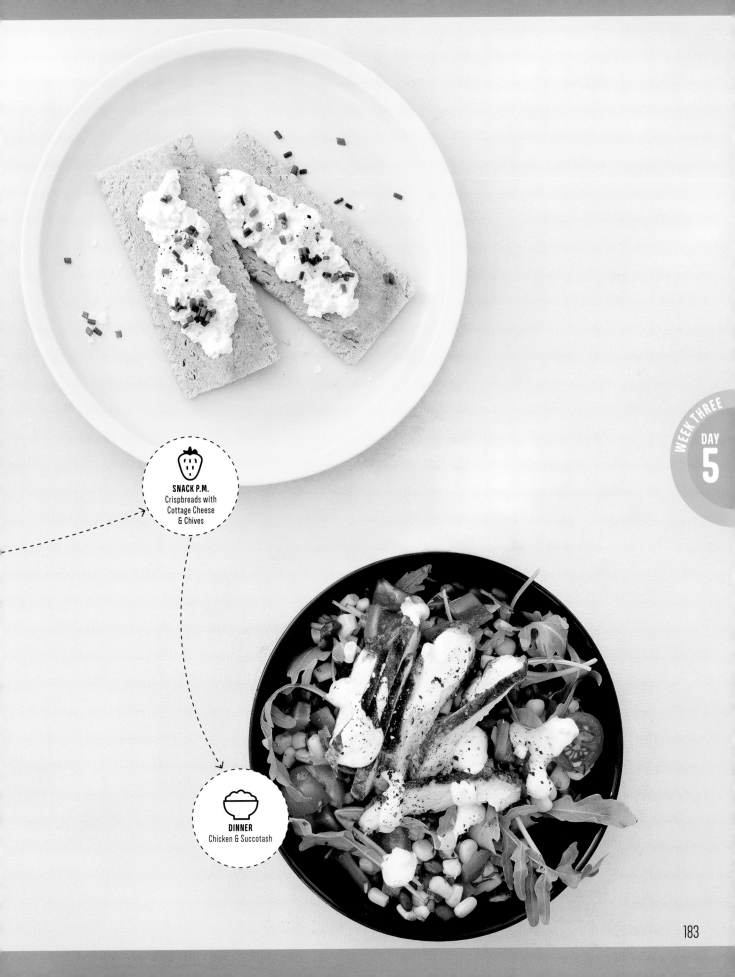

SNACK P.M.
Crispbreads with
Cottage Cheese
& Chives

DINNER
Chicken & Succotash

Sweet Rice Breakfast Pudding

SERVES 1 | **PREP TIME** 5 MINUTES, PLUS 15 MINUTES STANDING AND COOLING TIME | **COOKING TIME** 40 MINUTES | **DIFFICULTY** EASY

2 oz brown rice
¼ cup (60 ml) low-fat milk
¼ teaspoon pure vanilla extract
pinch of ground cinnamon
pinch of ground ginger
2 teaspoons honey
3½ oz low-fat plain yoghurt
½ medium mango, peeled
  and sliced
2 teaspoons flaked almonds
2 teaspoons shredded coconut

Bring the rice and 1 cup (250 ml) of water to a boil in a small saucepan over high heat, stirring occasionally. Reduce the heat to low and simmer, covered, for 20–25 minutes or until the liquid has been absorbed and the rice is tender. Remove from the heat and leave to stand, covered, for 5 minutes. Set aside to cool completely. To save time, the rice can be cooked the night before and stored in an airtight container in the refrigerator.

Place the rice, milk, vanilla, cinnamon, ginger, and honey in a small saucepan over medium heat and cook for 10–12 minutes or until thickened, stirring occasionally.

To serve, spoon the rice pudding into a serving bowl and top with the yoghurt and mango. Scatter over the flaked almonds and coconut.

Lemon & Blueberry Parfait

SERVES 1 | **PREP TIME** 10 MINUTES, PLUS 10 MINUTES CHILLING TIME | **DIFFICULTY** EASY

1 medium banana, peeled
7 oz low-fat plain yoghurt
finely grated zest and juice
  of ½ lemon, plus extra zest
  to garnish
1 teaspoon honey
1 oz natural muesli
3 oz blueberries

Mash half the banana in a medium bowl. Add the yoghurt, lemon zest, lemon juice, and half the honey and mix until well combined. Slice the remaining banana.

Layer the muesli, lemon yoghurt, banana, and blueberries in a glass.

Place in the refrigerator to chill for 10 minutes.

To serve, drizzle over the remaining honey and sprinkle over the extra lemon zest.

Chicken & Salad Roll

SERVES 1 | **PREP TIME** 10 MINUTES, PLUS 15 MINUTES COOLING TIME | **COOKING TIME** 15 MINUTES | **DIFFICULTY** EASY

2 cups (500 ml) salt-reduced
  vegetable stock
3½ oz boneless, skinless
  chicken breast
½ medium carrot, grated
½ Lebanese cucumber,
  cut into matchsticks
1 oz Chinese cabbage
  (wombok), shredded
¼ small red onion, thinly sliced
1 tablespoon chopped
  fresh cilantro
sea salt and ground black
  pepper, to taste
1 medium whole wheat roll,
  halved

DRESSING

3 teaspoons lemon juice
2 teaspoons salt-reduced
  tamari or soy sauce
1 teaspoon honey
½ garlic clove, crushed
¼ fresh red chilli, seeds
  removed, finely chopped

Heat the stock in a small saucepan over medium heat. Add the chicken and reduce the heat to medium–low. Cook for 10–12 minutes or until the chicken is cooked through. Drain off the excess liquid, then coarsely shred the chicken using two forks and set aside to cool completely. To save time, the chicken can be cooked the night before and stored in an airtight container in the refrigerator.

To make the dressing, whisk the lemon juice, tamari or soy sauce, honey, garlic, chilli, and 1 teaspoon of water together in a small bowl and set aside.

Place the chicken, carrot, cucumber, cabbage, red onion, and cilantro in a mixing bowl. Drizzle over the dressing, season with salt and pepper, if desired, and toss gently to combine.

To serve, place the bread roll on a serving plate and fill with the chicken salad.

Crispbreads with Cottage Cheese & Chives

SERVES 1 | **PREP TIME** 5 MINUTES | **DIFFICULTY** EASY

2 rye crispbreads

1 oz low-fat cottage cheese

2 teaspoons finely chopped fresh chives

sea salt and ground black pepper, to taste

Place the crispbreads on a serving plate, spread with the cottage cheese, and sprinkle over the chives. Serve seasoned with salt and pepper, if desired.

Chicken & Succotash

SERVES 1 | **PREP TIME** 15 MINUTES, PLUS 30 MINUTES CHILLING TIME | **COOKING TIME** 15 MINUTES | **DIFFICULTY** EASY

5¼ oz boneless, skinless chicken breast

2 oz tinned black beans, drained and rinsed

3 oz frozen corn kernels, thawed

¼ small red onion, finely chopped

¼ medium red bell pepper, seeds removed, chopped

3 cherry tomatoes, halved

1 small handful arugula leaves

sea salt and ground black pepper, to taste

CAJUN SPICE MIX

1 teaspoon ground cumin

1 teaspoon ground coriander

1 teaspoon sweet paprika

½ teaspoon cayenne pepper

¾ teaspoon olive oil

DRESSING

3½ oz low-fat plain yoghurt

2 teaspoons red wine vinegar

2 tablespoons chopped fresh basil

To make the Cajun spice mix, whisk the cumin, coriander, paprika, cayenne pepper, and oil together in a small bowl.

Add the chicken and rub with the spice mix. Cover with plastic wrap and refrigerate for 30 minutes.

Meanwhile, to make the dressing, whisk the yoghurt, vinegar, and half the basil together in a small bowl. If the dressing is a little thick, add 1 tablespoon of water at a time until the desired consistency is reached. Set aside.

Heat a barbecue grill-plate or chargrill pan over medium–high heat.

Add the chicken and grill for 4–6 minutes on each side or until cooked through. Set aside to cool slightly. When the chicken is cool enough to handle, cut into slices.

Place the black beans, corn, onion, bell pepper, tomatoes, and arugula in a bowl and top with the sliced chicken. Drizzle over the dressing and season with salt and pepper, if desired. Serve sprinkled with the remaining basil.

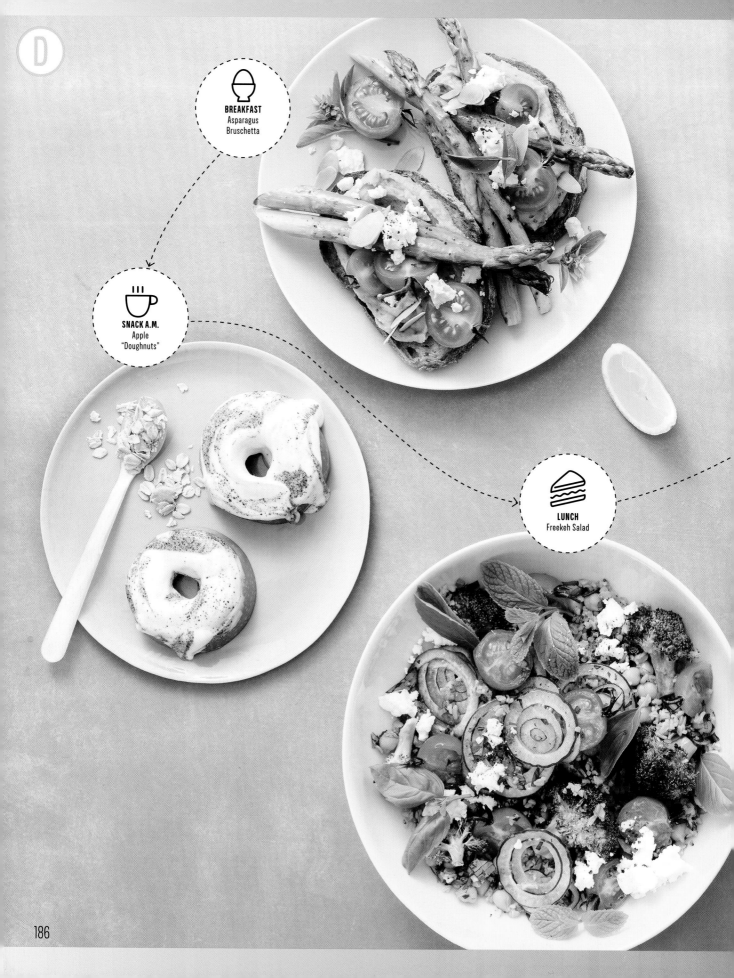

D

BREAKFAST
Asparagus
Bruschetta

SNACK A.M.
Apple
"Doughnuts"

LUNCH
Freekeh Salad

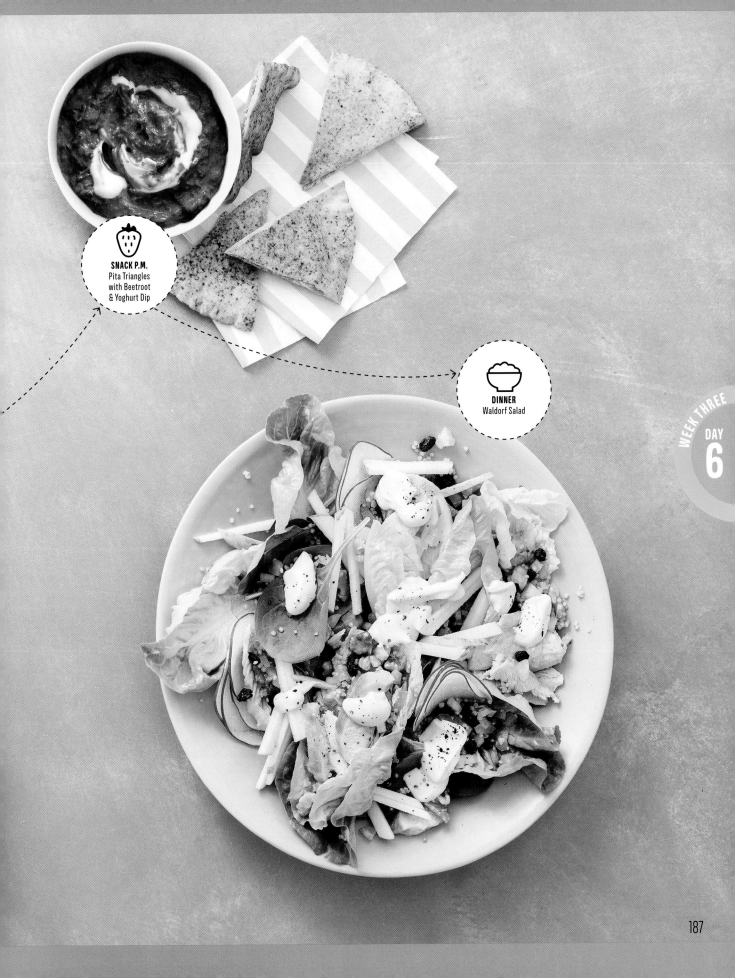

SNACK P.M.
Pita Triangles
with Beetroot
& Yoghurt Dip

DINNER
Waldorf Salad

Asparagus Bruschetta

SERVES 1 | **PREP TIME** 10 MINUTES | **COOKING TIME** 10 MINUTES | **DIFFICULTY** EASY

2 teaspoons flaked almonds

5 asparagus spears, trimmed

2 slices whole wheat bread

3 cherry tomatoes, halved

2 teaspoons chopped fresh basil

½ teaspoon lemon juice

sea salt and ground black pepper, to taste

1 oz low-fat goat's cheese, crumbled

WHITE BEAN PUREE

5¼ oz tinned cannellini beans, drained and rinsed

¼ garlic clove, crushed

lemon juice, to taste

2 teaspoons chopped fresh parsley

sea salt and ground black pepper, to taste

To make the bean puree, place the cannellini beans, garlic, lemon juice, parsley, salt, pepper, and 1 tablespoon of water in a food processor and pulse until smooth.

Heat a medium non-stick fry pan over medium heat. Add the almonds and cook for 2–3 minutes or until lightly toasted, stirring constantly. Transfer to a bowl and cool.

Heat the fry pan over medium–high heat. Add the asparagus spears and cook for 3–5 minutes or until tender. Remove from the heat and cut in half. Meanwhile, toast the bread to your liking.

Place the asparagus, tomatoes, and basil in a mixing bowl. Drizzle over the lemon juice and toss gently to combine. Season with salt and pepper, if desired.

To serve, spread the white bean puree on the toast, top with the asparagus mixture, and sprinkle over the goat's cheese and toasted almonds.

Apple "Doughnuts"

SERVES 1 | **PREP TIME** 10 MINUTES | **DIFFICULTY** EASY

3½ oz low-fat plain yoghurt

½ teaspoon acai berry powder

½ teaspoon honey

1 medium green apple, cored and halved

1 oz natural muesli

Place the yoghurt, acai berry powder, and honey in a small bowl and swirl together. To serve, spread the yoghurt mix over the apple halves and garnish with the muesli.

Freekeh Salad

SERVES 1 | **PREP TIME** 10 MINUTES | **COOKING TIME** 25 MINUTES | **DIFFICULTY** EASY

1½ oz cracked freekeh

2½ oz broccoli, cut into florets

oil spray

5 cherry tomatoes, halved

½ teaspoon balsamic vinegar

1 teaspoon finely grated lemon zest

1 teaspoon lemon juice

¼ small red onion, thinly sliced

2¾ oz tinned chickpeas, drained and rinsed

1 tablespoon each chopped mint, basil, and parsley

sea salt and ground black pepper, to taste

1 oz low-fat goat's cheese

Bring the freekeh and 1 cup (250 ml) of water to a boil in a small saucepan over high heat, stirring occasionally. Reduce the heat to low and simmer, covered, for 20–25 minutes or until the freekeh is tender. Remove from the heat and drain. Refresh under cold running water and drain well.

Meanwhile, preheat the oven to 400°F (350°F convection) and line a baking sheet with baking paper. Spread the broccoli over the lined baking sheet and spray lightly with oil. Bake in the oven for 5 minutes. Add the tomatoes and cook for a further 8–10 minutes or until the broccoli is tender and the tomatoes have softened. Remove from the oven and set aside.

Whisk the vinegar, lemon zest, lemon juice, and 2 teaspoons of water together in a small bowl. Place the freekeh, broccoli, tomatoes, onion, chickpeas, mint, basil, and parsley in a mixing bowl. Drizzle over the dressing, season with salt and pepper, if desired, and toss gently to combine.

To serve, place the freekeh salad in a serving bowl and crumble over the goat's cheese.

Pita Triangles with Beetroot & Yoghurt Dip

SERVES 1 | **PREP TIME** 5 MINUTES | **COOKING TIME** 15 MINUTES | **DIFFICULTY** EASY

½ whole wheat pita bread, cut into wedges

oil spray

BEETROOT & YOGHURT DIP

½ small beetroot, peeled and grated

pinch of ground cumin

pinch of ground coriander

lemon juice, to taste

3½ oz low-fat plain yoghurt

sea salt and ground black pepper, to taste

Preheat the oven to 400°F (350°F convection) and line a baking sheet with baking paper.

Lay the pita wedges in a single layer on the lined baking sheet and spray lightly with oil spray. Bake in the oven for 5 minutes or until they began to colour. Turn the wedges over and bake for a further 5–8 minutes or until both sides are lightly coloured, then set aside to cool.

Meanwhile, to make the beetroot and yoghurt dip, place the beetroot, cumin, coriander, lemon juice, yoghurt, salt, and pepper in a small bowl and mix until well combined.

Serve the pita triangles with beetroot and yoghurt dip.

Waldorf Salad

DINNER **SERVES** 1 | **PREP TIME** 15 MINUTES, PLUS 10 MINUTES COOLING TIME | **COOKING TIME** 15 MINUTES | **DIFFICULTY** EASY

1 oz quinoa

oil spray

3½ oz boneless, skinless chicken breast or 3½ oz tinned tuna in springwater, drained

⅓ oz walnut halves

½ medium apple, cored, cut into matchsticks

⅔ oz dried currants

1 celery stalk, finely chopped

1 medium radish, thinly sliced

1 large handful lettuce leaves

1 small handful baby spinach leaves

sea salt and ground black pepper, to taste

DRESSING

3½ oz low-fat plain yoghurt

½ teaspoon Dijon mustard

juice of ¼ lemon

Bring the quinoa and ½ cup (125 ml) of water to a boil in a small saucepan over high heat, stirring occasionally. Reduce the heat to low and simmer, covered, for 10–12 minutes or until the quinoa is tender. Drain off any excess liquid and set aside to cool.

Meanwhile, if using chicken, lightly spray a non-stick fry pan with oil and heat over medium heat. Add the chicken and cook for 3–4 minutes on each side or until cooked through. Set aside to cool.

To save time, the quinoa and chicken can be cooked the night before and stored in an airtight container in the refrigerator.

Heat a small non-stick fry pan over medium heat. Add the walnuts and toast for 1–2 minutes or until lightly browned and fragrant, stirring constantly. Set aside to cool. When cool enough to handle, roughly chop the nuts into small pieces.

To make the dressing, whisk the yoghurt, mustard, and lemon juice together in a small bowl.

Place the quinoa, chicken (or tuna, if using), apple, currants, celery, radish, lettuce, spinach, and walnuts on a serving plate. To serve, drizzle over the dressing and season with salt and pepper, if desired.

WEEK THREE DAY 6

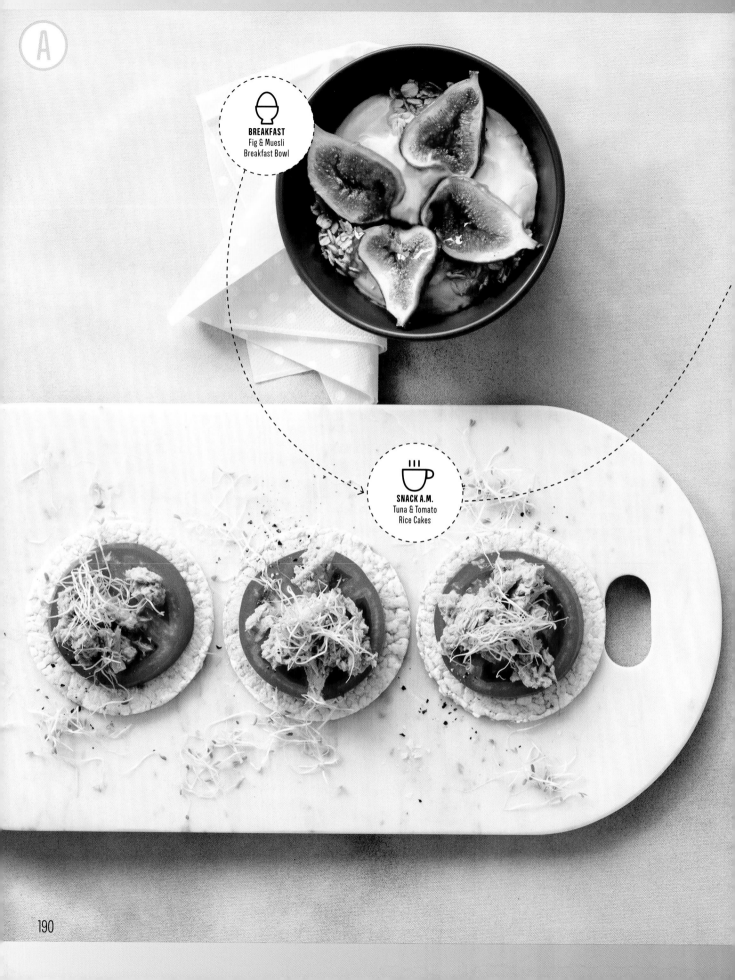

A

BREAKFAST
Fig & Muesli
Breakfast Bowl

SNACK A.M.
Tuna & Tomato
Rice Cakes

190

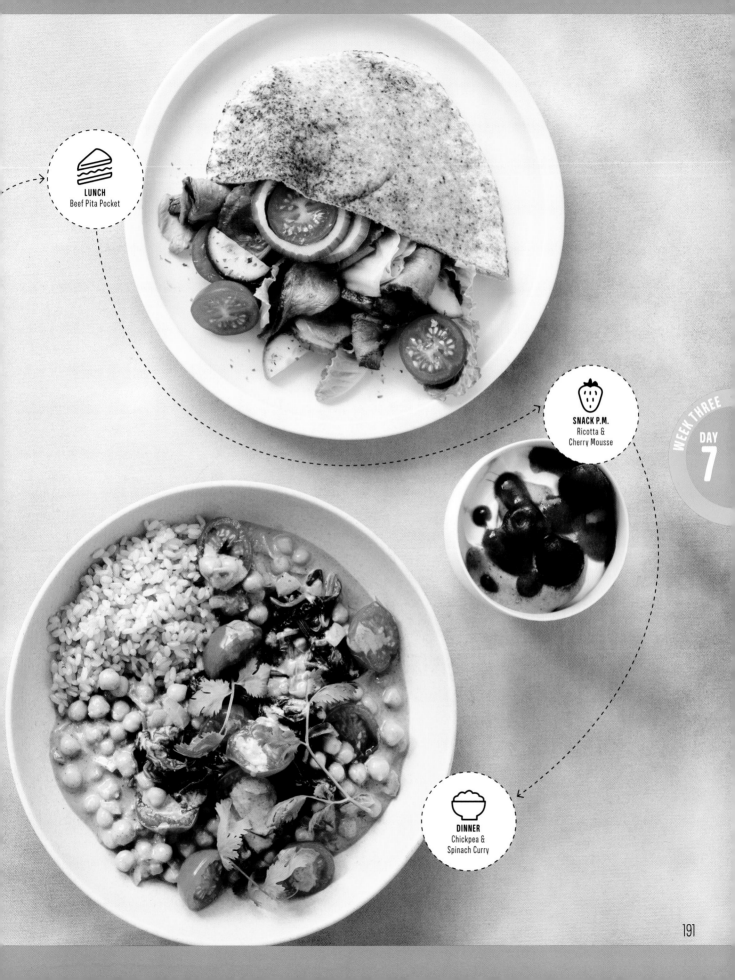

LUNCH
Beef Pita Pocket

SNACK P.M.
Ricotta &
Cherry Mousse

WEEK THREE

DAY
7

DINNER
Chickpea &
Spinach Curry

191

Fig & Muesli Breakfast Bowl

SERVES 1 | **PREP TIME** 5 MINUTES, PLUS 10 MINUTES COOLING TIME | **COOKING TIME** 15 MINUTES | **DIFFICULTY** EASY

1 tablespoon 100% orange juice

pinch of ground nutmeg

1 teaspoon honey, plus extra
  to serve

¼ teaspoon pure vanilla extract

2 medium figs, halved

2 oz natural muesli

7 oz low-fat plain yoghurt

Preheat the oven to 400°F (350°F convection) and line a baking sheet with baking paper.

Whisk the orange juice, nutmeg, honey, and vanilla together in a small bowl.

Place the fig halves on the lined baking sheet, cut side up, and spoon over the orange juice mixture. Roast the figs in the oven for 12–15 minutes or until tender and sticky. Remove from the oven and set aside to cool.

To serve, place the muesli in a serving bowl. Top with the yoghurt and roasted figs, and drizzle over some extra honey.

Tuna & Tomato Rice Cakes

SERVES 1 | **PREP TIME** 5 MINUTES | **DIFFICULTY** EASY

3 rice cakes

½ medium tomato, sliced

1¾ oz tinned tuna in
  springwater, drained

sea salt and ground black
  pepper, to taste

1 small handful alfalfa sprouts

To serve, place the rice cakes on a serving plate and top with the tomato and tuna. Season with salt and pepper, if desired, and top with alfalfa sprouts.

Beef Pita Pocket

SERVES 1 | **PREP TIME** 10 MINUTES, PLUS 10 MINUTES MARINATING TIME | **COOKING TIME** 10 MINUTES | **DIFFICULTY** EASY

¼ teaspoon dried oregano

1 teaspoon Dijon mustard, plus
  extra to serve (optional)

sea salt and ground black
  pepper, to taste

lemon juice, to taste

3½ oz lean beef steak

oil spray

5 cherry tomatoes, halved

½ Lebanese cucumber,
  halved and sliced

½ small red onion, thinly sliced

1 small handful lettuce leaves

½ whole wheat pita bread

Whisk the oregano, mustard, salt, pepper, and lemon juice together in a medium bowl. Place the steak in the bowl and rub with the marinade until well coated. Leave to marinate for 10 minutes, turning once during that time.

Lightly spray a chargrill pan with oil and heat over high heat. Grill the steak for 4–5 minutes on each side for medium or continue until cooked to your liking. Transfer to a heatproof plate and set aside to rest for 2 minutes. Slice the steak thinly against the grain.

Place the tomatoes, cucumber, red onion, and lettuce in a mixing bowl and toss gently to combine.

To serve, spread some additional mustard (if using) on the inside of the pita pocket. Fill the pita pocket with the sliced beef and salad.

Ricotta & Cherry Mousse

SERVES 1 | **PREP TIME** 5 MINUTES, PLUS 1 HOUR STANDING AND CHILLING TIME | **DIFFICULTY** EASY

20 cherries, pitted

finely grated zest and juice
of ½ lemon

2 teaspoons honey

3½ oz low-fat ricotta cheese

3½ oz low-fat plain yoghurt

¼ teaspoon pure vanilla extract

Place the cherries, lemon zest, lemon juice, and honey in a small bowl and stir to combine. Set aside for 30 minutes at room temperature. This will cause the cherries to soften a little and become syrupy.

Place the ricotta, yoghurt, vanilla extract, and half the cherries in a high-powered blender and blend until smooth. Pour the mixture into a glass, cover with plastic wrap, and refrigerate for 30 minutes to chill.

To serve, top the ricotta and cherry mousse with the remaining cherries. Drizzle over the remaining syrup.

Chickpea & Spinach Curry

SERVES 1 | **PREP TIME** 10 MINUTES | **COOKING TIME** 25 MINUTES | **DIFFICULTY** EASY

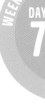

WEEK THREE
DAY
7

2 oz brown rice

oil spray

¼ small brown onion, chopped

½ teaspoon grated fresh ginger

½ garlic clove, crushed

¼ teaspoon ground coriander

½ teaspoon ground cumin

1 teaspoon ground turmeric

½ teaspoon curry powder

pinch of dried chilli flakes

½ teaspoon garam masala

½ cup (120 ml) light coconut milk

5½ oz tinned chickpeas,
drained and rinsed

8 cherry tomatoes, halved

1 large handful baby
spinach leaves

1 tablespoon fresh
cilantro leaves

Bring the rice and 1 cup (250 ml) of water to a boil in a small saucepan over high heat, stirring occasionally. Reduce the heat to low and simmer, covered, for 20–25 minutes or until the liquid has been absorbed and the rice is tender. Remove from the heat and leave to stand, covered, for 5 minutes.

Meanwhile, spray a medium saucepan with oil and heat over medium heat. Add the onion, ginger, and garlic and cook for 5 minutes or until the onion is soft and translucent, stirring occasionally. Add the ground coriander, cumin, turmeric, curry powder, chilli flakes, and garam masala and cook for a further 1–2 minutes or until fragrant, stirring constantly.

Stir in the coconut milk and chickpeas and bring to the boil over medium–high heat. Reduce the heat to low and simmer for 10 minutes, stirring occasionally. Add the tomatoes and spinach and cook for 3–5 minutes or until the tomatoes are warmed through and the spinach has wilted, stirring occasionally.

To serve, place the rice in a serving bowl and top with the chickpea and spinach curry. Sprinkle over the cilantro.

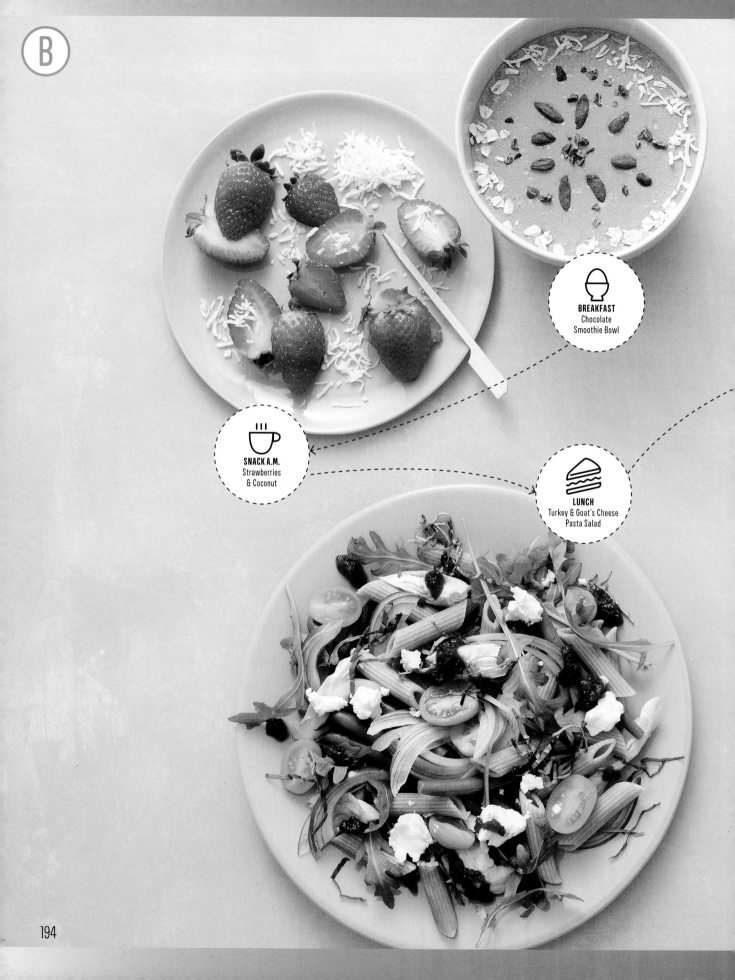

B

BREAKFAST
Chocolate
Smoothie Bowl

SNACK A.M.
Strawberries
& Coconut

LUNCH
Turkey & Goat's Cheese
Pasta Salad

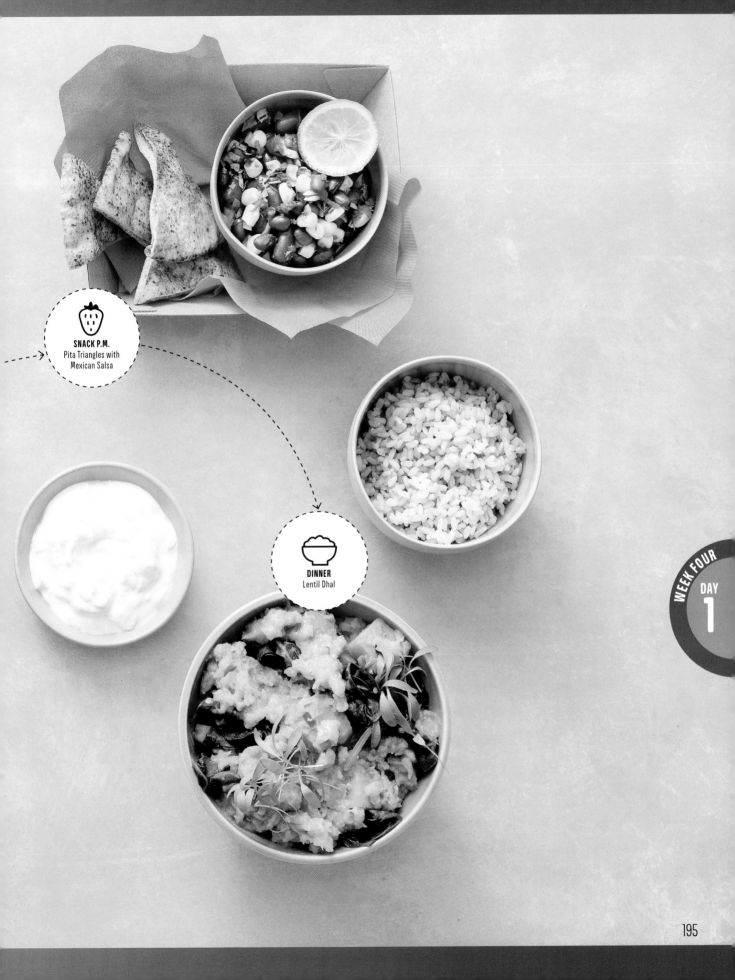

DINNER
Lentil Dhal

WEEK FOUR

DAY

1

195

Chocolate Smoothie Bowl

BREAKFAST **SERVES** 1 | **PREP TIME** 10 MINUTES, PLUS 30 MINUTES SOAKING TIME | **DIFFICULTY** EASY

1½ medjool dates, pitted

1 small handful kale, roughly chopped

½ medium banana, peeled

1 tablespoon raw cacao powder or 1½ tablespoons carob powder

¾ cup (190 ml) low-fat milk

5¼ oz low-fat plain yoghurt

TOPPINGS

1 oz natural muesli

1 tablespoon goji berries

2 teaspoons raw cacao nibs

1 tablespoon shredded coconut

Place the dates in a heatproof bowl, cover with boiling water, and leave to soak for 30 minutes to soften. Drain.

Place the dates, kale, banana, cacao or carob powder, milk, and yoghurt in a high-powered blender and blend until smooth.

To serve, pour the smoothie mixture into a serving bowl and top with the muesli, goji berries, cacao nibs, and shredded coconut.

Strawberries & Coconut

SNACK A.M. **SERVES** 1 | **PREP TIME** 5 MINUTES | **DIFFICULTY** EASY

4½ oz strawberries, halved or hulled and sliced

1 tablespoon shredded coconut

To serve, place the strawberries on a serving plate and sprinkle over the coconut.

Turkey & Goat's Cheese Pasta Salad

LUNCH **SERVES** 1 | **PREP TIME** 10 MINUTES | **COOKING TIME** 15 MINUTES | **DIFFICULTY** EASY

3 oz whole wheat pasta

oil spray

5 cherry tomatoes, halved

8 green beans, ends trimmed

¼ small red onion, thinly sliced

1 small handful arugula leaves

3¼ oz roast turkey, shredded

1 oz low-fat goat's cheese, crumbled

2 teaspoons shredded fresh basil

DRESSING

1 teaspoon cranberry sauce

1 teaspoon balsamic vinegar

½ teaspoon finely grated lemon zest

Fill a large saucepan with water, add a pinch of salt, and bring to a boil. Add the pasta and cook until al dente (see the pasta packet for the recommended cooking time). To save time, the pasta can be cooked the night before, drained and rinsed, then stored in an airtight container in the refrigerator.

Meanwhile, lightly spray a non-stick fry pan with oil and heat over medium–high heat. Add the tomatoes and cook for 1–3 minutes or until they start to soften and the skin begins to wrinkle, stirring frequently. Remove from the heat and set aside to cool.

Fill a medium saucepan with water and bring to a boil. Add the beans and blanch for 1 minute or until bright green and tender-crisp. Drain and refresh under cold running water. Drain and set aside.

To make the dressing, whisk the cranberry sauce, vinegar, lemon zest, and 2 teaspoons of water together in a small bowl and set aside.

Place the pasta, tomatoes, beans, onion, arugula, turkey, goat's cheese, and basil on a serving plate. Drizzle over the dressing and serve.

Pita Triangles with Mexican Salsa

SERVES 1 | **PREP TIME** 10 MINUTES | **COOKING TIME** 15 MINUTES | **DIFFICULTY** EASY

½ whole wheat pita bread, cut into wedges

oil spray

1½ oz tinned black beans, drained and rinsed

1½ oz tinned red kidney beans, drained and rinsed

½ medium tomato, diced

1 oz frozen corn kernels, thawed

2 teaspoons chopped fresh cilantro

2 teaspoons finely diced red onion

½ teaspoon chopped fresh red chilli (optional)

lime juice, to taste

sea salt and ground black pepper, to taste

Preheat the oven to 400°F (350°F convection) and line a baking sheet with baking paper.

Lay the pita wedges in a single layer on the lined baking sheet and spray lightly with oil spray. Bake in the oven for 5 minutes or until they begin to colour. Turn the wedges over and bake for a further 5–8 minutes or until both sides are lightly coloured, then set aside to cool.

Place the black beans, kidney beans, tomato, corn, cilantro, onion and chilli (if using), in a small serving bowl. Season with lime juice, salt, and pepper, if desired, and stir the salsa until well combined.

Serve the pita triangles with the salsa.

Lentil Dhal

SERVES 1 | **PREP TIME** 15 MINUTES | **COOKING TIME** 25 MINUTES | **DIFFICULTY** EASY

2 oz brown rice

oil spray

¼ small brown onion, finely chopped

½ garlic clove, crushed

½ teaspoon grated fresh ginger

¼ fresh red chilli, finely chopped

¼ teaspoon ground turmeric

¼ teaspoon ground cumin

½ medium sweet potato, cut into ¾ inch cubes

2 oz dried red lentils

⅔ cup (150 ml) salt-reduced vegetable stock

sea salt and ground black pepper, to taste

1 small handful baby spinach leaves

½ scallion, sliced

fresh micro cilantro leaves or regular cilantro, to garnish

CUCUMBER YOGHURT

¼ Lebanese cucumber

3½ oz low-fat plain yoghurt

lemon juice, to taste

½ garlic clove, crushed

sea salt and ground black pepper, to taste

Bring the rice and about 1 cup (200 ml) of water to a boil in a small saucepan over high heat, stirring occasionally. Reduce the heat to low and simmer, covered, for 20–25 minutes or until the liquid has been absorbed and the rice is tender. Remove from the heat and leave to stand, covered, for 5 minutes.

Meanwhile, lightly spray a medium saucepan with oil and heat over medium heat. Add the onion and cook for 5 minutes or until soft and translucent, stirring occasionally. Add the garlic, ginger, chilli, turmeric, and cumin and cook for 1 minute or until fragrant, stirring constantly.

Add the sweet potato and stir to coat with the spice mixture. Add the lentils and stock and bring to a boil. Reduce the heat to medium–low and cook, covered, for 20 minutes or until the lentils are tender and the sweet potato is cooked through. Season with salt and pepper, if desired. Just before serving, stir through the spinach and cook for 1–2 minutes or until wilted.

To make the cucumber yoghurt, peel the cucumber, cut in half horizontally and remove the seeds by scraping a spoon down the middle. Grate the flesh and squeeze out any excess water. Place the yoghurt, cucumber, lemon juice, garlic, salt, and pepper in a small bowl and mix until well combined. To save time, the cucumber yoghurt can be prepared the night before and stored in an airtight container in the refrigerator.

Stir the sliced scallion through the dhal, then place in a serving bowl, with the rice and cucumber yoghurt in separate bowls alongside. Sprinkle with cilantro and serve.

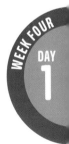

WEEK FOUR
DAY 1

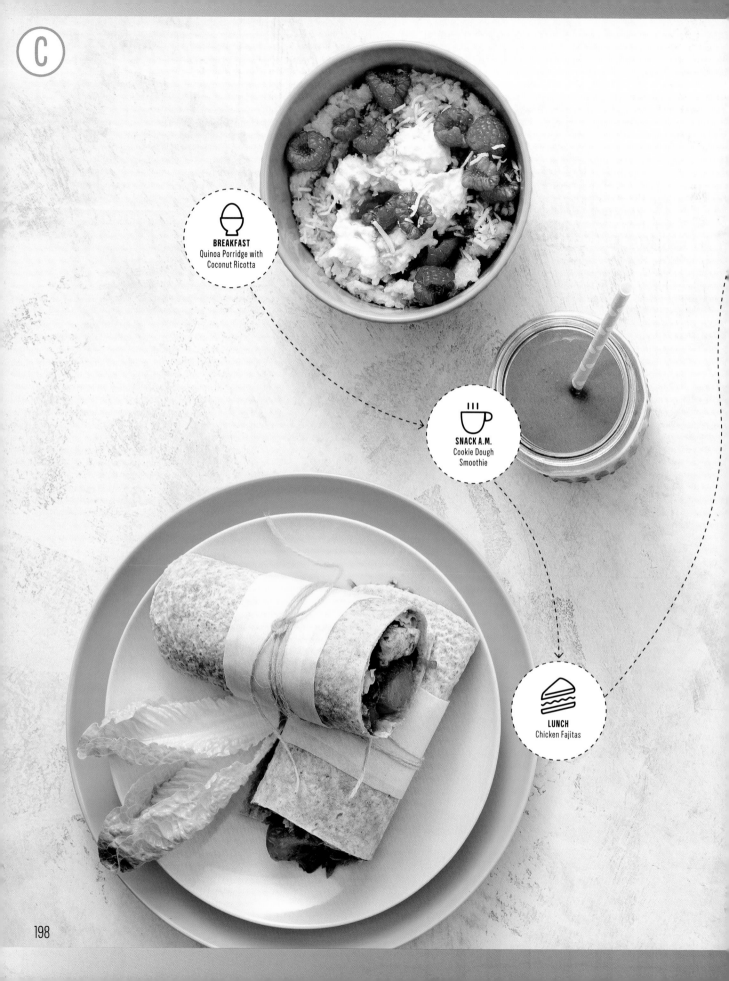

C

BREAKFAST
Quinoa Porridge with
Coconut Ricotta

SNACK A.M.
Cookie Dough
Smoothie

LUNCH
Chicken Fajitas

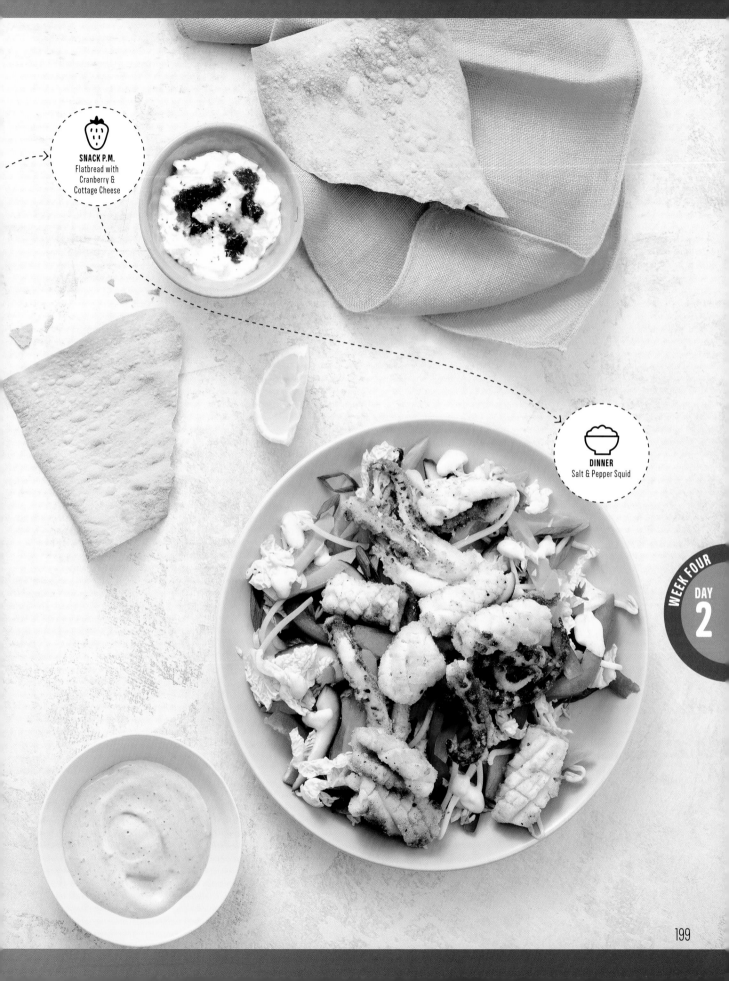

SNACK P.M.
Flatbread with
Cranberry &
Cottage Cheese

DINNER
Salt & Pepper Squid

WEEK FOUR

DAY
2

199

Quinoa Porridge with Coconut Ricotta

BREAKFAST **SERVES** 1 | **PREP TIME** 5 MINUTES, PLUS 30 MINUTES CHILLING TIME | **COOKING TIME** 10 MINUTES | **DIFFICULTY** EASY

¼ cup (60 ml) low-fat milk
¼ teaspoon pure vanilla extract
2 oz quinoa flakes
3 oz raspberries
2 teaspoons shredded coconut

COCONUT RICOTTA
1¾ oz low-fat ricotta cheese
1½ tablespoons light coconut milk
1 teaspoon pure maple syrup
2 teaspoons shredded coconut

To make the coconut ricotta, place the ricotta, coconut milk, maple syrup, and shredded coconut in a small bowl and mix until well combined. Cover with plastic wrap and chill in the refrigerator for 30 minutes or overnight.

Meanwhile, in a small saucepan, bring the milk, vanilla, and ½ cup (125 ml) of water to a boil over high heat. Add the quinoa and reduce the heat to low. Simmer for 5 minutes or until thickened, stirring occasionally.

To serve, spoon the quinoa porridge into a bowl. Top with the coconut ricotta, raspberries, and shredded coconut.

Cookie Dough Smoothie

SNACK A.M. **SERVES** 1 | **PREP TIME** 5 MINUTES, PLUS 30 MINUTES SOAKING TIME | **DIFFICULTY** EASY

3 medjool dates, pitted
½ medium banana, peeled
¾ cup (190 ml) low-fat milk
1¾ oz low-fat plain yoghurt
1 oz rolled oats
¼ teaspoon 100% natural peanut butter

½ teaspoon raw cacao powder
1 scoop (1 oz) chocolate-flavoured protein powder (optional)

Place the dates in a heatproof bowl, cover with boiling water and leave to soak for 30 minutes to soften. Drain.

Place the dates, banana, milk, yoghurt, oats, peanut butter, cacao and protein powder (if using), in a high-powered blender and blend until smooth.

To serve, pour into a glass or jar.

Chicken Fajitas

LUNCH **SERVES** 1 | **PREP TIME** 10 MINUTES, PLUS 30 MINUTES MARINATING TIME | **COOKING TIME** 10 MINUTES | **DIFFICULTY** EASY

½ teaspoon smoked paprika
pinch of ground cumin
pinch each of dried chilli flakes and dried oregano
sea salt and ground black pepper, to taste
lemon juice, to taste
3½ oz boneless, skinless chicken breast, thinly sliced
oil spray
¼ small red onion, thinly sliced
½ garlic clove, crushed
¼ medium red bell pepper, seeds removed, sliced
5 cherry tomatoes, halved
1 teaspoon finely chopped fresh cilantro, plus extra to garnish
1 whole wheat wrap
1 small handful romaine lettuce leaves

Place the paprika, cumin, chilli flakes, oregano, salt, and lemon juice in a small bowl and mix until well combined. Add the chicken and toss to coat, ensuring that all the chicken is evenly coated in the spice mix. Cover with plastic wrap and refrigerate for 30 minutes to marinate.

Lightly spray a non-stick fry pan with oil and heat over medium–high heat. Add the chicken and cook for 3–4 minutes or until browned and cooked through. Transfer to a bowl and set aside.

Remove the pan from the heat, re-spray with oil then return to a medium heat. Add the onion and cook for 2–3 minutes or until it starts to soften, stirring occasionally. Add the garlic and cook for 1 minute or until fragrant, stirring frequently. Increase the heat to medium–high, add the bell pepper and tomatoes and cook for 2–3 minutes or until softened, stirring occasionally. Stir in the chicken and cilantro and season with salt and pepper, if desired. Remove from the heat.

Warm the wrap in a large dry fry pan over medium–high heat for 30 seconds on each side.

Place the warmed wrap on a serving plate. Place the lettuce, chicken fajita mixture, and extra cilantro on the wrap, roll up, and secure. Cut in half and serve.

Flatbread with Cranberry & Cottage Cheese

SERVES 1 | **PREP TIME** 5 MINUTES | **COOKING TIME** 10 MINUTES | **DIFFICULTY** EASY

½ whole wheat lavash
oil spray
1 oz low-fat cottage cheese
½ teaspoon cranberry sauce
sea salt and ground black
    pepper, to taste

Preheat the oven to 350°F (325°F convection) and line a baking sheet with baking paper.

Place the lavash on the lined baking sheet and spray lightly with oil. Bake in the oven for 8–10 minutes or until golden and crispy.

Place the cottage cheese and cranberry sauce in a small bowl. Season with salt and pepper, if desired, and serve with the toasted lavash.

Salt & Pepper Squid

SERVES 1 | **PREP TIME** 20 MINUTES | **COOKING TIME** 5 MINUTES | **DIFFICULTY** EASY

8½ oz squid tube, cleaned
1 tablespoon brown rice flour
¾ teaspoon sea salt
¾ teaspoon ground black
    pepper
¼ teaspoon sweet paprika
oil spray
3½ oz Chinese cabbage
    (wombok), shredded
1 small handful bean sprouts
½ Lebanese cucumber, thinly
    sliced on an angle
½ medium carrot, thinly sliced
    on an angle
¼ medium red bell pepper,
    seeds removed, thinly sliced
    on an angle
1 scallion, thinly sliced
    on an angle
lemon wedges, to serve

**AVOCADO
YOGHURT DRESSING**
⅓ oz avocado
1 tablespoon roughly chopped
    fresh cilantro
3½ oz low-fat plain yoghurt
½ garlic clove, crushed
2 teaspoons finely grated
    lime zest
sea salt and ground black
    pepper, to taste

To make the avocado yoghurt dressing, place the avocado, cilantro, yoghurt, garlic, lime zest, salt, pepper, and 1 tablespoon of water in a high-powered blender and blend until smooth. If the dressing is a little too thick, add 2 teaspoons of water at a time until the desired consistency is reached.

Cut the squid tube in half lengthways and open out flat. Score the inside of the squid in a criss-cross pattern with a sharp knife and cut into 2 inch pieces. Dry the squid pieces with a paper towel.

Place the flour, salt, pepper, and paprika in a large bowl and mix until well combined. Add the squid pieces and toss gently to coat.

Lightly spray the squid pieces with oil and heat a large non-stick fry pan over high heat. Add half the squid and cook for 1–2 minutes or until just cooked through. Transfer to a plate and repeat with the remaining squid.

Place the cabbage, bean sprouts, cucumber, carrot, bell pepper, scallion, and salt and pepper squid on a serving plate. Serve with the dressing on the side and lemon wedges.

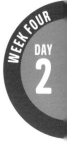

WEEK FOUR
DAY
2

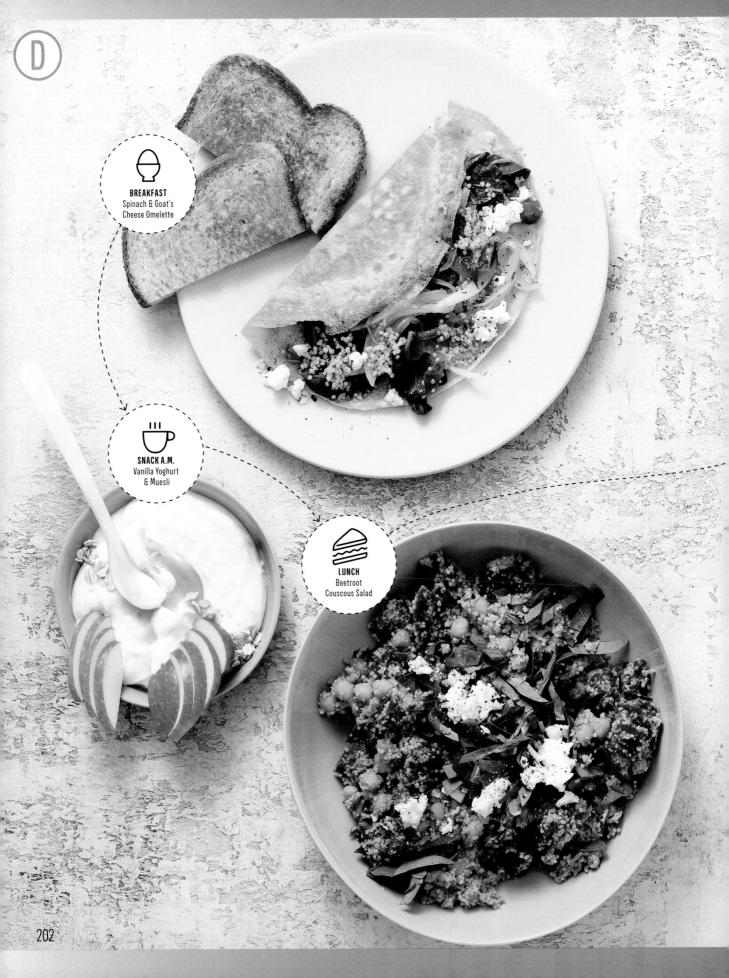

D

BREAKFAST
Spinach & Goat's
Cheese Omelette

SNACK A.M.
Vanilla Yoghurt
& Muesli

LUNCH
Beetroot
Couscous Salad

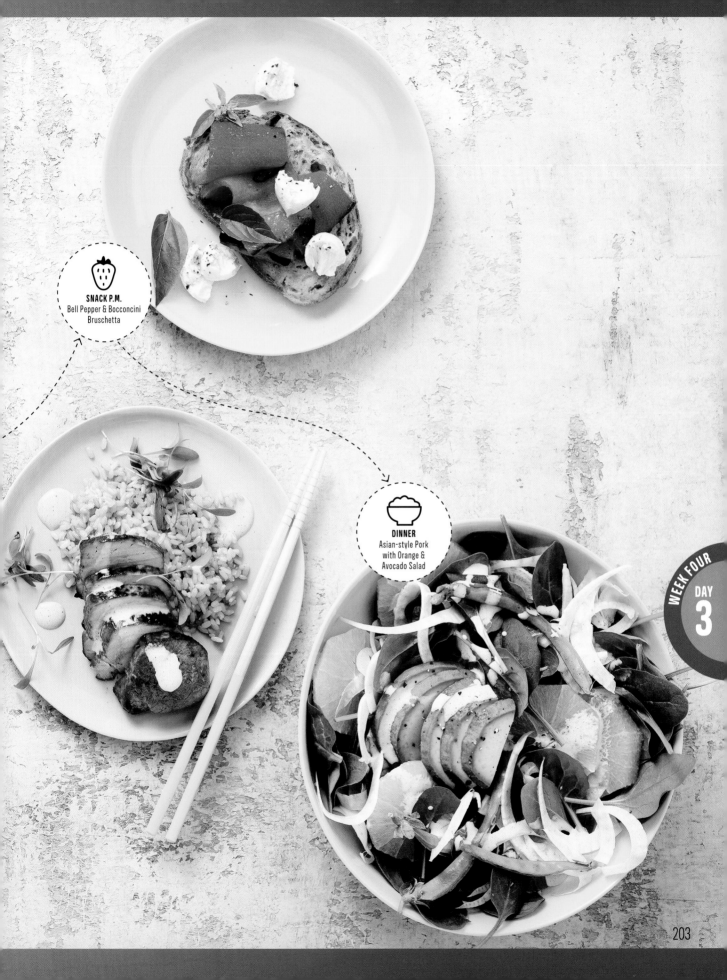

SNACK P.M.
Bell Pepper & Bocconcini
Bruschetta

DINNER
Asian-style Pork
with Orange &
Avocado Salad

WEEK FOUR

DAY 3

Spinach & Goat's Cheese Omelette

SERVES 1 | **PREP TIME** 10 MINUTES | **COOKING TIME** 15 MINUTES | **DIFFICULTY** EASY

1 oz quinoa

1½ teaspoons olive oil

¼ small brown onion, thinly sliced

½ garlic clove, crushed

3 semi-dried tomatoes, thinly sliced

1 small handful baby spinach leaves

sea salt and ground black pepper, to taste

2 large eggs

1 oz low-fat goat's cheese, crumbled

1 slice whole wheat bread, toasted

Bring the quinoa and ½ cup (125 ml) of water to a boil in a small saucepan over high heat, stirring occasionally. Reduce the heat to low and simmer, covered, for 10–12 minutes or until the quinoa is tender. Drain off any excess liquid.

Meanwhile, heat half the oil in a non-stick fry pan over medium–high heat. Add the onion and cook for 3–4 minutes or until soft, stirring frequently. Add the garlic and semi-dried tomato and cook for 1 minute or until fragrant, stirring frequently. Add the spinach and cook for a further 1–2 minutes or until wilted. Season with salt and pepper, if desired. Transfer the mixture to a bowl.

Whisk the eggs, salt, and pepper together in a small bowl. Wipe the fry pan clean and heat the remaining oil over medium heat. Pour in the egg mixture and swirl to cover the base of the pan. Cook for 1–2 minutes or until the egg starts to set and the underside is golden in colour. Reduce the heat to medium–low.

Sprinkle the quinoa, tomato, and spinach mixture and the goat's cheese over half the omelette. Cook for 1 minute or until the egg is set. Fold in half to cover the filling and, using a spatula, transfer to a serving plate and serve with the toast.

Vanilla Yoghurt & Muesli

SERVES 1 | **PREP TIME** 5 MINUTES | **DIFFICULTY** EASY

3½ oz low-fat plain yoghurt

¼ teaspoon pure vanilla extract

½ teaspoon honey

1 oz natural muesli

1 medium red apple, cored and sliced or 1 medium banana, peeled and sliced

Place the yoghurt and vanilla in a small bowl and mix until well combined.

To serve, top with the honey, muesli, and apple or banana.

Beetroot Couscous Salad

SERVES 1 | **PREP TIME** 10 MINUTES, PLUS 10 MINUTES COOLING TIME | **COOKING TIME** 40 MINUTES | **DIFFICULTY** EASY

1 small beetroot

¼ teaspoon olive oil

1⅓ oz couscous

2¾ oz tinned chickpeas, drained and rinsed

sea salt and ground black pepper, to taste

1 oz low-fat goat's cheese

1 small handful baby spinach leaves, shredded

DRESSING

1 teaspoon lemon juice

½ teaspoon finely grated lemon zest

2 teaspoons chopped fresh parsley

Preheat the oven to 350°F (325°F convection). Wrap the beetroot in foil with 1 tablespoon of water, place into a small roasting pan, and bake for 30–40 minutes or until tender. Test the beetroot with a skewer—it is cooked if the skewer pierces the flesh easily. Set aside to cool, reserving the roasting juices. Peel under cold running water, then cut into ½ inch cubes.

Meanwhile, in a small saucepan, bring the olive oil and ½ cup (125 ml) of water to the boil. Add the couscous and remove the pan from the heat. Leave to stand, covered, for 2–3 minutes before fluffing with a fork to help separate the grains.

To make the dressing, whisk the lemon juice, lemon zest, parsley, and 2 teaspoons of water together in a small bowl and set aside.

Place the couscous, beetroot, reserved beetroot juice, and chickpeas in a mixing bowl. Drizzle over the dressing and toss gently to combine. Season with salt and pepper, if desired. To serve, place the beetroot couscous salad in a serving bowl, crumble the goat's cheese and sprinkle over, then top with the shredded spinach.

Bell Pepper & Bocconcini Bruschetta

SERVES 1 | **PREP TIME** 5 MINUTES, PLUS 5 MINUTES RESTING TIME | **COOKING TIME** 10 MINUTES | **DIFFICULTY** EASY

¼ medium red bell pepper, seeds removed

⅔ oz baby bocconcini, torn

fresh basil leaves

lemon juice, to taste

sea salt and ground black pepper, to taste

1 slice whole wheat bread

oil spray

½ garlic clove

Heat a small non-stick fry pan over high heat. Place the bell pepper, skin side down, in the hot pan. Cook for 5–7 minutes or until the skin starts to blister and turn brown.

Transfer to a bowl and cover with plastic wrap. Leave to sweat for 5 minutes, then peel off the skin and cut into ¾ inch pieces.

Place the bell pepper, bocconcini, basil, lemon juice, salt, and pepper in a small bowl and toss gently to combine.

Toast the bread to your liking. Lightly spray the toast with oil and rub with the cut side of the garlic.

To serve, place the toast on a serving plate and top with the bell pepper and bocconcini mixture. Season with pepper, if desired.

Asian-style Pork with Orange & Avocado Salad

SERVES 1 | **PREP TIME** 15 MINUTES, PLUS 4 HOURS MARINATING TIME | **COOKING TIME** 25 MINUTES | **DIFFICULTY** EASY

3 oz pork tenderloin

1 oz brown rice

1 medium orange, peeled and sliced

¾ oz avocado

1 large handful baby spinach leaves

½ small fennel bulb, thinly sliced

1½ oz snow peas, trimmed and thinly sliced on an angle

micro herbs, to garnish (optional)

ASIAN-STYLE MARINADE

1 teaspoon honey

1 teaspoon salt-reduced tamari or soy sauce

2 teaspoons hoisin sauce

¼ teaspoon grated fresh ginger

1 teaspoon lemon juice

½ garlic clove, crushed

DRESSING

3½ oz low-fat plain yoghurt

1 tablespoon chopped fresh cilantro

1 teaspoon lime juice

1 teaspoon honey

1 teaspoon salt-reduced tamari or soy sauce

½ garlic clove, crushed

To make the marinade, place the honey, tamari or soy sauce, hoisin sauce, ginger, lemon juice, and garlic in a bowl and mix until well combined. Add the pork and rub with the marinade. Cover with plastic wrap and refrigerate for 4 hours or overnight.

Bring the rice and ½ cup (125 ml) of water to the boil in a small saucepan over high heat, stirring occasionally. Reduce the heat to low and simmer, covered, for 20–25 minutes or until the liquid has been absorbed and the rice is tender. Remove from the heat and leave to stand, covered, for 5 minutes.

Meanwhile, preheat the oven to 400°F (350°F convection) and line a baking sheet with baking paper.

Heat a non-stick fry pan over medium–high heat. Add the pork, reserving the marinade, and cook for 6–7 minutes or until lightly browned on all sides, turning every 2 minutes. Transfer to the lined baking sheet.

Pour the reserved marinade over the pork and roast in the oven for 8–10 minutes or until cooked to your liking, basting and turning once during the cooking time. Transfer to a plate and leave to rest for 2 minutes. When cool enough to handle, cut into thick slices.

To make the dressing, place the yoghurt, cilantro, lime juice, honey, tamari or soy sauce, and garlic in a high-powered blender and blend until smooth, then set aside.

Place the orange, avocado, spinach, fennel, and snow peas in a mixing bowl. Drizzle over half the dressing and toss gently to combine.

To serve, place the rice on a serving plate and top with the Asian-style pork. Serve with the orange and avocado salad on the side. Drizzle over the remaining dressing and garnish with micro herbs (if using).

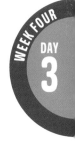

WEEK FOUR
DAY
3

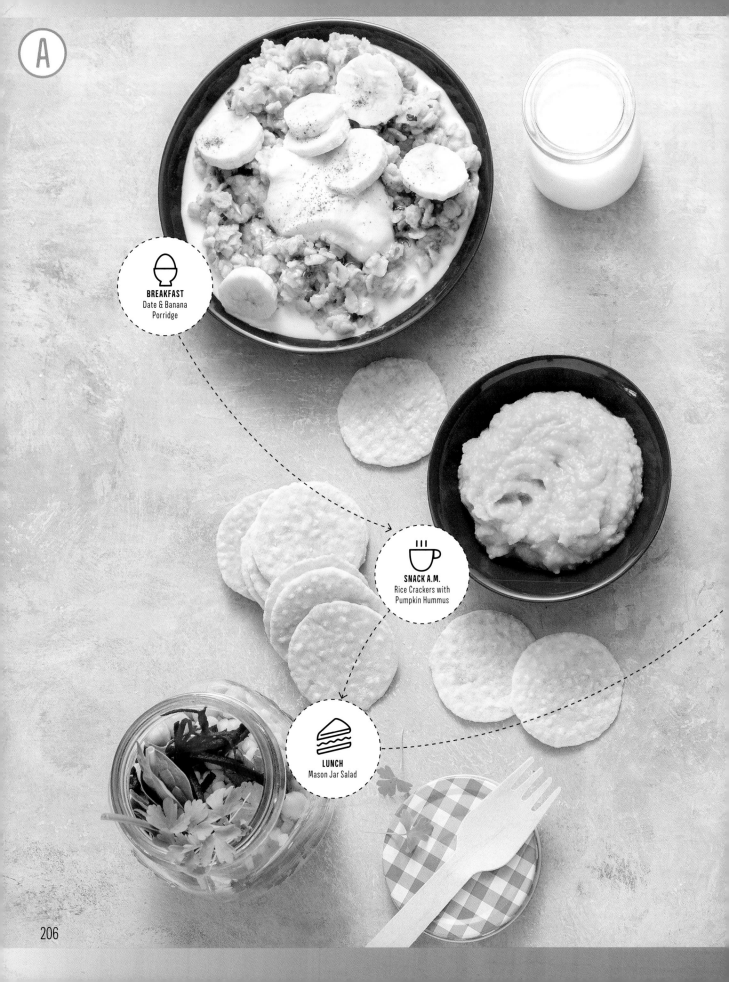

A

BREAKFAST
Date & Banana
Porridge

SNACK A.M.
Rice Crackers with
Pumpkin Hummus

LUNCH
Mason Jar Salad

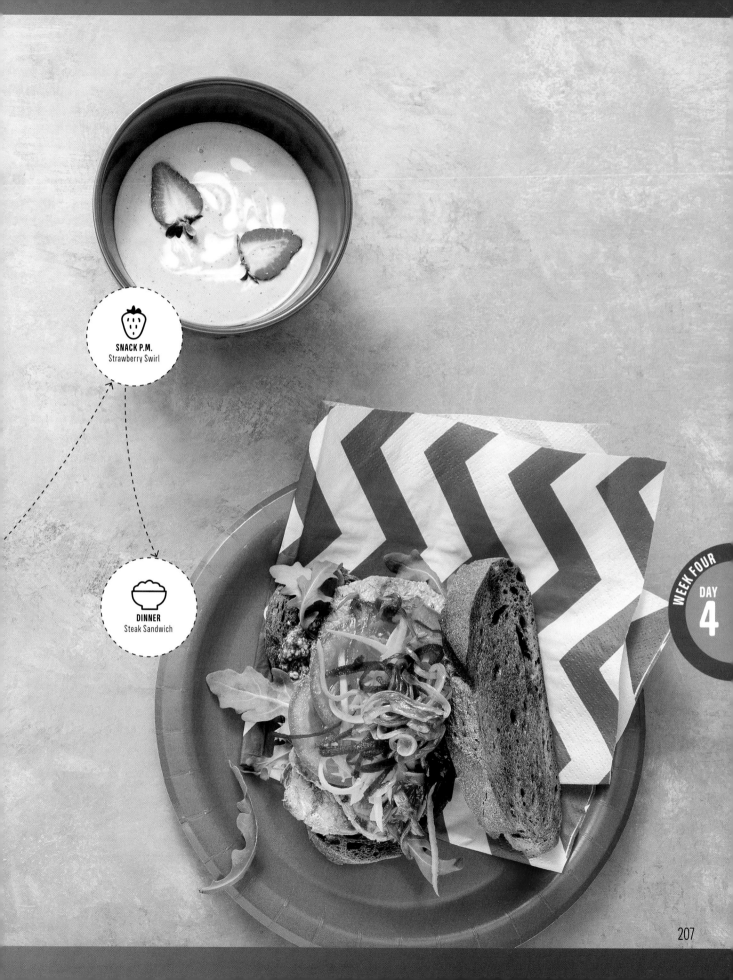

SNACK P.M.
Strawberry Swirl

DINNER
Steak Sandwich

WEEK FOUR
DAY
4

207

Date & Banana Porridge

BREAKFAST **SERVES** 1 | **PREP TIME** 5 MINUTES | **COOKING TIME** 10 MINUTES | **DIFFICULTY** EASY

1½ medjool dates, pitted and chopped

2 oz rolled oats

½ cup (125 ml) low-fat milk

3½ oz low-fat plain yoghurt

½ medium banana, peeled and sliced

½ teaspoon honey

ground cinnamon, to dust (optional)

In a small saucepan, bring about 1 cup (200 ml) of water to the boil over high heat. Add the dates and cook for 5 minutes or until soft.

Stir in the oats and half the milk and reduce the heat to medium–low. Simmer for 5 minutes or until thickened, stirring occasionally.

To serve, spoon the porridge into a serving bowl. Top with the remaining milk, yoghurt, and banana and drizzle over the honey. Dust with cinnamon (if using).

Rice Crackers with Pumpkin Hummus

SNACK A.M. **SERVES** 1 | **PREP TIME** 5 MINUTES, PLUS 10 MINUTES COOLING TIME | **COOKING TIME** 15 MINUTES | **DIFFICULTY** EASY

12 plain rice crackers

PUMPKIN HUMMUS

4½ oz pumpkin, peeled and cut into ¾ in cubes

2¾ oz tinned chickpeas, drained and rinsed

¼ garlic clove, crushed

lemon juice, to taste

pinch of smoked paprika

sea salt, to taste

To make the pumpkin hummus, add 2 inches of water to a saucepan and insert a steamer basket. Cover with a lid and bring the water to the boil over high heat, then reduce the heat to medium. Add the pumpkin and steam, covered, for 12–15 minutes or until soft. Alternatively, microwave on high for 8–10 minutes. Set aside to cool.

Place the pumpkin, chickpeas, garlic, lemon juice, paprika, and salt in a food processor and pulse until smooth and creamy. To save time, the pumpkin hummus can be made the night before and stored in an airtight container in the refrigerator.

Serve the rice crackers with the pumpkin hummus.

Mason Jar Salad

LUNCH **SERVES** 1 | **PREP TIME** 10 MINUTES | **COOKING TIME** 15 MINUTES | **DIFFICULTY** EASY

1 oz pearl couscous

5¼ oz tinned chickpeas, drained and rinsed

½ small beetroot, grated

½ Lebanese cucumber, sliced

1 scallion, sliced

1 small handful baby spinach leaves

2 teaspoons chopped fresh parsley

DRESSING

½ teaspoon Dijon mustard

½ teaspoon apple cider vinegar

1 teaspoon lemon juice

sea salt and ground black pepper, to taste

Fill a saucepan with water and bring to a boil. Stir in the pearl couscous and simmer over medium heat for 10–12 minutes or until al dente. Drain and set aside to cool.

Meanwhile, to make the dressing, whisk the mustard, vinegar, lemon juice, salt, pepper, and 2 teaspoons of water together in a small bowl. Pour into the bottom of a mason jar.

Place the chickpeas in the jar on top of the dressing.

Layer the beetroot, pearl couscous, cucumber, scallion, spinach, and parsley into the mason jar and serve. Mix through before eating.

Strawberry Swirl

SERVES 1 | **PREP TIME** 5 MINUTES | **DIFFICULTY** EASY

10¾ oz low-fat plain yoghurt
9 oz strawberries, halved

Place half the yoghurt and half the strawberries in a high-powered blender and blend until smooth.

To serve, place the remaining yoghurt in a serving bowl. Add the strawberry yoghurt and swirl through with a spoon. Top with the remaining strawberries.

Steak Sandwich

SERVES 1 | **PREP TIME** 10 MINUTES, PLUS 10 MINUTES COOLING TIME | **COOKING TIME** 35 MINUTES | **DIFFICULTY** EASY

oil spray
½ small brown onion,
  thinly sliced
2 teaspoons pure maple syrup
2 teaspoons balsamic vinegar
3 oz lean beef minute steak
sea salt and ground black
  pepper, to taste
2 slices whole wheat bread
1 teaspoon whole grain
  mustard
1 small handful arugula leaves
½ medium tomato, sliced
¼ medium carrot, grated
½ small beetroot, grated

Spray a small non-stick fry pan with oil and heat over low heat. Add the onion and cook slowly for 15–20 minutes or until soft and golden, stirring occasionally. Don't be tempted to increase the heat as this can cause the onion to burn. Add the maple syrup and balsamic vinegar and cook for a further 5–10 minutes or until sticky and caramelised, stirring occasionally. Set aside to cool.

Season the steak with salt and pepper, if desired. Spray a chargrill pan with oil and heat over medium–high heat. Add the steak and cook for 1 minute on each side or until cooked to your liking.

Meanwhile, toast the bread to your liking.

To serve, place one piece of toast on a serving plate. Spread over the mustard and top with the arugula and steak. Layer on the tomato, carrot, beetroot, and caramelised onion and top with the other slice of toast.

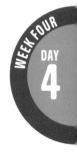

WEEK FOUR
DAY
4

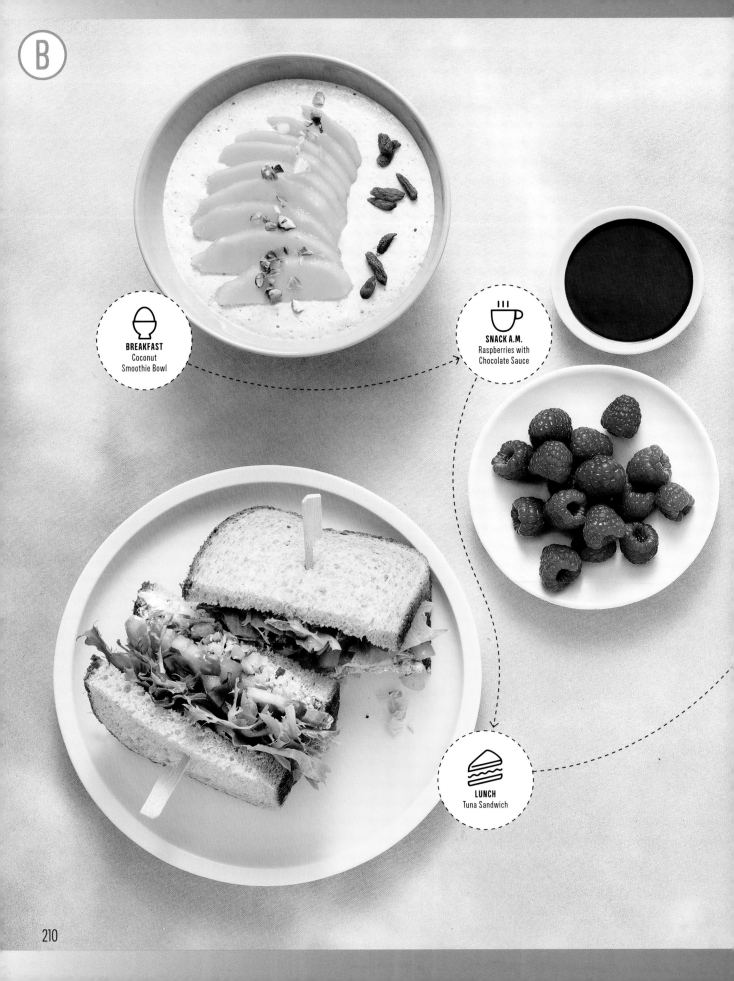

B

BREAKFAST
Coconut
Smoothie Bowl

SNACK A.M.
Raspberries with
Chocolate Sauce

LUNCH
Tuna Sandwich

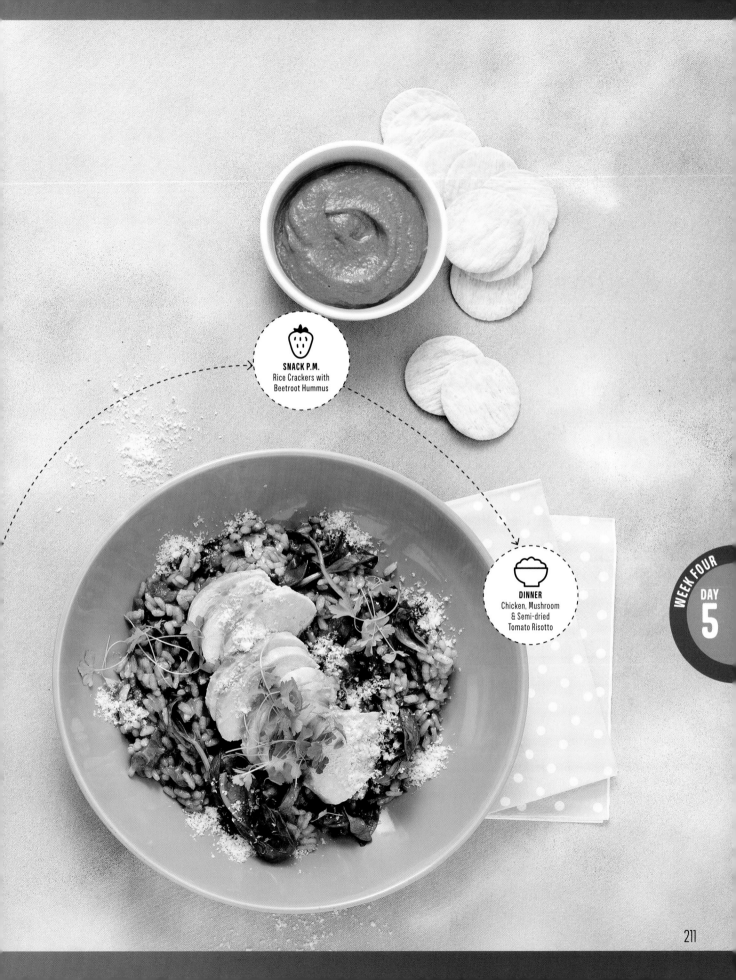

SNACK P.M.
Rice Crackers with
Beetroot Hummus

DINNER
Chicken, Mushroom
& Semi-dried
Tomato Risotto

WEEK FOUR
DAY
5

Coconut Smoothie Bowl

SERVES 1 | **PREP TIME** 5 MINUTES | **DIFFICULTY** EASY

½ medium banana, peeled

1½ oz tinned chickpeas, drained and rinsed

1½ tablespoons light coconut milk

¾ cup (190 ml) low-fat milk

5¼ oz low-fat plain yoghurt

1 oz rolled oats

¼ teaspoon pure vanilla extract

TOPPINGS

½ medium mango, peeled and sliced

⅓ oz unsalted pistachio kernels, roughly chopped

1 tablespoon goji berries

Place the banana, chickpeas, coconut milk, milk, yoghurt, oats, and vanilla in a high-powered blender and blend until smooth.

To serve, pour the smoothie mixture into a serving bowl and top with the mango, pistachios, and goji berries.

Raspberries with Chocolate Sauce

SERVES 1 | **PREP TIME** 5 MINUTES | **COOKING TIME** 5 MINUTES | **DIFFICULTY** EASY

1½ teaspoons coconut oil

1 teaspoon pure maple syrup

2 teaspoons raw cacao powder

2¾ oz raspberries

Heat the coconut oil and maple syrup in a small saucepan over low heat. Add the cacao powder and heat for 5 minutes or until the sauce is warmed through and well combined, stirring constantly.

To serve, place the raspberries on a small plate and serve the chocolate sauce on the side.

Tuna Sandwich

SERVES 1 | **PREP TIME** 10 MINUTES | **DIFFICULTY** EASY

1¾ oz low-fat plain yoghurt

1 oz low-fat cottage cheese

1 teaspoon lemon juice

2 teaspoons chopped capers

1 teaspoon chopped fresh dill

3½ oz tinned tuna in springwater, drained

¼ small red onion, finely chopped

½ celery stalk, finely chopped

sea salt and ground black pepper, to taste

2 slices whole wheat bread

1 small handful lettuce leaves

½ medium tomato, sliced

Whisk the yoghurt, cottage cheese, lemon juice, capers, and dill together in a small bowl.

Add the tuna, onion, and celery and mix until well combined. Season with salt and pepper, if desired.

On one slice of bread, layer the lettuce, tomato, and tuna mixture. Top with the other slice of bread.

To serve, place the sandwich on a serving plate and cut in half.

Rice Crackers with Beetroot Hummus

SNACK P.M.   **SERVES** 1 | **PREP TIME** 5 MINUTES, PLUS 10 MINUTES COOLING TIME | **COOKING TIME** 40 MINUTES | **DIFFICULTY** EASY

12 plain rice crackers

BEETROOT HUMMUS

1 small beetroot

2¾ oz tinned chickpeas, drained and rinsed

¼ garlic clove, crushed

pinch of ground cumin

lemon juice, to taste

sea salt and ground black pepper, to taste

To make the beetroot hummus, wrap the beetroot in foil with 1 tablespoon of water (this helps the beetroot to steam). Place in a small roasting pan and bake in the oven for 30–40 minutes or until tender. Test the beetroot with a skewer—it is cooked if the skewer pierces the flesh easily. Set aside to cool. When cool enough to handle, peel the beetroot under cool running water, then cut into cubes. To save time, the beetroot can be roasted the night before and stored in an airtight container in the refrigerator.

Place the beetroot, chickpeas, garlic, cumin, and 2 teaspoons of water in a food processor and process until smooth. Season with lemon juice, salt and pepper, if desired.

Place the beetroot dip in a small bowl and serve with the rice crackers.

Chicken, Mushroom & Semi-dried Tomato Risotto

DINNER   **SERVES** 1 | **PREP TIME** 10 MINUTES | **COOKING TIME** 50 MINUTES | **DIFFICULTY** EASY

1⅔ oz cups (375 ml) salt-reduced vegetable stock

oil spray

¼ small brown onion, finely chopped

½ garlic clove, crushed

2¾ oz mushrooms, sliced

4 semi-dried tomatoes, sliced

2 oz arborio rice

½ teaspoon fresh thyme leaves

1 small handful baby spinach leaves

⅔ oz parmesan cheese, grated

sea salt and ground black pepper, to taste

3½ oz boneless, skinless chicken breast

fresh parsley leaves, to garnish (optional)

Heat the stock in a small saucepan over medium heat.

Spray a medium saucepan with oil and heat over medium heat. Add the onion and garlic and cook for 5 minutes or until the onion is soft and translucent, stirring occasionally. Add the mushrooms and cook for 4–5 minutes or until they start to soften. Add the tomato and cook for a further 2 minutes, stirring frequently.

Add the rice and thyme and cook for 2–3 minutes or until lightly toasted, stirring frequently. Pour one-quarter of the warmed stock into the pan with the rice and cook for 6–8 minutes or until most of the stock has been absorbed, stirring constantly.

Continue adding the stock a ladleful at a time, allowing all the liquid to be absorbed before adding the next ladleful, stirring frequently. Cook for 15–20 minutes or until all the stock has been used and the rice is cooked but still al dente. If all the stock has been used and the rice is not ready, add ¼ cup (60 ml) of hot water at a time until cooked.

Stir in the spinach and half the parmesan cheese and cook for 1–2 minutes or until the spinach has wilted. Season with salt and pepper, if desired.

Meanwhile, spray a non-stick fry pan with oil and heat over medium heat. Add the chicken and cook for 4–6 minutes on each side or until cooked through. Set aside to cool slightly. When cool enough to handle, cut the chicken into thick slices.

To serve, place the risotto in a serving bowl, top with the chicken and sprinkle over the remaining parmesan cheese. Garnish with the parsley (if using).

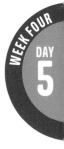

WEEK FOUR DAY 5

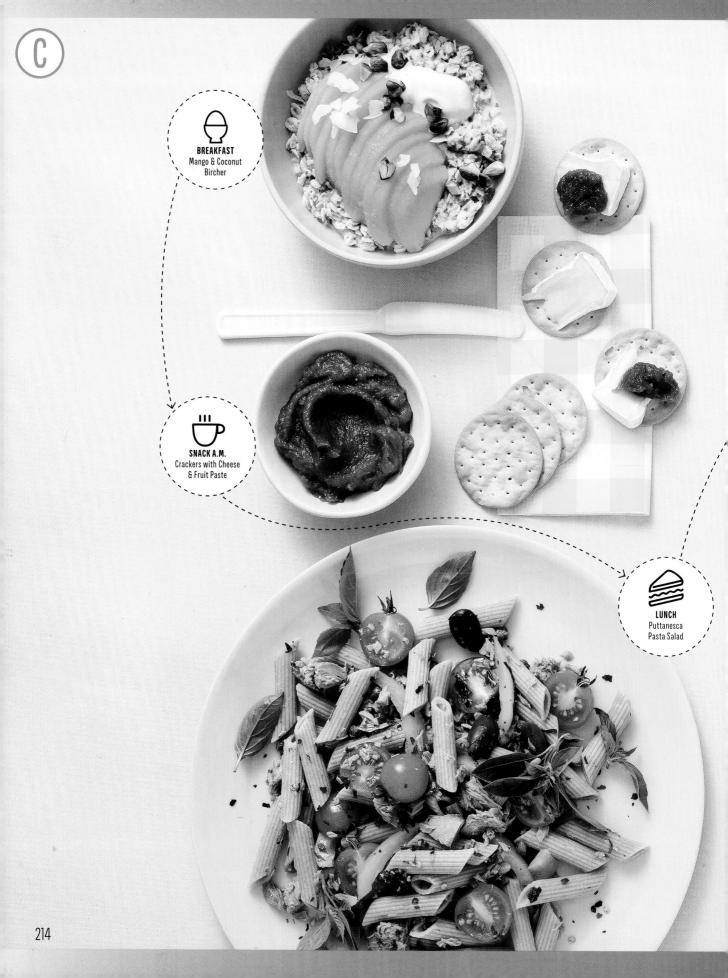

C

BREAKFAST
Mango & Coconut
Bircher

SNACK A.M.
Crackers with Cheese
& Fruit Paste

LUNCH
Puttanesca
Pasta Salad

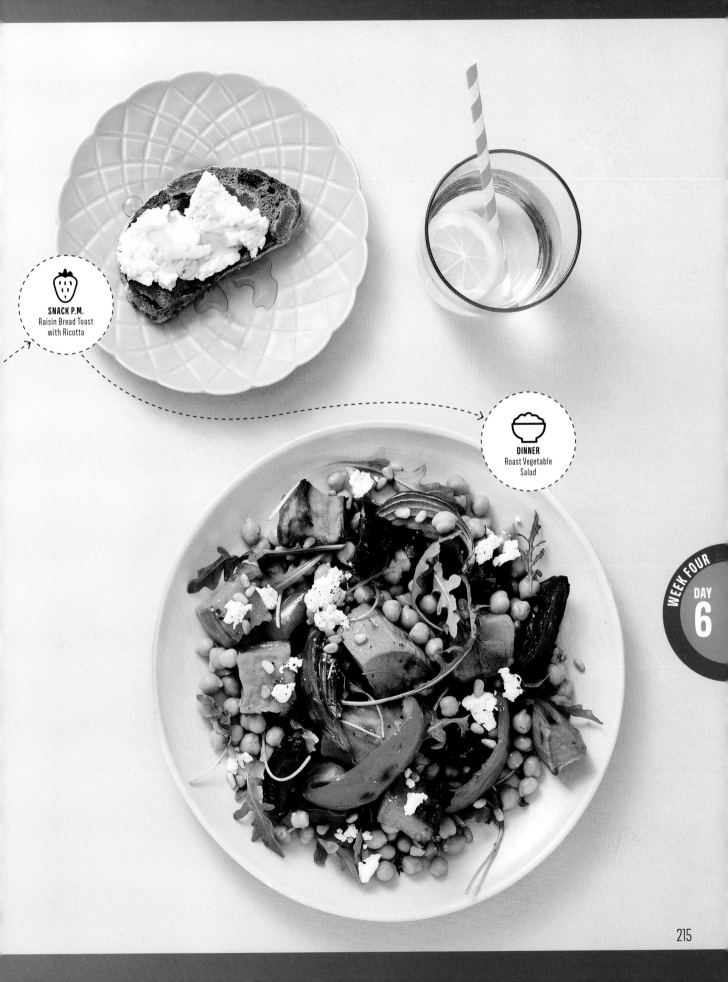

SNACK P.M.
Raisin Bread Toast
with Ricotta

DINNER
Roast Vegetable
Salad

WEEK FOUR

DAY
6

Mango & Coconut Bircher

BREAKFAST **SERVES** 1 | **PREP TIME** 5 MINUTES, PLUS OVERNIGHT SOAKING | **DIFFICULTY** EASY

2 oz rolled oats

1 teaspoon chia seeds

½ cup (125 ml) low-fat milk

1 teaspoon honey

¼ teaspoon pure vanilla extract (optional)

½ medium mango

1¾ oz low-fat plain yoghurt

⅓ oz unsalted pistachio kernels, roughly chopped

2 teaspoons coconut flakes

Place the oats, chia seeds, milk, honey, and vanilla (if using), in a bowl and mix until well combined. Cover with plastic wrap and place in the refrigerator to soak overnight.

The next morning, peel and slice the mango.

To serve, transfer the bircher to a serving bowl. Top with the yoghurt, mango, pistachios, and coconut.

Crackers with Cheese & Fruit Paste

SNACK A.M. **SERVES** 1 | **PREP TIME** 5 MINUTES, PLUS 15 MINUTES COOLING TIME | **COOKING TIME** 20 MINUTES | **DIFFICULTY** EASY

6 plain water crackers

1½ oz camembert cheese, sliced

FRUIT PASTE

2 dried figs, sliced

1 small pear, cored, peeled, and chopped

2 tablespoons apple cider vinegar

1 tablespoon honey

pinch of ground cinnamon

1 clove

To make the fruit paste, place the fig, pear, vinegar, honey, cinnamon, clove and 2 teaspoons of water in a small saucepan and bring to the boil over medium heat. Reduce the heat to low and simmer for 15–20 minutes or until the mixture is thick, stirring occasionally. Discard the clove. Remove the pan from the heat and set aside to cool, then blend the mixture in a high-powered blender until smooth. To save time, the paste can be made the night before and stored in an airtight container in the refrigerator.

To serve, top the crackers with the camembert cheese and fruit paste.

Puttanesca Pasta Salad

LUNCH **SERVES** 1 | **PREP TIME** 10 MINUTES, PLUS 10 MINUTES COOLING TIME | **COOKING TIME** 15 MINUTES | **DIFFICULTY** EASY

3 oz whole wheat pasta

5 cherry tomatoes, quartered

4 kalamata olives, pitted and sliced

¼ medium yellow bell pepper, seeds removed, thinly sliced

1 tablespoon capers, rinsed

3½ oz tinned tuna in springwater, drained

sea salt and ground black pepper, to taste

dried chilli flakes (optional)

DRESSING

2 teaspoons finely chopped fresh basil, plus extra to garnish (optional)

2 teaspoons finely chopped fresh parsley

½ garlic clove, crushed

1 teaspoon balsamic vinegar

Fill a large saucepan with water, add a pinch of salt, and bring to the boil. Add the pasta and cook until al dente (see the pasta packet for the recommended cooking time). Drain and refresh under cool running water. Set aside to cool. To save time, the pasta can be cooked the night before and stored in an airtight container in the refrigerator.

To make the dressing, whisk the basil, parsley, garlic, vinegar, and 2 teaspoons of water together in a small bowl and set aside.

Place the pasta, tomatoes, olives, bell pepper, capers and tuna in a mixing bowl. Drizzle over the dressing, season with salt and pepper, if desired, and toss gently to combine.

To serve, place the salad in a serving bowl and garnish with chilli and extra basil (if using).

Raisin Bread Toast with Ricotta

SERVES 1 | **PREP TIME** 5 MINUTES | **COOKING TIME** 2 MINUTES | **DIFFICULTY** EASY

1 slice raisin bread
1 oz low-fat ricotta cheese
¼ teaspoon honey

Toast the bread to your liking.

To serve, spread the ricotta over the toast and drizzle the honey on top.

Roast Vegetable Salad

DINNER **SERVES** 1 | **PREP TIME** 10 MINUTES | **COOKING TIME** 40 MINUTES | **DIFFICULTY** EASY

½ medium sweet potato, peeled and cut into 1 in cubes
1 small beetroot, peeled and cut into wedges
1 garlic clove
oil spray
sea salt and ground black pepper, to taste
½ medium red bell pepper, seeds removed, thickly sliced
¼ small red onion, cut into wedges
8 oz tinned chickpeas, drained and rinsed
1 teaspoon pine nuts
1 small handful arugula leaves
1 oz low-fat goat's cheese, crumbled

DRESSING
2 teaspoons lemon juice
2 teaspoons chopped fresh oregano
½ teaspoon whole grain mustard

Preheat the oven to 400°F (350°F convection) and line a baking sheet with baking paper.

Place the sweet potato, beetroot and garlic on the lined baking sheet, spray lightly with oil and season with salt and pepper, if desired. Roast in the oven for 20 minutes. Remove from the oven and turn the vegetables with tongs. Add the bell pepper, onion, and chickpeas and spray lightly with oil. Return to the oven and roast for 10–15 minutes, turning with tongs after 10 minutes. Add the pine nuts and roast for a further 5 minutes or until the vegetables are tender and browned.

Meanwhile, to make the dressing, whisk the lemon juice, oregano, mustard, and 2 teaspoons of water together in a small bowl and set aside.

Place the roast vegetables, chickpeas, pine nuts, and arugula in a mixing bowl. Drizzle over the dressing and toss gently to combine.

To serve, place the roast vegetable salad on a serving plate and top with the crumbled goat's cheese.

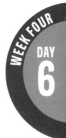

WEEK FOUR
DAY
6

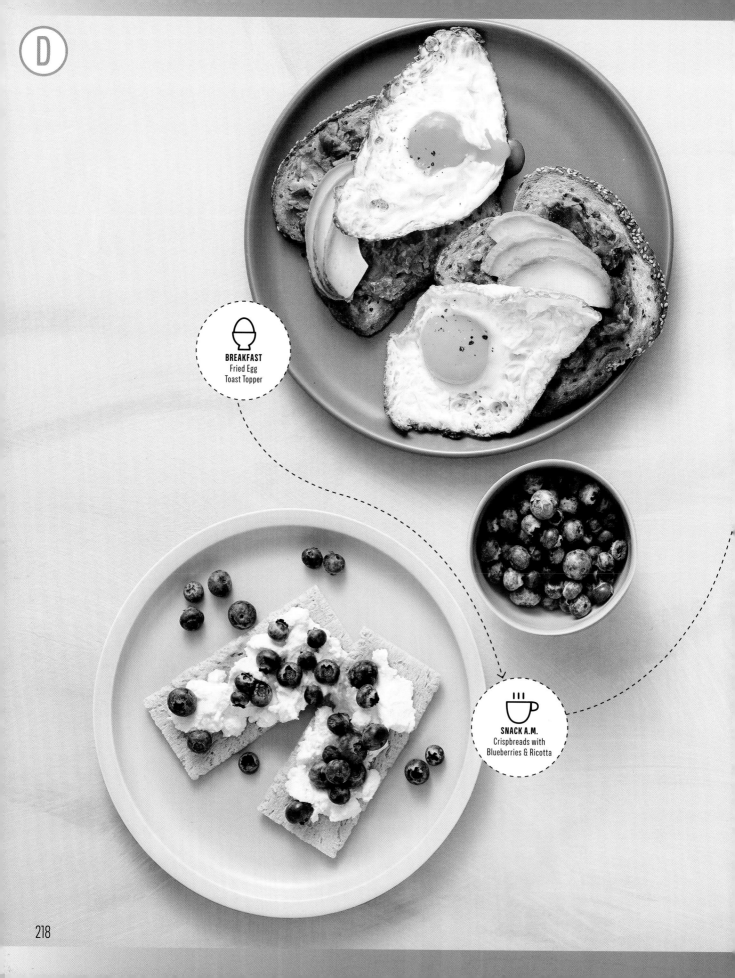

D

BREAKFAST
Fried Egg
Toast Topper

SNACK A.M.
Crispbreads with
Blueberries & Ricotta

218

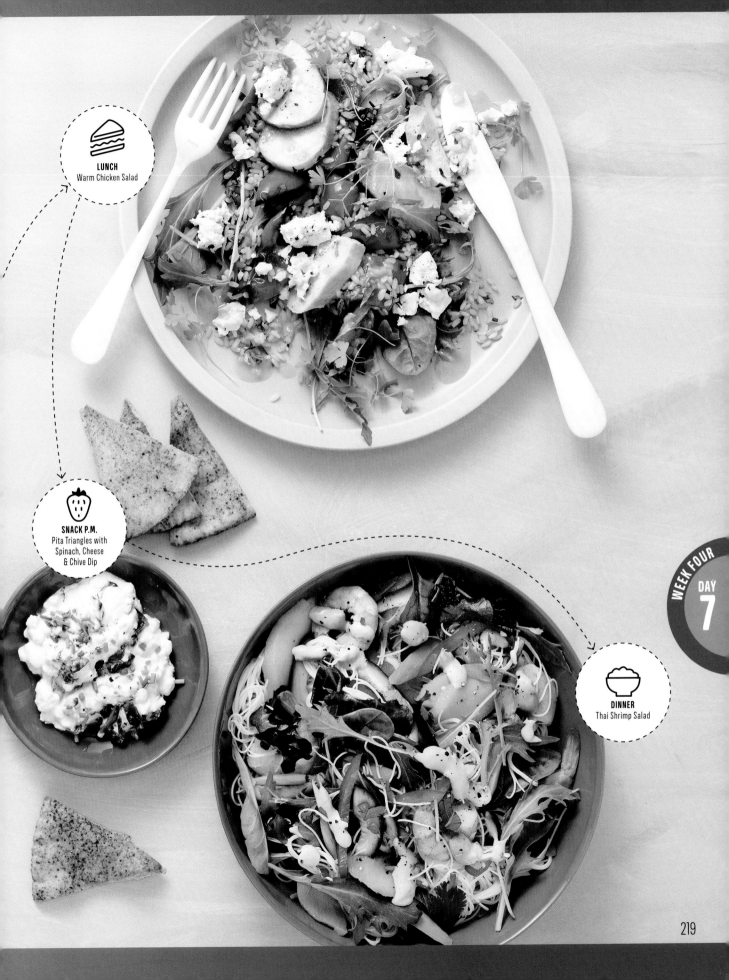

LUNCH
Warm Chicken Salad

SNACK P.M.
Pita Triangles with
Spinach, Cheese
& Chive Dip

DINNER
Thai Shrimp Salad

WEEK FOUR

DAY
7

Fried Egg Toast Topper

SERVES 1 | **PREP TIME** 10 MINUTES | **COOKING TIME** 15 MINUTES | **DIFFICULTY** EASY

oil spray

1 tablespoon finely diced
    brown onion

¼ garlic clove, crushed

¼ teaspoon each ground
    cumin, chilli powder, and
    ground coriander

2 oz tinned red kidney beans,
    drained and rinsed

1½ oz tinned crushed tomatoes

⅔ oz low-fat cheddar cheese

sea salt and ground black
    pepper, to taste

2 slices whole wheat bread

2 large eggs

1 oz avocado, sliced

Lightly spray a non-stick fry pan with oil and heat over medium heat. Add the onion and cook for 5 minutes or until soft and translucent, stirring occasionally. Add the crushed garlic, cumin, chilli powder, and coriander and cook for 1 minute, stirring frequently. Add the beans and tomatoes and cook for 5 minutes or until heated through, stirring frequently.

Remove from the heat and, using a fork or potato masher, mash the beans and tomatoes until almost smooth. Grate the cheese in and mix until melted and well combined. Season with salt and pepper, if desired. Cover with foil and set aside.

Toast the bread to your liking.

Meanwhile, lightly spray a non-stick fry pan with oil and heat over medium–low heat. Crack one egg into a small bowl and gently pour the egg into the fry pan. Repeat with the second egg. Cook the eggs for 1–2 minutes or until the white is opaque and the yolk has set.

To serve, spread the bean mixture over the toast and top with the avocado and fried eggs.

Crispbreads with Blueberries & Ricotta

SERVES 1 | **PREP TIME** 5 MINUTES | **DIFFICULTY** EASY

1¾ oz low-fat ricotta cheese

2 rye crispbreads

5¾ oz blueberries

To serve, spread the ricotta over the crispbreads and top with the blueberries.

Warm Chicken Salad

SERVES 1 | **PREP TIME** 10 MINUTES, PLUS 10 MINUTES COOLING TIME | **COOKING TIME** 25 MINUTES | **DIFFICULTY** EASY

1 oz brown rice

¼ medium red bell pepper,
    seeds removed

oil spray

1¾ oz boneless, skinless
    chicken breast

1 handful mixed lettuce leaves

1 oz salt-reduced low-fat
    feta cheese, crumbled

sea salt and ground black
    pepper, to taste

2 teaspoons chopped fresh
    parsley

DRESSING

1 teaspoon Dijon mustard

1 teaspoon honey

½ garlic clove, crushed

lemon juice, to taste

Bring the rice and ½ cup (125 ml) of water to the boil in a small saucepan over high heat, stirring occasionally. Reduce the heat to low and simmer, covered, for 20–25 minutes or until the liquid has been absorbed and the rice is tender. Remove from the heat and leave to stand, covered, for 5 minutes. Set aside to cool. To save time, the rice can be cooked the night before and stored in an airtight container in the refrigerator.

Meanwhile, heat a small non-stick fry pan over high heat. Place the bell pepper, skin side down, in the hot pan. Cook for 5–7 minutes or until the skin starts to blister and turn brown. Transfer to a bowl, cover with plastic wrap, and leave to sweat for 5 minutes. Peel off the skin and cut into ¾ inch pieces.

Wipe the pan clean, spray lightly with oil and reheat over medium–high heat. Add the chicken and cook for 4–6 minutes on each side or until cooked through. Set aside to cool slightly, then cut the chicken into thick slices.

To make the dressing, whisk the mustard, honey, garlic, lemon juice, and 2 teaspoons of water together in a small bowl and set aside.

Place the rice, bell pepper, chicken, lettuce, and feta in a mixing bowl. Drizzle over the dressing, season with salt and pepper, if desired, and toss gently to combine. To serve, place the warm chicken salad in a serving bowl and garnish with the parsley.

Pita Triangles with Spinach, Cheese & Chive Dip

SERVES 1 | **PREP TIME** 10 MINUTES, PLUS 5 MINUTES COOLING TIME | **COOKING TIME** 15 MINUTES | **DIFFICULTY** EASY

½ whole wheat pita bread,
  cut into wedges

oil spray

**SPINACH, CHEESE
& CHIVE DIP**

oil spray

½ garlic clove, crushed

1 small handful baby spinach
  leaves, finely chopped

2 oz low-fat cottage cheese

lemon juice, to taste

sea salt and ground black
  pepper, to taste

finely chopped fresh chives,
  to taste

Preheat the oven to 400°F (350°F convection) and line a baking sheet with baking paper.

Lay the pita wedges in a single layer on the lined baking sheet and spray lightly with oil spray. Bake in the oven for 5 minutes or until they begin to colour. Turn the wedges over and bake for a further 5–8 minutes or until both sides are lightly coloured. Set aside to cool.

Meanwhile, to make the spinach dip, lightly spray a non-stick fry pan with oil and heat over medium–high heat. Add the garlic and cook for 15 seconds, stirring constantly. Add the spinach and cook for 1–2 minutes or until wilted, stirring frequently. Remove from the heat and set aside to cool.

Place the cooled spinach mixture, cottage cheese, and lemon juice in a bowl and gently mix together. Season with salt and pepper, if desired, and top with the chives.

Serve the pita triangles with the spinach, cheese, and chive dip.

Thai Shrimp Salad

SERVES 1 | **PREP TIME** 20 MINUTES, PLUS 10 MINUTES SOAKING TIME | **COOKING TIME** 5 MINUTES | **DIFFICULTY** EASY

1¾ oz rice vermicelli noodles

oil spray

10 medium raw shrimp,
  peeled and deveined,
  tails intact

1 medium mango, peeled
  and sliced

½ Lebanese cucumber, thinly
  sliced on an angle

½ medium carrot, thinly sliced
  on an angle

¼ medium red bell pepper,
  seeds removed, thinly sliced
  on an angle

½ scallion, thinly sliced
  on an angle

1 small handful mixed
  lettuce leaves

½ fresh red chilli, seeds
  removed, thinly sliced

1 tablespoon chopped
  fresh cilantro

1 tablespoon chopped
  fresh mint

AVOCADO DRESSING

1 oz avocado

1 tablespoon chopped
  fresh cilantro

3½ oz low-fat plain yoghurt

½ garlic clove, crushed

2 teaspoons lemon juice

sea salt and ground black
  pepper, to taste

Place the noodles in a heatproof bowl and cover with boiling water. Leave for 10 minutes, then loosen the noodles with a fork. Drain and refresh under cool running water. Drain well and set aside to cool slightly. When cool enough to handle, cut into shorter lengths.

Lightly spray a non-stick fry pan with oil and heat over medium–high heat. Add the shrimp and cook for 2–3 minutes or until they change colour and are cooked through, stirring frequently. Transfer to a plate and set aside to rest.

To make the dressing, place the avocado, cilantro, yoghurt, garlic, lemon juice, salt, pepper, and 1 tablespoon of water in a high-powered blender and blend until smooth. If the dressing is too thick, add 2 teaspoons of water at a time until the desired consistency is reached.

Place the noodles, shrimp, mango, cucumber, carrot, bell pepper, scallion, lettuce, chilli, cilantro, and mint in a mixing bowl. Drizzle over half the dressing and toss gently to combine.

To serve, place the Thai shrimp salad in a serving bowl and drizzle over the remaining dressing.

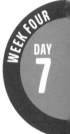

WEEK FOUR
DAY
7

SWAP-OUT RECIPES

I love seeing you make some of my favourite recipes, so make sure you take a photo of your finished dish! Share it with me by posting it to social media, using **#kaylaitsines** so I can see it!

Berry Parfait with Maple Yoghurt

SERVES 1 | **PREP TIME** 5 MINUTES | **DIFFICULTY** EASY

6 oz frozen mixed
  berries, thawed
7 oz low-fat plain yoghurt

1 teaspoon pure
  maple syrup
2 oz natural muesli

Place half the mixed berries in a high-powered blender and blend to a smooth puree.

To serve, place the berry puree in a cup or small bowl, and top with the yoghurt, maple syrup, muesli, and remaining berries.

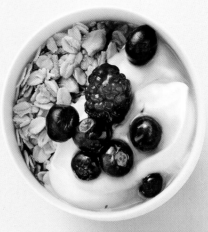

Banana Split Overnight Oats

SERVES 1 | **PREP TIME** 5 MINUTES, PLUS OVERNIGHT CHILLING TIME
COOKING TIME 5 MINUTES | **DIFFICULTY** EASY

2 oz rolled oats
½ cup (125 ml) low-fat milk
3½ oz low-fat plain yoghurt
1 teaspoon honey
½ teaspoon ground
  cinnamon
oil spray
1 medium banana, peeled
  and halved lengthwise

2 teaspoons raw
  cacao powder
2 teaspoons pure
  vanilla extract
1½ tablespoons pure
  maple syrup
raw cacao nibs, to garnish

Place the oats, milk, and half the yoghurt in a bowl and mix well to combine. Cover with plastic wrap and place in the refrigerator to chill overnight. If you like, remove the oats from the refrigerator 10 minutes before you wish to serve them to bring to room temperature.

Whisk the honey, cinnamon, and 1 teaspoon of water together in a small bowl.

Heat a non-stick fry pan over medium–high heat and spray lightly with oil spray. Add the banana halves, cut side down, and cook for 1–2 minutes or until lightly golden and a little crispy. Carefully flip the bananas and cook for a further minute. Reduce the heat to medium–low, add the honey mixture, and cook for 30–60 seconds. Remove from the heat.

Whisk the cacao powder, vanilla, and maple syrup together in a small bowl.

To serve, top the oats with the grilled banana halves and their syrup. Dollop over the remaining yoghurt, then drizzle over the chocolate sauce. Garnish with cacao nibs.

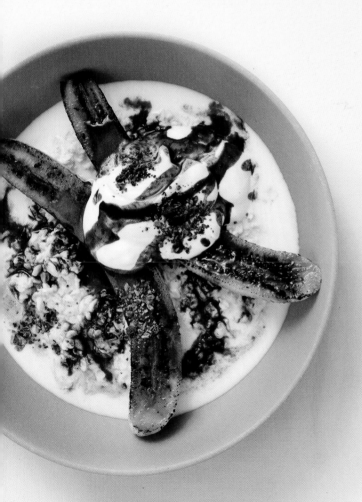

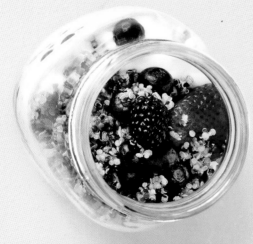

Spiced Ricotta Toast with Pear

SERVES 1 | **PREP TIME** 5 MINUTES
COOKING TIME 2 MINUTES | **DIFFICULTY** EASY

2 slices raisin bread
3½ oz low-fat ricotta cheese
¼ teaspoon ground cinnamon
pinch of ground nutmeg
pinch of ground cardamom

1 small pear,
  cored and sliced
2 teaspoons honey
finely grated lemon
  zest and juice, to taste

Toast the raisin bread to your liking.

Spread the ricotta on the toast, sprinkle with
cinnamon, nutmeg, and cardamom, then layer
over the sliced pear. Drizzle with the honey,
and add lemon zest and juice to taste.

Mixed Berry Quinoa Parfait

SERVES 1 | **PREP TIME** 5 MINUTES, PLUS 20 MINUTES
COOLING TIME **COOKING TIME** 40 MINUTES | **DIFFICULTY** EASY

2 oz quinoa
2 teaspoons pure
  maple syrup

7 oz low-fat plain yoghurt
6 oz frozen mixed
  berries, thawed

Preheat the oven to 325°F (280°F convection) and line a
baking sheet with baking paper.

Bring the quinoa and 1 cup (250 ml) of water to the boil
in a small saucepan over high heat, stirring occasionally.
Reduce the heat to low and simmer, covered, for
10–12 minutes or until the liquid has been absorbed
and the quinoa is tender. Add the maple syrup and stir
to combine. Set aside to cool. To save time, the quinoa
can be cooked the night before and stored in an airtight
container in the refrigerator.

Spread half the cooked quinoa evenly over the lined
baking sheet and bake in the oven for 15 minutes. Stir
the quinoa and spread out evenly again, then bake for a
further 8–10 minutes or until crispy. Remove from the
oven and set aside to cool.

Meanwhile, place the yoghurt and the remaining cooked
quinoa in a bowl and stir to combine.

To serve, layer the berries, yoghurt mixture, and crispy
quinoa in a glass or jar.

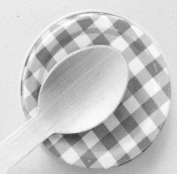

Acai Smoothie Bowl

SERVES 1 | **PREP TIME** 10 MINUTES, PLUS 10 MINUTES COOLING TIME
COOKING TIME 15 MINUTES | **DIFFICULTY** EASY

2 oz pumpkin, peeled and
   cut into ¾ inch cubes
1 teaspoon acai berry powder
6 oz frozen mixed berries
¾ cup (190 ml) low-fat milk
5¼ oz low-fat plain yoghurt

TOPPINGS

1 oz natural muesli
   or rolled oats
2 teaspoons coconut flakes
1 teaspoon chia seeds
2 oz strawberries, hulled
   and halved
1 teaspoon goji berries

Add 2 inches of water to a saucepan and insert a steamer basket. Cover with a lid and bring the water to the boil over high heat, then reduce the heat to medium. Add the pumpkin and steam, covered, for 12–15 minutes or until soft. Alternatively, microwave on high for 8–10 minutes. Set aside to cool.

Place the pumpkin, acai powder, berries, milk, and yoghurt in a high-powered blender and blend until smooth.

To serve, pour the smoothie mixture into a serving bowl and top with the muesli, coconut flakes, chia seeds, strawberries, and goji berries.

Green Smoothie Bowl

SERVES 1 | **PREP TIME** 5 MINUTES | **DIFFICULTY** EASY

½ medium zucchini,
   chopped
1 medium banana, peeled
   and chopped
½ teaspoon spirulina
   powder, plus extra
   to garnish (optional)
7 oz low-fat plain yoghurt
½ cup (125 ml) low-fat milk

TOPPINGS

1 oz natural muesli
   or rolled oats
1 tablespoon coconut flakes
1½ oz blueberries
1¾ oz frozen blackberries,
   thawed
1 teaspoon raw cacao nibs

Place the zucchini, banana, spirulina, yoghurt, and milk in a high-powered blender and blend until smooth.

To serve, pour the smoothie mixture into a serving bowl and top with the muesli, coconut flakes, blueberries, blackberries, and cacao nibs. Garnish with more spirulina powder, if desired.

Cherry Smoothie Bowl

SERVES 1 | **PREP TIME** 10 MINUTES | **DIFFICULTY** EASY

10 cherries, pitted

1¼ oz tinned chickpeas, drained and rinsed

½ medium banana, peeled

¾ cup (190 ml) low-fat milk

5¼ oz low-fat plain yoghurt

3 oz raspberries

TOPPINGS

1 oz natural muesli or rolled oats

1 teaspoon coconut flakes

½ teaspoon chia seeds

1 teaspoon pumpkin seeds (pepitas)

Place the cherries, chickpeas, banana, milk, yoghurt, and half the raspberries in a high-powered blender and blend until smooth.

To serve, pour the smoothie mixture into a serving bowl and top with the muesli, coconut, chia seeds, pumpkin seeds, and remaining raspberries.

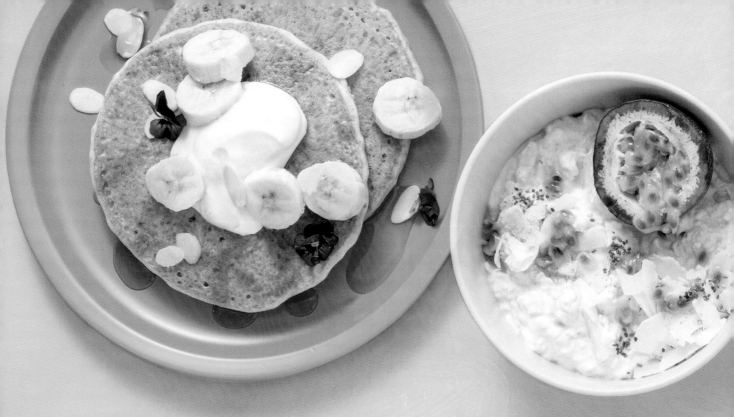

Banana & Almond Pancakes

SERVES 1 | **PREP TIME** 10 MINUTES, PLUS 10 MINUTES RESTING TIME
COOKING TIME 15 MINUTES | **DIFFICULTY** EASY

2½ oz whole wheat plain flour

1 teaspoon baking powder

pinch of ground cinnamon

2 teaspoons almond butter

¼ cup (60 ml) low-fat milk

1 tablespoon pure
  maple syrup

oil spray

3½ oz low-fat plain yoghurt

½ medium banana,
  peeled and sliced

1 teaspoon flaked almonds

Place the flour, baking powder, and cinnamon in a
mixing bowl and mix until well combined. Whisk the
almond butter, milk, 2 teaspoons of the maple syrup, and
2 tablespoons of water together in a second bowl until
well combined. Pour into the dry ingredients and whisk
thoroughly until smooth.

Lightly spray a non-stick fry pan with oil spray and heat
over medium–high heat. Pour half the batter into the pan.
Cook for 1–2 minutes or until bubbles rise to the surface
and the underside is golden brown. Using a spatula, flip
it over and cook for a further 1–2 minutes or until golden
brown and cooked through. Transfer to a plate and cover
loosely with foil to keep warm, then repeat with the
remaining batter to make two pancakes in total.

Serve the pancakes topped with the yoghurt, banana,
and almonds, and drizzled with the remaining syrup.

Tropical Overnight Oats

SERVES 1 | **PREP TIME** 5 MINUTES, PLUS OVERNIGHT CHILLING TIME
DIFFICULTY EASY

2 oz rolled oats

¼ cup (60 ml) light
  coconut milk

3½ oz low-fat plain yoghurt

¼ cup (60 ml) low-fat milk

½ teaspoon chia seeds,
  plus extra to garnish

1¾ oz pineapple, peeled
  and chopped

1 passionfruit

1 teaspoon coconut flakes

pinch of ground cinnamon

Place the oats, coconut milk, yoghurt, milk, chia seeds,
and pineapple in a bowl and mix until well combined.
Cover with plastic wrap and place in the refrigerator to
chill overnight.

To serve, stir the overnight oats, top with the passionfruit
pulp, and sprinkle over the coconut flakes, cinnamon, and
extra chia seeds.

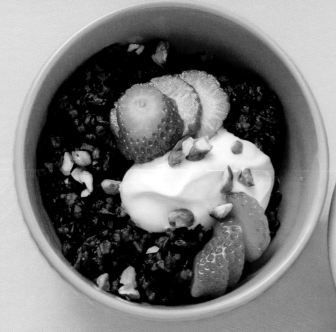

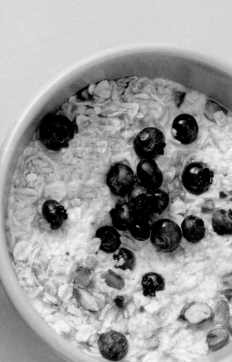

Black Rice Breakfast Pudding

SERVES 1 | **PREP TIME** 5 MINUTES
COOKING TIME 40 MINUTES | **DIFFICULTY** EASY

2 oz black rice

1½ tablespoons light
coconut milk

¼ cup (60 ml) low-fat milk

¼ teaspoon pure
vanilla extract

2 teaspoons pure
maple syrup

3½ oz low-fat plain yoghurt

4¾ oz strawberries, hulled
and sliced

⅓ oz unsalted pistachio
kernels, roughly chopped

Place the rice, coconut milk, milk, vanilla, maple syrup,
and ¾ cup (175 ml) of water in a medium saucepan and
bring to the boil over medium–high heat. Reduce the
heat to medium–low and simmer for 35–40 minutes or
until the liquid is absorbed and the rice is tender, stirring
occasionally. Check the rice during the last 10 minutes
of cooking time. If all the liquid is absorbed and the rice
is not ready, add ¼ cup (60 ml) of hot water at a time
until cooked, stirring frequently.

To serve, spoon the rice pudding into a serving bowl and
top with the yoghurt and sliced strawberries. Scatter over
the chopped pistachios.

DIY Muesli

SERVES 1 | **PREP TIME** 15 MINUTES | **DIFFICULTY** EASY

¾ cup (190 ml) low-fat milk

½ teaspoon honey

3 oz blueberries

MUESLI (MAKES ENOUGH FOR 4 SERVES)

4¼ oz rolled oats

4¼ oz quinoa flakes

⅓ oz unsalted
pistachio kernels,
roughly chopped

2 teaspoons
sunflower seeds

1½ oz shredded coconut

1 tablespoon chia seeds

½ teaspoon
ground cinnamon

½ teaspoon ground nutmeg

To make the muesli, place all the ingredients in a mixing
bowl and mix until well combined.

To serve, place one-quarter of the muesli in a serving
bowl and pour over the milk. Drizzle with the honey and
top with the blueberries.

Pumpkin Smash on Toast

SERVES 1 | **PREP TIME** 10 MINUTES
COOKING TIME 25 MINUTES | **DIFFICULTY** EASY

2 oz pumpkin, peeled and cut into 1 in cubes
oil spray
pinch of ground allspice (optional)
sea salt and ground black pepper, to taste
1 oz salt-reduced low-fat feta cheese, crumbled
1¾ oz mushrooms, sliced
1 garlic clove, crushed

¼ teaspoon white vinegar
2 large eggs
2 slices whole wheat bread
⅓ oz unsalted pistachio kernels,
  roughly chopped
1 small handful chopped fresh parsley
  or micro herbs

Preheat the oven to 350°F (325°F convection) and line a baking sheet with baking paper.

Place the pumpkin on the lined baking sheet and spray lightly with oil. Season with allspice, salt, and pepper, if desired. Bake in the oven for 20–25 minutes or until lightly browned and tender, using tongs to turn the pumpkin halfway through the cooking time.

Place the pumpkin in a small bowl and roughly mash using a potato masher or fork. Add the feta and mix gently to combine.

Meanwhile, spray a non-stick fry pan with oil and heat over medium–low heat. Add the mushrooms and garlic and cook for 6–7 minutes or until the mushrooms are tender and juicy, stirring occasionally. Season with salt and pepper, if desired.

Add 3 inches of water to a saucepan. Add the vinegar and bring to the boil over medium heat, then reduce the heat to medium–low.

Break the eggs into the water and cook for 2–3 minutes for a semi-soft yolk or 3–4 minutes for a firm yolk. Remove the eggs from the water using a slotted spoon and allow to drain on paper towel.

Toast the bread to your liking.

To serve, place the toast on a serving plate, spread over the pumpkin and feta smash, and top with the mushroom mixture and poached eggs. Sprinkle over the pistachios and parsley or micro herbs.

Zucchini & Feta Fritter Burger

SERVES 1 | **PREP TIME** 10 MINUTES, PLUS 30 MINUTES CHILLING TIME
COOKING TIME 10 MINUTES | **DIFFICULTY** EASY

½ medium zucchini

2¾ oz tinned cannellini beans, drained and rinsed

1 oz salt-reduced low-fat feta cheese, crumbled

1 large egg, lightly whisked

½ teaspoon finely grated lemon zest

¼ teaspoon baking powder

1 teaspoon chopped fresh dill

sea salt and ground black pepper, to taste

oil spray

1 oz avocado

1 medium whole wheat roll

1 small handful lettuce leaves

¼ small red onion, thinly sliced

Grate the zucchini and, using your hands, squeeze out as much liquid from the zucchini as possible. Transfer to a mixing bowl.

Place the cannellini beans in a small bowl and mash with a fork until a smooth paste has formed. Place the cannellini paste, feta, egg, lemon zest, baking powder, dill, salt, and pepper in the mixing bowl with the zucchini and mix until well combined.

Shape the zucchini mixture into two even patties. Place on a plate, cover with plastic wrap, and refrigerate for 30 minutes.

Lightly spray a non-stick fry pan with oil and heat over medium–high heat. Add the patties and cook for 2–3 minutes on each side or until golden and cooked through. Remove from the heat. Cover with foil and set aside.

Meanwhile, place the avocado in a small bowl and roughly mash using a fork. Season with salt and pepper, if desired.

To serve, cut the bread roll in half and toast lightly in a toaster or under a hot oven grill. On the bottom half of the roll, layer the smashed avocado, lettuce, zucchini and feta fritters, and onion. Top with the other half of the roll.

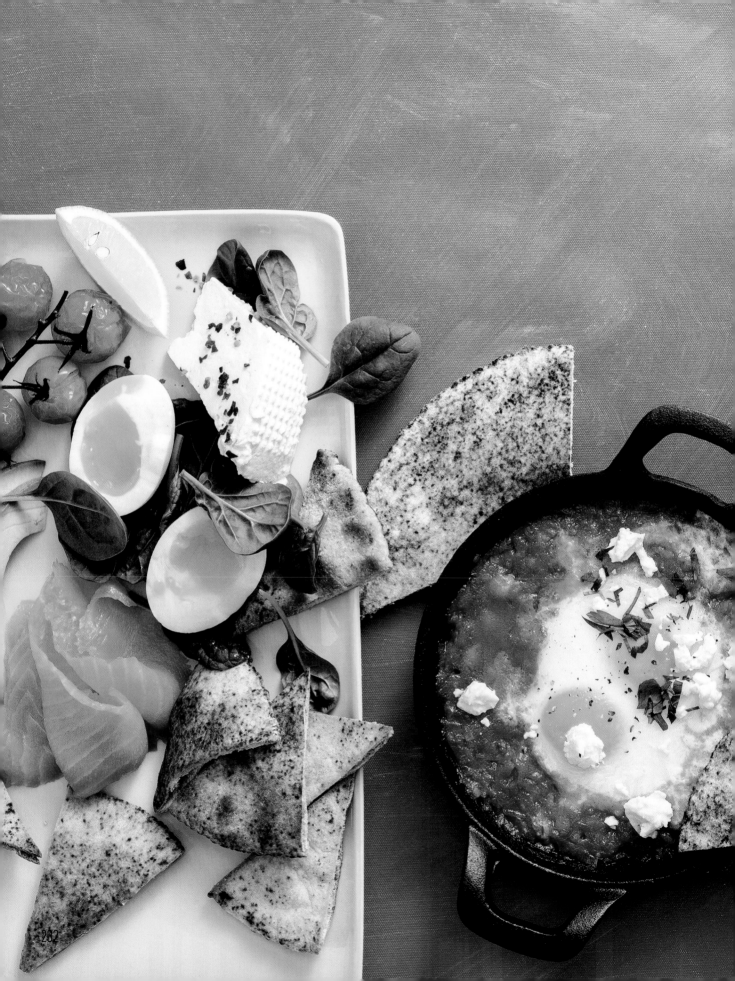

Breakfast Mezze

SERVES 1 | **PREP TIME** 5 MINUTES
COOKING TIME 15 MINUTES | **DIFFICULTY** EASY

1 whole wheat pita bread,
 cut into wedges
oil spray
1 teaspoon ground sumac
1 large egg
5 cherry tomatoes
½ garlic clove, crushed
1 tablespoon chopped
 fresh basil leaves

1 oz avocado, sliced
1 small handful baby
 spinach leaves
1½ oz smoked salmon
1¾ oz low-fat ricotta cheese
pinch of dried chilli flakes
lemon wedge, to serve

Preheat the oven to 400°F (350°F convection) and line a baking sheet with baking paper. Lay the pita wedges in a single layer on the lined baking sheet and spray lightly with oil spray. Bake in the oven for 5 minutes or until they begin to colour. Turn the wedges over, lightly spray with oil and sprinkle with the sumac. Bake for a further 5–8 minutes or until both sides are lightly coloured. Set aside to cool.

Meanwhile, place the egg in a small saucepan and fill with cold water until it is covered by 1 inch. Bring the water to the boil over high heat. Reduce the heat to low and simmer, covered, for 4–5 minutes. Remove the egg from the pan with a slotted spoon and place in a bowl of iced water. Leave for 1 minute. Tap the egg gently on the bench to crack the shell and peel. Cut the egg in half.

Lightly spray a non-stick fry pan with oil and heat over medium–high heat. Add the tomatoes and cook for 2–3 minutes or until they start to soften and the skin begins to wrinkle, shaking the pan frequently. Add the garlic and cook for 1 minute or until fragrant, shaking the pan frequently. Remove from the heat and gently stir in the basil.

To serve, place the spiced pita wedges, egg, tomatoes, avocado, spinach, salmon, and ricotta on a serving plate. Sprinkle the chilli flakes over the ricotta and serve with a lemon wedge on the side.

Baked Eggs

SERVES 1 | **PREP TIME** 10 MINUTES
COOKING TIME 35 MINUTES | **DIFFICULTY** EASY

oil spray
1½ teaspoons olive oil
¼ small brown onion,
 finely diced
½ garlic clove, crushed
½ teaspoon smoked paprika
¼ teaspoon ground cumin
2¾ oz tinned crushed
 tomatoes
⅔ oz tinned chickpeas,
 drained and rinsed

sea salt and ground
 black pepper, to taste
2 large eggs
1 whole wheat pita bread
1 oz salt-reduced low-fat
 feta cheese, crumbled
2 teaspoons chopped
 fresh parsley

Preheat the oven to 350°F (325°F convection) and spray a 6 inch ramekin with oil.

Heat the olive oil in a non-stick fry pan over medium heat. Add the onion and cook for 5–7 minutes or until soft and translucent, stirring frequently. Add the garlic, paprika, and ground cumin and cook for 1 minute or until fragrant, stirring constantly.

Add the crushed tomatoes, chickpeas, and ¼ cup (60 ml) of water and bring to the boil. Reduce the heat to medium–low and simmer for 12–15 minutes or until thickened, stirring occasionally. Season with salt and pepper, if desired, and transfer to the prepared ramekin.

Make two indents in the sauce mixture and gently crack an egg into each.

Bake in the oven for 8–10 minutes or until the eggs are cooked to your liking. Remove from the oven and set aside to cool slightly.

Meanwhile, wrap the pita bread in foil and place in the oven for 5 minutes to warm through. Cut into wedges.

To serve, sprinkle the feta and chopped parsley over the baked eggs and serve with the pita wedges on the side.

Quinoa Sushi

SERVES 1 | **PREP TIME** 15 MINUTES, PLUS 15 MINUTES COOLING AND STANDING TIME
COOKING TIME 15 MINUTES | **DIFFICULTY** MEDIUM

1 oz quinoa

¼ teaspoon ground turmeric

2 nori sheets

3½ oz tinned tuna in springwater,
 drained

½ Lebanese cucumber, cut into
 matchsticks (julienned)

½ medium carrot, cut into matchsticks
 (julienned)

½ small beetroot, cut into matchsticks
 (julienned)

1 small handful snow pea sprouts

salt-reduced tamari or soy sauce,
 for dipping

Bring the quinoa, turmeric, and ½ cup (125 ml) of water to the boil in a small
saucepan over high heat, stirring occasionally. Reduce the heat to low and
simmer, covered, for 10–12 minutes or until the quinoa is tender. Set aside
to cool.

Place a sushi mat on a clean chopping board with the slats running
horizontally. Place one nori sheet on the mat, shiny side down. Spoon half the
cooked quinoa onto the bottom two-thirds of the nori sheet, leaving a small
border around the edge. Top with half the tuna, cucumber, carrot, beetroot,
and snow pea sprouts. Hold the filling in place while rolling the mat over to
enclose the filling, gently pulling the mat as you go. Continue to roll until the
filling is covered with the nori sheet. Shape your hands around the mat to
gently tighten the roll.

Repeat with the remaining nori sheet and filling ingredients to make two rolls
in total. Leave the rolls to sit for 2 minutes, then cut into thick rounds with
a sharp knife.

To serve, place the sushi on a serving plate and serve with a small dish of
tamari or soy sauce for dipping.

Vietnamese Shrimp Salad

SERVES 1 | **PREP TIME** 15 MINUTES, PLUS 10 MINUTES SOAKING TIME
COOKING TIME 5 MINUTES | **DIFFICULTY** EASY

1¾ oz rice vermicelli noodles
oil spray
10 medium raw shrimp, peeled and deveined, tails intact
½ medium carrot, cut into matchsticks
½ Lebanese cucumber, cut into matchsticks
1 small handful bean sprouts
8 green beans, ends trimmed, finely chopped
1 tablespoon chopped fresh cilantro
1 tablespoon chopped fresh mint

NUOC CHAM DRESSING
2 teaspoons honey
2 teaspoons fish sauce
juice of ½ lime
¼ fresh red chilli, seeds removed, finely chopped
¼ garlic clove, crushed

To make the nuoc cham dressing, whisk the honey, fish sauce, lime juice, chilli, and garlic together in a small bowl.

Place the noodles in a heatproof bowl and cover with boiling water. Leave for 10 minutes, then loosen the noodles with a fork. Drain and refresh under cool running water. Drain well.

Heat a non-stick fry pan over medium–high heat and spray lightly with oil spray. Add the shrimp and cook for 2–3 minutes or until they change colour and are cooked through, stirring frequently. Transfer to a plate and set aside to rest.

Place the noodles, shrimp, carrot, cucumber, bean sprouts, beans, cilantro, and mint in a large bowl. Drizzle over the dressing and toss gently to combine, then serve.

Chicken Pita Pocket

SERVES 1 | **PREP TIME** 5 MINUTES
COOKING TIME 20 MINUTES | **DIFFICULTY** EASY

oil spray
3½ oz boneless, skinless chicken breast, thinly sliced
¼ small brown onion, thinly sliced
4½ oz mushrooms, sliced
½ teaspoon dried thyme
1 small handful arugula leaves
sea salt and ground black pepper, to taste
1 tablespoon chopped fresh parsley
½ whole wheat pita bread

Heat a small non-stick fry pan over medium heat and spray lightly with oil spray. Add the chicken and cook for 3–4 minutes or until browned and cooked through. Transfer to a heatproof bowl and set aside.

Wipe the fry pan clean, reheat over medium heat and spray lightly with oil spray. Add the onion and cook for 3–5 minutes or until soft and translucent. Add the mushrooms and thyme and cook for 5–6 minutes or until tender and juicy. Add the arugula and cook for a further minute or until slightly wilted. Season with salt and pepper, if desired.

Place the arugula and mushroom mixture, chicken, and parsley in a mixing bowl and toss gently to combine.

To serve, fill the pita pocket with the chicken and mushroom mixture.

Moroccan Lamb & Chickpea Salad

SERVES 1 | **PREP TIME** 20 MINUTES, PLUS 5 MINUTES RESTING TIME
COOKING TIME 10 MINUTES | **DIFFICULTY** EASY

3 oz lean lamb leg steaks
5 cherry tomatoes, halved
1¼ oz tinned chickpeas, drained and rinsed
¼ small red onion, thinly sliced
1 small handful baby spinach leaves
⅔ oz salt-reduced low-fat feta cheese, crumbled
1 tablespoon chopped fresh cilantro
1 tablespoon chopped fresh mint
1 whole wheat pita bread

MOROCCAN SEASONING
¼ teaspoon cayenne pepper
¼ teaspoon ground cinnamon
¼ teaspoon ground cumin
¼ teaspoon ground coriander
¼ teaspoon smoked paprika
sea salt, to taste
½ garlic clove, crushed
lemon juice, to taste

TZATZIKI
¼ Lebanese cucumber
1¾ oz low-fat plain yoghurt
lemon juice, to taste
½ garlic clove, crushed
½ teaspoon finely chopped fresh dill
sea salt and ground black pepper, to taste

To make the Moroccan seasoning, whisk the ground spices, salt, garlic, and lemon juice together in a small bowl.

Place the lamb and the Moroccan seasoning in a bowl and gently toss to combine. Ensure that the lamb is well coated in the seasoning.

Heat a barbecue grill-plate or chargrill pan over high heat. Add the lamb and grill for 4–5 minutes on each side or until cooked to your liking. Transfer to a plate, cover with foil, and allow to rest for 5 minutes. Slice the lamb against the grain.

To make the tzatziki, peel the cucumber, cut in half horizontally and remove the seeds by scraping a spoon down the middle. Grate the flesh and squeeze out any excess water. Place the cucumber, yoghurt, lemon juice, garlic, dill, salt, and pepper in a small bowl and mix until well combined.

Place the tomatoes, chickpeas, onion, spinach, feta, cilantro, and mint in a mixing bowl and toss gently to combine.

Meanwhile, warm the pita bread on a chargrill over medium–high heat for 30 seconds on each side. Remove from the heat and cut in half.

To serve, place the chickpea salad on a serving plate and top with the lamb. Drizzle over the tzatziki and serve with the pita bread on the side.

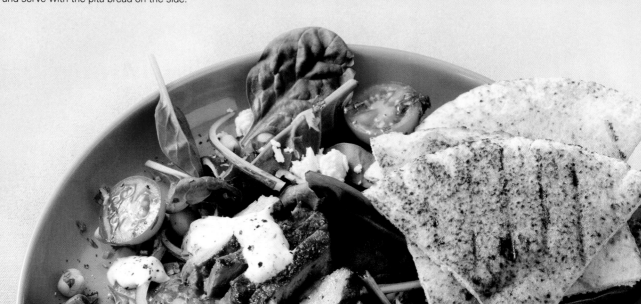

Club Sandwich

SERVES 1 | **PREP TIME** 10 MINUTES | **COOKING TIME** 10 MINUTES | **DIFFICULTY** EASY

3½ oz boneless, skinless chicken breast, thinly sliced

sea salt and ground black pepper, to taste

oil spray

2 slices whole wheat bread

2 oz low-fat cottage cheese

2 teaspoons chopped fresh chives

1 small handful lettuce leaves

¼ medium carrot, grated

½ medium tomato, sliced

¼ small red onion, chopped

Place the chicken between two pieces of plastic wrap and tenderise using a meat tenderiser. Season with salt and pepper, if desired.

Lightly spray a non-stick fry pan with oil spray and heat over medium heat. Add the chicken and cook for 3–4 minutes on each side or until cooked through. Transfer to a plate and rest for 2–3 minutes. Cut into thin slices.

Meanwhile, toast the bread to your liking. Cut each slice in half to form two triangles.

Place the cottage cheese and chives in a small bowl and mix to combine.

To serve, place one of the toasted triangles on a serving plate and add the lettuce and carrot, followed by another toasted triangle. Spread over half the cottage cheese and add the chicken, followed by another toasted triangle. Layer the tomato and onion. Spread the remaining cottage cheese over the remaining toasted triangle and place on top of the assembled club sandwich, cheese side down. Pierce the sandwich with a bamboo skewer to hold it together.

B

Mini Quiche & Salad

SERVES 1 | **PREP TIME** 10 MINUTES, PLUS 5 MINUTES COOLING TIME
COOKING TIME 25 MINUTES | **DIFFICULTY** EASY

oil spray
2 slices whole wheat bread
¼ small brown onion, finely diced
¼ medium red bell pepper,
  seeds removed, diced
1 oz mushroom sliced
2 large eggs
¼ cup (60 ml) low-fat milk
sea salt and ground black pepper,
  to taste

⅓ oz low-fat cheddar cheese, grated
1 small handful lettuce leaves,
  chopped

DRESSING

¼ teaspoon Dijon mustard
¼ teaspoon white vinegar
lemon juice, to taste

Preheat the oven to 325°F (285°F convection) and lightly spray 2 cups in
a 6-cup muffin tin with oil spray.

Trim the crusts off the bread and, using a rolling pin, gently roll out until
⅛ inch thick. Use a 4 or 5 inch round pastry cutter to cut out disks from the
bread slices. Line the prepared muffin cups with the bread disks.

Lightly spray a non-stick fry pan with oil and heat over medium heat. Add
the onion, bell pepper, and mushroom and cook for 6–7 minutes or until the
pepper is soft and the mushroom is tender. Remove from the heat and
set aside to cool slightly.

Whisk the eggs, milk, salt, and pepper together in a small bowl.

Divide the mushroom mixture and cheese evenly between the bread cups
and pour over the egg mixture. Bake in the oven for 15 minutes or until golden
brown and just set.

To make the dressing, whisk the mustard, vinegar, lemon juice, and
1 tablespoon of water together in a small bowl.

Place the lettuce in a mixing bowl, drizzle over the dressing, and toss gently
to combine.

To serve, place the mini quiches on a plate with the lettuce salad on the side.

Roast Pumpkin Pasta Salad

SERVES 1 | **PREP TIME** 10 MINUTES, PLUS 10 MINUTES COOLING TIME
COOKING TIME 25 MINUTES | **DIFFICULTY** EASY

2 oz pumpkin, peeled and cut into
 1 in cubes
oil spray
sea salt and ground black pepper,
 to taste
3 oz whole wheat pasta
¼ small red onion, finely chopped
5 cherry tomatoes, halved
1 small handful arugula leaves
5¼ oz tinned chickpeas,
 drained and rinsed
1 oz salt-reduced low-fat feta cheese,
 crumbled

DRESSING

1 teaspoon white vinegar
½ garlic clove, crushed
2 teaspoons finely chopped
 fresh basil
2 teaspoons finely chopped
 fresh parsley
sea salt and ground black pepper,
 to taste

Preheat the oven to 350°F (325°F convection) and line a baking sheet with baking paper.

Place the pumpkin on the lined baking sheet and spray lightly with oil spray. Season with salt and pepper, if desired. Roast in the oven for 20–25 minutes or until the pumpkin is tender and lightly browned, turning with tongs every 10 minutes. Set aside to cool.

Meanwhile, fill a large saucepan with water, add a pinch of salt, and bring to a boil. Add the pasta and cook until al dente (see the pasta packet for the recommended cooking time). Drain and refresh under cool running water. Set aside to cool.

To save time, the pasta and pumpkin can be cooked the night before and stored in an airtight container in the refrigerator.

To make the dressing, whisk the vinegar, garlic, basil, parsley, salt, pepper, and 1 tablespoon of water together in a small bowl.

Place the pumpkin, onion, tomatoes, arugula, chickpeas, and pasta in a mixing bowl. Drizzle over the dressing and toss gently to combine.

To serve, place the roast pumpkin pasta salad in a serving bowl and sprinkle over the feta.

Chicken & Couscous Salad

SERVES 1 | **PREP TIME** 10 MINUTES | **COOKING TIME** 15 MINUTES | **DIFFICULTY** EASY

2 oz pearl couscous

3 asparagus spears, trimmed

3 oz roast chicken, chopped

1 scallion, thinly sliced

1 small handful baby spinach leaves

finely grated zest and juice of ½ lemon

1 tablespoon chopped fresh mint

1 tablespoon chopped fresh basil

sea salt and ground black pepper,
 to taste

Fill a saucepan with water and bring to a boil. Stir in the pearl couscous and simmer over medium heat for 10–12 minutes or until al dente. Drain and set aside to cool.

Meanwhile, heat a non-stick fry pan over medium–high heat. Add the asparagus and cook for 3–5 minutes or until it starts to change colour and is the desired tenderness. Allow to cool slightly, then cut the spears in half.

Place the couscous, asparagus, chicken, scallion, spinach, lemon zest, and lemon juice, mint and basil in a mixing bowl. Season with salt and pepper, if desired, and toss gently to combine.

To serve, place the chicken and couscous salad in a serving bowl.

Chicken Skewers with Vietnamese Noodle Salad

SERVES 1 | **PREP TIME** 15 MINUTES, PLUS 40 MINUTES SOAKING AND MARINATING TIME
COOKING TIME 10 MINUTES | **DIFFICULTY** EASY

2 teaspoons rice wine vinegar

1 teaspoon fish sauce

1 teaspoon honey

3½ oz boneless, skinless chicken breast, cut into strips

3½ oz rice vermicelli noodles

oil spray

¼ medium carrot, cut into matchsticks

¼ Lebanese cucumber, cut into matchsticks

¼ medium red bell pepper, seeds removed, thinly sliced

½ scallion, thinly sliced

⅔ oz snow peas, trimmed and thinly sliced

1 small handful fresh cilantro leaves

1 small handful fresh mint leaves

DRESSING

2 teaspoons honey

2 teaspoons fish sauce

juice of ½ lime

¼ fresh red chilli, seeds removed, finely chopped

½ garlic clove, crushed

Soak two wooden skewers in cold water for 30 minutes. This will help stop the skewers from burning during cooking.

Whisk the vinegar, fish sauce, and honey together in a bowl, add the chicken and turn to coat. Cover with plastic wrap and place in the refrigerator for 10 minutes.

Meanwhile, place the noodles in a heatproof bowl and cover with boiling water. Leave for 10 minutes, then loosen the noodles with a fork. Drain and refresh under cool running water. Drain well and set aside to cool.

Preheat a barbecue grill-plate or chargrill pan over medium–high heat. Thread the chicken onto the skewers. Lightly spray with oil and grill for 6–8 minutes or until cooked through, turning frequently.

To make the dressing, whisk the ingredients together in a small bowl.

Place the noodles, carrot, cucumber, bell pepper, scallion, snow peas, cilantro, and mint in a mixing bowl. Drizzle over the dressing and toss gently to combine. To serve, place the noodle salad on a serving plate and top with the chicken skewers.

Moroccan Beef Bowl

SERVES 1 | **PREP TIME** 15 MINUTES, PLUS 10 MINUTES COOLING TIME
COOKING TIME 20 MINUTES | **DIFFICULTY** EASY

3 oz lean beef strips

2 oz pearl couscous

oil spray

½ medium carrot, grated

¼ small red onion, thinly sliced

1 small handful baby spinach leaves

¼ small fennel bulb, thinly sliced

3 cherry tomatoes, halved

1 tablespoon fresh cilantro leaves

1 lemon wedge

MOROCCAN SEASONING

¼ teaspoon cayenne pepper

¼ teaspoon ground cinnamon

¼ teaspoon ground cumin

¼ teaspoon ground coriander

¼ teaspoon smoked paprika

1 teaspoon sea salt

½ garlic clove, crushed

juice of ½ lemon

DRESSING

finely grated zest and juice of ½ medium orange

juice of ½ lemon

1 tablespoon chopped fresh cilantro

sea salt and ground black pepper, to taste

To make the Moroccan seasoning, whisk the ground spices, salt, garlic, and lemon juice together in a medium bowl. Place the beef in the bowl and rub with the spice mix. Ensure that all the beef is coated. Cover with plastic wrap and refrigerate for 30 minutes to marinate. Alternatively, leave to marinate overnight.

To make the dressing, whisk the orange zest and juice, lemon juice, cilantro, salt, pepper, and 1 teaspoon of water together in a small bowl.

Fill a saucepan with water and bring to a boil. Stir in the pearl couscous and simmer over medium heat for 10–12 minutes or until al dente. Drain and set aside to cool. Once cooled, drizzle over half the dressing and toss gently to combine.

Lightly spray a non-stick fry pan with oil and heat over medium–high heat. Add the beef strips and cook for 3–5 minutes or until browned and cooked to your liking, stirring frequently. Set aside to cool slightly.

To serve, arrange the carrot, onion, spinach, fennel, and tomatoes in a serving bowl and drizzle over the remaining dressing. Top with the pearl couscous and Moroccan spiced beef and scatter over the cilantro. Serve with a lemon wedge on the side.

Chicken & Soba Noodle Soup

SERVES 1 | **PREP TIME** 10 MINUTES, PLUS 5 MINUTES COOLING TIME
COOKING TIME 25 MINUTES | **DIFFICULTY** EASY

3½ oz soba noodles
1 cup (250 ml) salt-reduced chicken stock
3½ oz boneless, skinless chicken breast
½ in piece fresh ginger, peeled and grated
¼ lemongrass stalk, halved lengthways

1 tablespoon fish sauce
1¾ oz shiitake mushrooms
1 scallion, thinly sliced
1½ oz snow peas, trimmed and thinly sliced
1 nori sheet, finely shredded

Fill a large saucepan with water, add a pinch of salt, and bring to a boil. Add the noodles and cook for 7–8 minutes. Drain and place in a bowl of cold water. Using your hands, vigorously rub the noodles together—this will help to wash off the excess starch and separate the noodles. Refresh under cold water and drain well.

Place the stock and 1 cup (250 ml) of water in a medium saucepan and bring to the boil over medium–high heat. Add the chicken and return to the boil. Reduce the heat to medium–low and simmer for 10–12 minutes or until cooked through. Remove the chicken using a slotted spoon and set aside to cool slightly. When cool enough to handle, cut into thick slices.

Add the ginger, lemongrass, fish sauce, mushroom, scallion, and snow peas to the stock and simmer for 5 minutes or until the vegetables are cooked, stirring occasionally.

Meanwhile, pour boiling water over the noodles to reheat. Drain well.

To serve, place the warmed noodles in a serving bowl and top with the sliced chicken. Carefully pour over the vegetables and broth. Scatter over the nori.

Savoury French Toast

SERVES 1 | **PREP TIME** 5 MINUTES | **COOKING TIME** 15 MINUTES | **DIFFICULTY** EASY

oil spray

8 cherry tomatoes, halved

1 large egg

¼ cup (60 ml) low-fat milk

½ garlic clove, crushed

2 teaspoons chopped fresh parsley

sea salt and ground black pepper, to taste

1 slice whole wheat bread

1 large handful baby spinach leaves

⅓ oz parmesan cheese, grated

Lightly spray a non-stick fry pan with oil and heat over medium–high heat. Add the tomatoes and cook for 2–3 minutes or until they start to soften and the skin begins to wrinkle, shaking the pan frequently. Transfer to a bowl, cover with foil, and set aside.

Whisk the egg, milk, garlic, parsley, salt, and pepper together in a bowl.

Wipe the pan clean. Lightly spray with oil spray and reheat over medium heat.

Dip the bread in the egg mixture, coating evenly. Shake off any excess mixture. Add to the pan and cook for 4–5 minutes on each side or until lightly browned.

To serve, top the French toast with the spinach and tomatoes. Sprinkle over the parmesan cheese.

Chicken Salad Basket

SERVES 1 | **PREP TIME** 10 MINUTES, PLUS 10 MINUTES COOLING TIME
COOKING TIME 15 MINUTES | **DIFFICULTY** EASY

1 medium corn tortilla

oil spray

1½ oz roast chicken, shredded

1 small handful lettuce leaves, chopped

1½ oz tinned red kidney beans, drained and rinsed

¼ small red onion, finely diced

3 cherry tomatoes, quartered

¾ oz tinned corn kernels, drained and rinsed

¾ oz low-fat cheddar cheese, grated

DRESSING

1 teaspoon lemon juice, to taste

pinch of dried chilli flakes

2 teaspoons finely chopped fresh cilantro

Preheat the oven to 375°F (340°F convection).

Wrap the tortilla in foil and place in the oven for 10 minutes to warm. (Alternatively, wrap the tortilla in a damp paper towel and warm it for 30 seconds in the microwave.) Lightly spray both sides of the warmed tortilla with oil. Turn a muffin tin upside down. Nestle the tortilla between 4 cups to form a basket. Bake in the oven for 10–12 minutes or until firm and lightly toasted. Remove from the oven and transfer to a wire rack to cool.

To make the dressing, whisk the lemon juice, chilli flakes, cilantro, and 2 teaspoons of water together in a small bowl.

Place the chicken, lettuce, kidney beans, onion, tomatoes, corn, and cheese in a mixing bowl. Drizzle over the dressing and toss gently to combine.

To serve, place the tortilla basket on a plate and fill with the chicken salad.

Zesty Jar Salad

SERVES 1 | **PREP TIME** 10 MINUTES | **COOKING TIME** 15 MINUTES | **DIFFICULTY** EASY

1 oz quinoa

1 medium carrot, spiralised

2¾ oz tinned chickpeas, drained
and rinsed

1 oz salt-reduced low-fat feta
cheese, crumbled

1 small handful baby spinach leaves

DRESSING

2 teaspoons lime juice

2 teaspoons finely chopped fresh mint

2 teaspoons finely chopped fresh
cilantro, plus extra to garnish

1 teaspoon honey

sea salt and ground black pepper,
to taste

Bring the quinoa and ½ cup (125 ml) of water to a boil in a small
saucepan over high heat, stirring occasionally. Reduce the heat to low
and simmer, covered, for 10–12 minutes or until the quinoa is tender.
Drain off any excess liquid. To save time, the quinoa can be cooked the
night before and stored in an airtight container in the refrigerator.

Meanwhile, to make the dressing, whisk the lime juice, mint, cilantro,
honey, and 1 tablespoon of water together in a small bowl. Season with
salt and pepper, if desired, and pour into the bottom of a mason jar.

Place the carrot and chickpeas in a bowl and toss gently to combine.
Place in the jar on top of the dressing.

Layer the quinoa, feta, spinach, and extra cilantro into the mason jar.

To serve, pour the contents of the mason jar into a serving bowl
and toss gently to combine.

Tuna & Chickpea Salad

SERVES 1 | **PREP TIME** 10 MINUTES, PLUS 10 MINUTES COOLING TIME **COOKING TIME** 25 MINUTES | **DIFFICULTY** EASY

1 oz brown rice

1½ oz tinned chickpeas, drained
   and rinsed

¼ small red onion, diced

¼ Lebanese cucumber, chopped

1 small handful arugula leaves

1¾ oz tinned tuna in springwater, drained

DRESSING

½ garlic clove, crushed

1 tablespoon finely chopped
   fresh parsley

2 teaspoons lemon juice

1½ oz low-fat sour cream

sea salt and ground black pepper, to taste

Bring the rice and ½ cup (125 ml) of water to the boil in a small saucepan over high heat, stirring occasionally. Reduce the heat to low and simmer, covered, for 20–25 minutes or until the liquid has been absorbed and the rice is tender. Remove from the heat and leave to stand, covered, for 5 minutes. Set aside to cool. To save time, the rice can be cooked the night before and stored in an airtight container in the refrigerator.

To make the dressing, whisk the garlic, parsley, lemon juice, and sour cream together in a small bowl. Season with salt and pepper, if desired.

Place the rice, chickpeas, onion, cucumber, arugula, and tuna in a serving bowl. Drizzle over the dressing to serve.

Pumpkin & Shrimp Laksa

SERVES 1 | **PREP TIME** 10 MINUTES, PLUS 10 MINUTES SOAKING TIME
COOKING TIME 20 MINUTES | **DIFFICULTY** EASY

3½ oz rice vermicelli noodles

1½ teaspoons olive oil

2 tablespoons laksa paste

4¼ oz pumpkin, peeled and cut
into ¾ in pieces

1 cup (250 ml) salt-reduced
vegetable stock

¼ cup (60 ml) light coconut milk

10 medium raw shrimp, peeled
and deveined, tails intact

1 teaspoon fish sauce

lime juice, to taste

1 small handful bean sprouts

1 scallion, sliced

1 small handful fresh cilantro

lime wedges, to serve

Place the noodles in a heatproof bowl and cover with boiling water. Leave for
10 minutes, then loosen the noodles with a fork. Drain and refresh under cool
running water. Drain well.

Meanwhile, heat the oil in a medium saucepan over medium heat. Add the
laksa paste and cook for 1 minute, stirring constantly. Add the pumpkin, stock,
and coconut milk and bring to a boil. Reduce the heat to medium–low and
simmer for 10–12 minutes or until the pumpkin is tender. If the laksa is too
thick towards the end of the cooking time, stir in a small amount of water.

Add the shrimp, fish sauce and lime juice and cook for 3–4 minutes or until the
shrimp change colour and are cooked through.

To serve, place the noodles in a serving bowl and pour over the pumpkin and
shrimp laksa. Top with the bean sprouts, scallion, and cilantro. Serve with lime
wedges on the side.

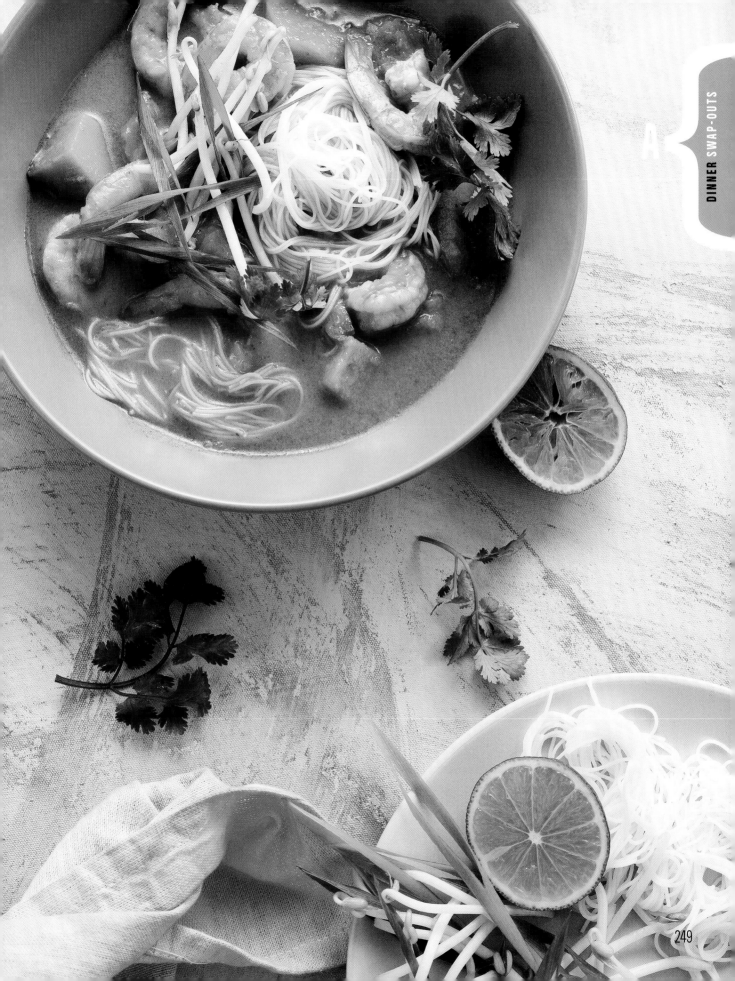

Greek Orzo & Chicken Salad

SERVES 1 | **PREP TIME** 15 MINUTES, PLUS 10 MINUTES COOLING TIME
COOKING TIME 20 MINUTES | **DIFFICULTY** EASY

3 oz orzo

3½ oz boneless, skinless chicken breast

¼ garlic clove, crushed

½ teaspoon dried oregano

finely grated zest and
  juice of ½ lemon

1½ teaspoons olive oil

oil spray

½ medium zucchini, thinly sliced
  into ribbons

1 small handful baby spinach leaves

3 cherry tomatoes, halved

¼ small red onion, chopped

4 kalamata olives, pitted, halved

DRESSING

1½ teaspoons olive oil

finely grated zest and juice of ½ lemon

¼ teaspoon Dijon mustard

sea salt and ground black pepper,
  to taste

Fill a large saucepan with water, add a pinch of salt, and bring to a boil. Add the orzo and cook until al dente (see the pasta packet for the recommended cooking time). Drain and refresh under cool running water. Set aside to cool. To save time, the orzo can be cooked the night before and stored in an airtight container in the refrigerator.

Meanwhile, slice the chicken in half horizontally to make two thin fillets and place in a medium bowl. Add the garlic, oregano, lemon zest and juice, and oil and toss to coat.

Heat a chargrill pan over medium–high heat and spray lightly with oil spray. Add the zucchini and cook for 1–2 minutes on each side or until tender and charred. Remove from the heat and set aside on a plate.

Cook the chicken in the same pan for 2–3 minutes each side or until cooked through and coloured. Remove from the heat and set aside to rest on a plate. When cool enough to handle, cut the chicken into slices.

To make the dressing, whisk the oil, lemon zest and juice, mustard, salt, and pepper together in a small bowl.

Place the orzo, zucchini, spinach, tomatoes, onion, and olives in a mixing bowl. Drizzle over the dressing and toss gently to combine.

To serve, place the orzo in a serving bowl and top with the sliced chicken.

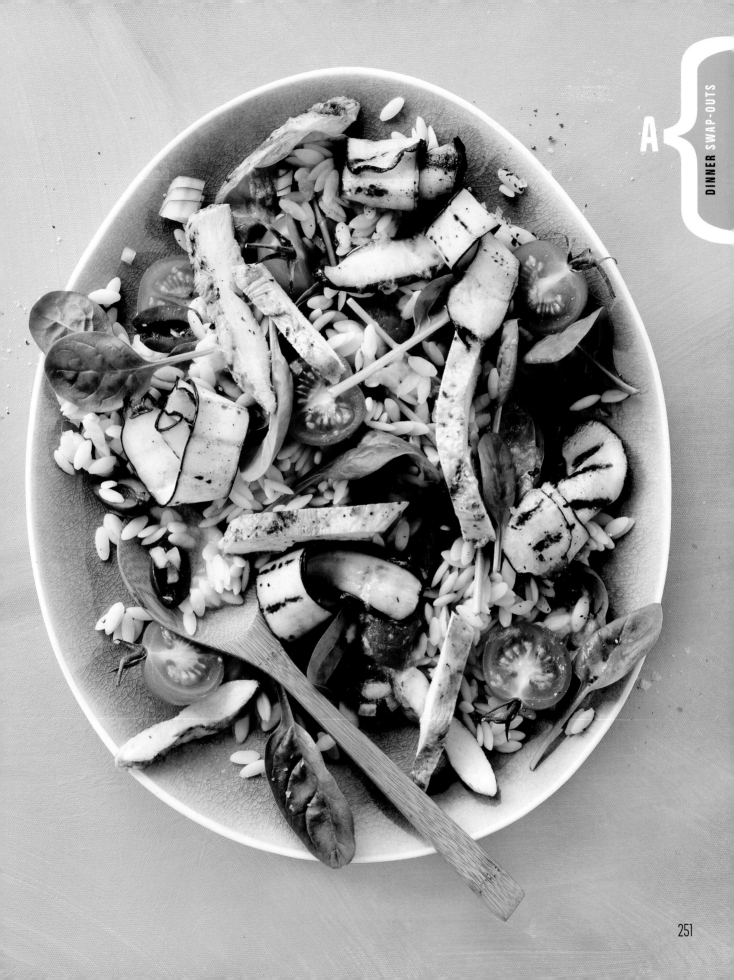

Gado Gado Bowl

SERVES 1 | **PREP TIME** 15 MINUTES, PLUS 10 MINUTES STANDING AND COOLING TIME
COOKING TIME 30 MINUTES | **DIFFICULTY** MEDIUM

2 oz brown rice

2 large eggs

8 green beans, trimmed

1 oz Chinese cabbage (wombok),
 shredded

fresh cilantro leaves, to garnish

½ medium carrot, cut into batons

¼ medium red bell pepper, seeds
 removed, thinly sliced

1 small handful bean sprouts

lime wedges, to serve

PEANUT SAUCE

1 tablespoon 100% natural peanut butter

½ teaspoon salt-reduced tamari
 or soy sauce

1 teaspoon pure maple syrup

½ garlic clove, crushed

lime juice, to taste

¼ teaspoon fish sauce

¼ fresh red chilli, seeds removed,
 finely chopped (optional)

sea salt and ground black pepper, to taste

Bring the rice and 1 cup (250 ml) of water to a boil in a small saucepan over high heat, stirring occasionally. Reduce the heat to low and simmer, covered, for 20–25 minutes or until the liquid has been absorbed and the rice is tender. Remove from the heat and leave to stand, covered, for 5 minutes. To save time, the rice can be cooked the night before and stored in an airtight container in the refrigerator.

Meanwhile, place the eggs in a small saucepan and fill with cold water until they are covered by ¾ inches. Bring the water to the boil over high heat. Reduce the heat to low and simmer, covered, for 7–8 minutes. Remove the eggs from the saucepan with a slotted spoon and place in a bowl of iced water. Leave for 1 minute. Tap the eggs gently on the bench to crack the shells, then peel and cut in half.

Add 2 inches of water to a saucepan and insert a steamer basket. Cover with a lid and bring the water to a boil over high heat, then reduce the heat to medium. Steam the beans and cabbage for 3–4 minutes or until just tender. Place in a bowl of iced water to stop them from cooking and set aside. When cool, drain and set aside.

To make the peanut sauce, whisk the peanut butter, tamari or soy sauce, maple syrup, garlic, lime juice, fish sauce, and chilli (if using) together in a small bowl. Season with salt and pepper, if desired. Add 2 teaspoons of water at a time until a thick but pourable consistency is reached. Adjust the seasoning if needed.

To serve, arrange the green beans, cilantro, cabbage, carrot, bell pepper, bean sprouts, and rice in a serving bowl and drizzle over the peanut sauce. Top with the egg and serve with lime wedges on the side.

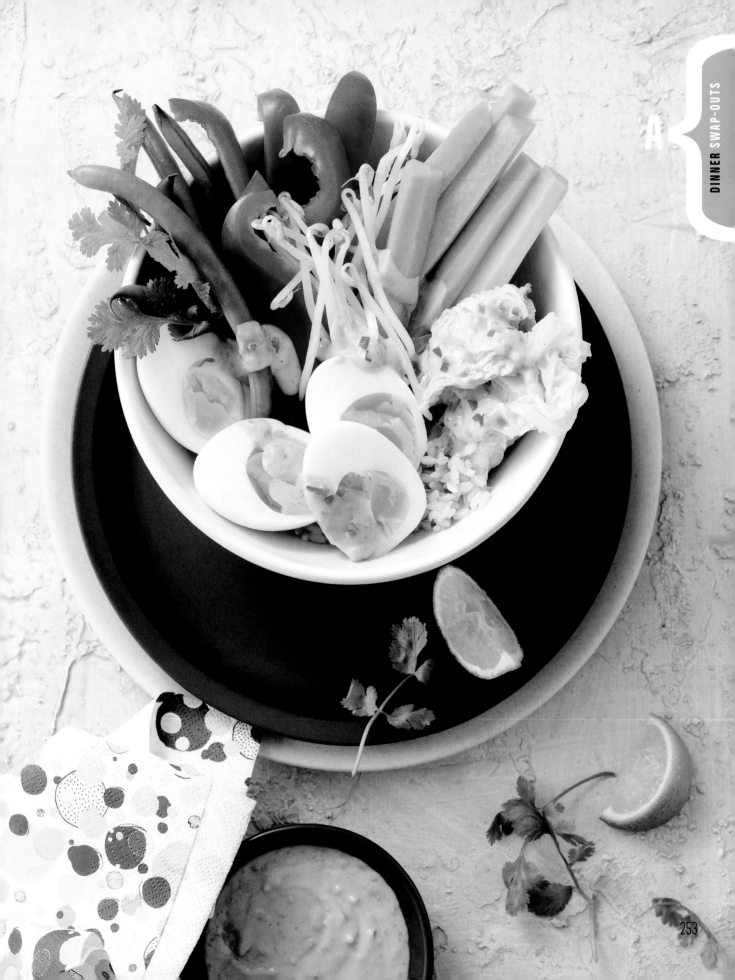

253

Seafood Stir-fry

SERVES 1 | **PREP TIME** 10 MINUTES, PLUS 15 MINUTES STANDING AND MARINATING TIME
COOKING TIME 25 MINUTES | **DIFFICULTY** EASY

2 oz brown rice
½ garlic clove, crushed
pinch of chilli powder
2 teaspoons salt-reduced tamari
  or soy sauce
1 teaspoon rice wine vinegar
2 teaspoons sesame seeds
4½ oz white fish fillet, skin removed,
  cut into 1 in cubes

1½ teaspoons sesame oil
1 scallion, sliced
¼ medium red bell pepper, seeds
  removed, thinly sliced
2 oz bok choy, chopped
1½ oz snow peas, trimmed and halved
fresh cilantro leaves, to garnish

Bring the rice and 1 cup (250 ml) of water to a boil in a small saucepan over high heat, stirring occasionally. Reduce the heat to low and simmer, covered, for 20–25 minutes or until the liquid has been absorbed and the rice is tender. Remove from the heat and leave to stand, covered, for 5 minutes.

Meanwhile, whisk the garlic, chilli powder, tamari or soy sauce, rice wine vinegar, half the sesame seeds, and 1 tablespoon of water together in a medium bowl. Add the fish cubes and turn to coat. Cover with plastic wrap and refrigerate for 10 minutes to marinate. Drain the fish and reserve the marinade.

Heat a large wok over high heat until hot. Add the oil and carefully swirl it around to coat the side of the wok. Add the fish and stir-fry for 1 minute. Add the scallion and bell pepper and stir-fry for 2 minutes. Add the reserved marinade, bok choy, and snow peas and continue to stir-fry for 2–3 minutes or until the fish is cooked through and the vegetables are tender.

To serve, place the rice in a serving bowl and top with the fish stir-fry. Garnish with cilantro leaves and the remaining sesame seeds.

Cauliflower & Lentil Pilaf

SERVES 1 | **PREP TIME** 10 MINUTES, PLUS 5 MINUTES STANDING TIME
COOKING TIME 30 MINUTES | **DIFFICULTY** EASY

oil spray
¼ small brown onion, diced
½ garlic clove, crushed
1 tablespoon korma curry paste
2 oz brown rice
3½ oz cauliflower, cut into florets
¾ cup (200 ml) salt-reduced vegetable
  stock

¾ oz frozen peas, thawed
5¼ oz tinned brown lentils,
  drained and rinsed
lemon juice, to taste
sea salt and ground black pepper,
  to taste
1 tablespoon chopped fresh parsley
¾ oz slivered almonds, toasted

Heat a large saucepan over medium heat and spray with oil spray. Add the
onion and cook for 5 minutes or until soft and translucent, stirring occasionally.

Add the garlic and korma curry paste and cook for 1 minute or until fragrant,
stirring constantly.

Add the rice and cauliflower and cook for 2 minutes, stirring frequently.

Stir in the stock and bring to a boil over high heat. Reduce the heat to low and
simmer, covered, for 15–20 minutes or until the liquid is absorbed and
the rice is tender. In the last 3–4 minutes of cooking time stir through the
peas and lentils. Remove from the heat and leave to stand for 5 minutes
before fluffing with a fork to separate the grains. Stir through the lemon juice
and season with salt and pepper, if desired.

To serve, place the pilaf in a serving bowl and sprinkle over the parsley and
slivered almonds.

Sweet Potato Gnocchi

SERVES 1 | **PREP TIME** 20 MINUTES, PLUS 15 MINUTES COOLING TIME
COOKING TIME 1 HOUR | **DIFFICULTY** MEDIUM

½ large sweet potato

pinch of ground nutmeg

sea salt and ground black pepper, to taste

⅓ oz whole wheat flour, plus extra
  for dusting

2¾ oz quinoa flour

oil spray

½ garlic clove, crushed

¼ teaspoon dried oregano

5¼ oz tinned lentils, drained and rinsed

2¾ oz tinned crushed tomatoes

¼ cup (65 ml) salt-reduced vegetable
  stock

1 small handful kale, chopped

juice of ¼ lemon

⅔ oz parmesan cheese, grated

Preheat the oven to 400°F (350°F convection) and line a baking sheet with baking paper.

Wrap the sweet potato in foil and place on the lined baking sheet. Roast for 45 minutes until tender. Once cool enough to handle, remove the foil carefully and peel the sweet potato. Transfer the flesh to a bowl and, using a potato masher, mash until smooth. Season with nutmeg, salt, and pepper, if desired, and mix until well combined. Set aside to cool completely.

Place the sweet potato on a clean work surface that has been lightly dusted with whole wheat flour. A little at a time, add the remaining whole wheat and quinoa flour and knead it in. Continue adding the flour and kneading until a firm dough has formed—it should not be sticky to the touch. Place half the dough on a lightly floured work surface and roll out to form a ¾-inch-thick log. Cut the log into ¾ inch pieces and gently press down on each piece with the back of a fork to make indents. Repeat with the remaining dough.

Fill a medium saucepan with water and bring to a boil. Add half the gnocchi to the water, wait until they float to the top and remove with a slotted spoon. Transfer to a lined baking sheet and repeat with the remaining gnocchi.

Meanwhile, lightly spray a small saucepan with oil and heat over medium heat. Add the garlic and oregano and cook for 1 minute or until fragrant, stirring constantly. Add the lentils, tomatoes, and stock, reduce the heat to medium–low and cook for 10–15 minutes or until the sauce reaches the desired consistency, stirring occasionally. Add the kale and lemon juice and cook, covered, for a further 5 minutes or until the kale has wilted, stirring occasionally. Season with salt and pepper, if desired.

To serve, place the sweet potato gnocchi in a serving bowl and top with the lentil and kale sauce. Sprinkle over the parmesan cheese.

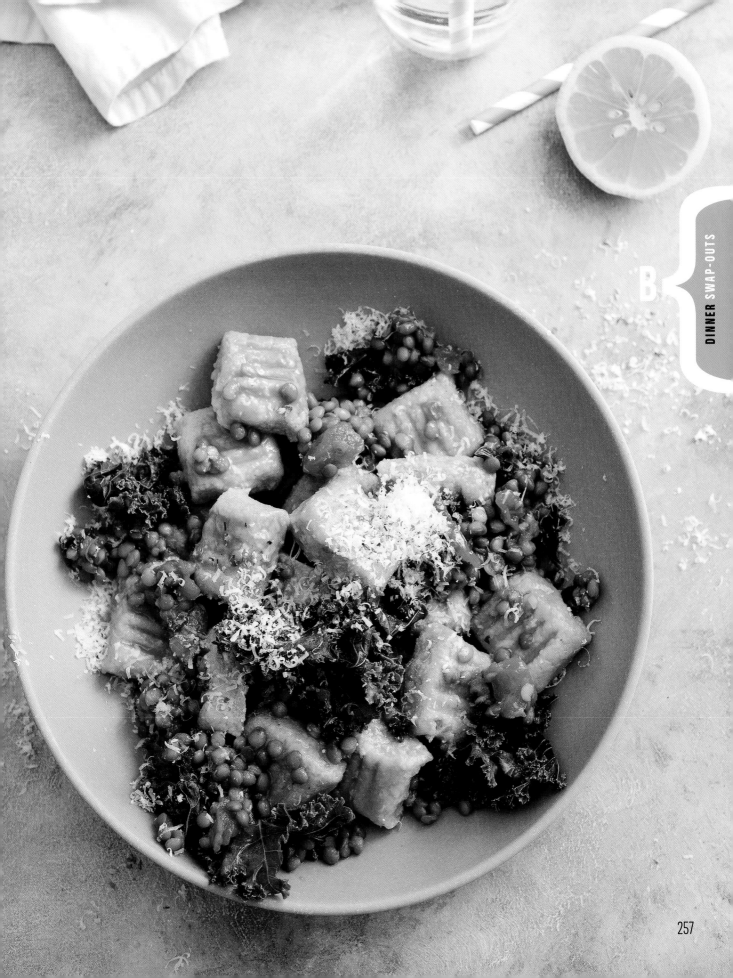

Beetroot & Goat's Cheese Tart

SERVES 1 | **PREP TIME** 10 MINUTES, PLUS 15 MINUTES COOLING TIME
COOKING TIME 50 MINUTES | **DIFFICULTY** MEDIUM

1¼ small beetroots
1 cup (225 ml) salt-reduced vegetable stock
2 oz polenta
2 large eggs, lightly whisked
1 teaspoon chopped fresh thyme
sea salt and ground black pepper, to taste
1 oz low-fat goat's cheese, crumbled
1 small handful arugula leaves

CARAMELISED ONION
oil spray
½ small red onion, sliced
2 teaspoons pure maple syrup
2 teaspoons balsamic vinegar

Preheat the oven to 350°F (325°F convection) and line a baking sheet with baking paper.

Wrap the beetroots in foil with 1 tablespoon of water (this helps the beetroot to steam). Place in a small roasting pan and bake in the oven for 30–40 minutes or until tender. Test the beetroot with a skewer—it is cooked if the skewer pierces the flesh easily. Set aside to cool. When cool enough to handle, peel the beetroot under cold running water, then slice.

Meanwhile, bring the stock to a simmer in a medium saucepan over medium heat. Pour in the polenta and cook for 5–7 minutes or until the polenta is very thick, stirring constantly with a wooden spoon. Ensure that all lumps have been beaten out. Remove from the heat, stir in the egg and thyme and season generously with salt and pepper. Allow to cool slightly.

Using a spatula, spread the polenta evenly into an oval shape on the lined baking sheet and bake for 15–20 minutes or until light golden and set.

Meanwhile, to make the caramelised onion, lightly spray a small non-stick fry pan with oil and heat over low heat. Add the sliced onion and cook slowly for 15–20 minutes or until soft and golden, stirring occasionally. Don't be tempted to increase the heat as this can cause the onion to burn. Add the maple syrup and balsamic vinegar and cook for a further 5–10 minutes or until sticky and caramelised, stirring occasionally. Set aside to cool.

Cover the polenta base with the cooked beetroot followed by the caramelised onion. Scatter over the goat's cheese and bake for a further 8–10 minutes or until the toppings are heated through and the cheese is softening and starting to colour.

To serve, place the beetroot and goat's cheese tart on a serving plate and top with the arugula.

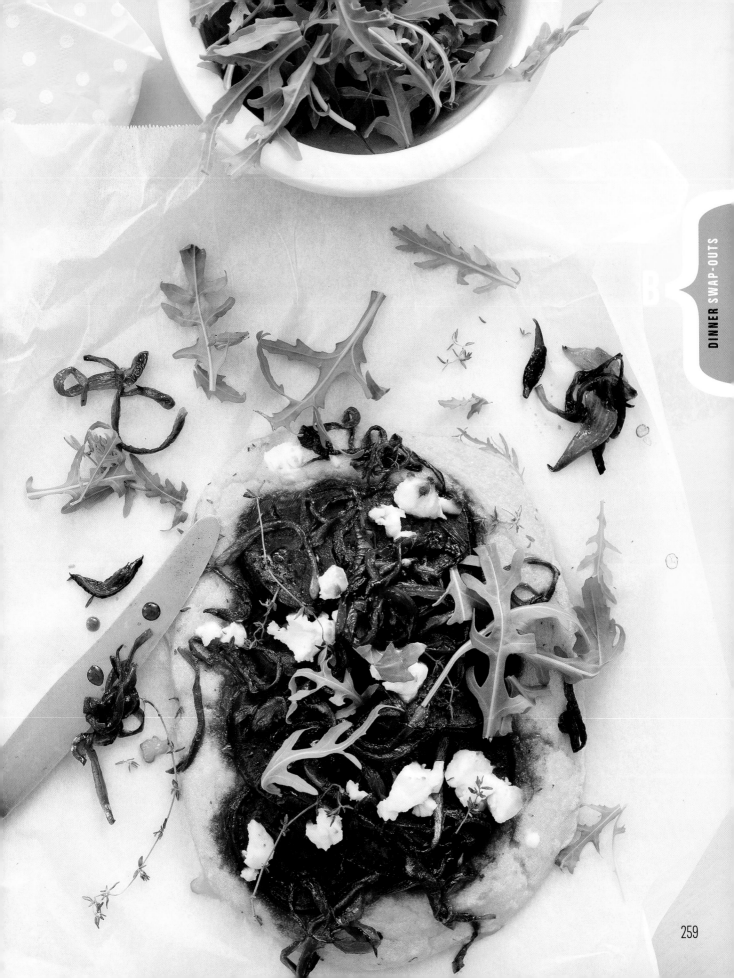

Pork & Corn Tacos

SERVES 1 | **PREP TIME** 10 MINUTES | **COOKING TIME** 25 MINUTES | **DIFFICULTY** EASY

3 oz pork tenderloin

oil spray

sea salt and ground black pepper, to taste

2 medium corn tortillas

3 oz red cabbage, shredded

2 teaspoons chopped fresh cilantro
 or micro herbs

lime wedges, to serve

3½ oz low-fat plain yoghurt, to serve

CORN SALSA

oil spray

2 oz frozen corn kernels, thawed

¼ small red onion, finely diced

1 tablespoon chopped fresh cilantro

juice of ¼ lime

¼ teaspoon jalapeño or fresh red chilli,
 seeds removed, chopped (optional)

sea salt and ground black pepper, to taste

Preheat the oven to 400°F (350°F convection) and line a baking sheet with baking paper.

Place the pork tenderloin on a plate and lightly spray with oil spray. Season with salt and pepper, if desired.

Heat a non-stick fry pan over medium–high heat. Add the pork and cook for 6–7 minutes or until lightly browned on all sides, turning every 2 minutes. Transfer to the lined baking sheet and roast in the oven for 8–10 minutes or until cooked to your liking, turning once during the cooking time. Transfer to a plate and leave to rest for 2 minutes. Cut into thin slices.

To make the corn salsa, wipe the fry pan clean, re-spray with oil spray and heat over medium heat. Add the corn kernels and cook for 3–5 minutes until lightly browned, stirring frequently. Remove from the heat and set aside to cool.

Place the corn, onion, cilantro, lime juice, and jalapeño or red chilli, if using, in a small bowl and toss gently to combine. Season with salt and pepper, if desired.

Warm the tortillas, one at a time, in a dry pan over medium heat for 15 seconds on each side.

To serve, place the tortillas on a serving plate. Top with the cabbage, pork, corn salsa, and cilantro or micro herbs. Serve with the lime wedges and yoghurt on the side.

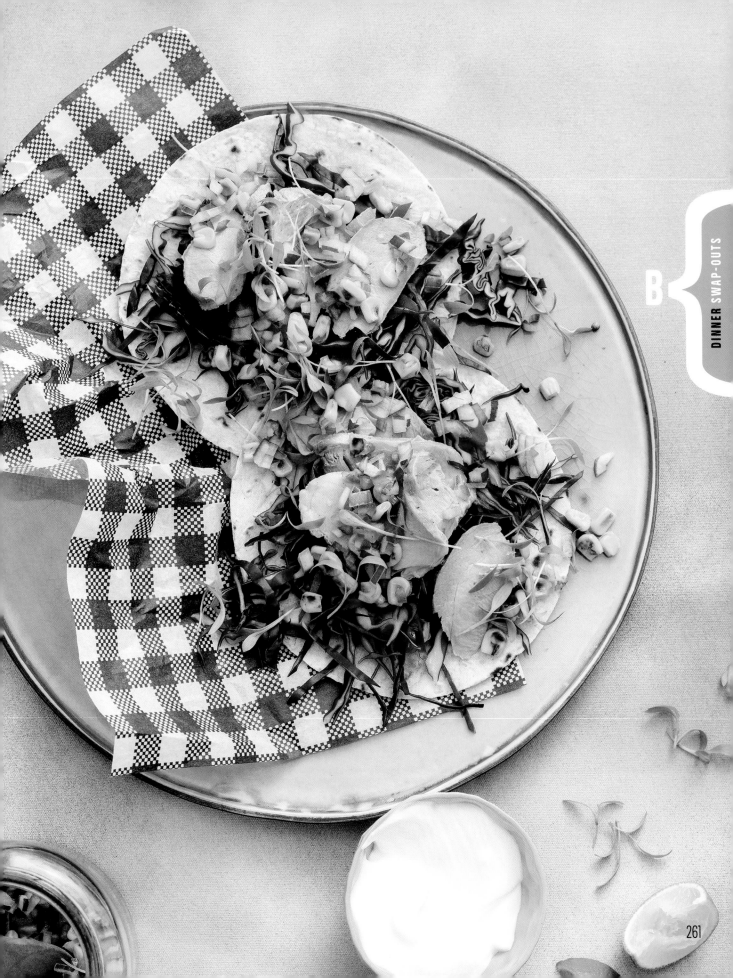

Pumpkin Soup with Cheesy Bread

SERVES 4 | **PREP TIME** 15 MINUTES, PLUS 10 MINUTES COOLING TIME
COOKING TIME 30 MINUTES | **DIFFICULTY** EASY

oil spray

1 large leek, halved and thinly sliced

2 garlic cloves, crushed

1 teaspoon dried sage

1 teaspoon ground cumin

½ teaspoon ground nutmeg

17 oz pumpkin, peeled and chopped

2 medium carrots, chopped

5 cups salt-reduced vegetable stock

21 oz tinned cannellini beans, drained and rinsed

sea salt and ground black pepper, to taste

2 medium whole wheat rolls, halved

3½ oz low-fat goat's cheese, crumbled

Lightly spray a large saucepan with oil and heat over medium heat. Add the leek and cook for 2–3 minutes until soft but not coloured, stirring occasionally.

Add the garlic, sage, cumin, and nutmeg and cook for 1 minute or until fragrant, stirring occasionally.

Add the pumpkin, carrot, and stock and bring to a boil over high heat. Reduce the heat to low and simmer, covered, for 15 minutes or until the pumpkin is soft. Add half the cannellini beans and simmer for 5 minutes or until heated through. Remove from the heat and set aside to cool slightly.

Meanwhile, preheat the oven to 350°F (325°F convection) and line a baking sheet with baking paper.

Transfer the soup, in batches, to a high-powered blender or food processor and blend until smooth (or use a stick blender). If using a blender, place a towel over the top of the lid before blending to avoid any accidents. Return the soup to the pan, add the remaining cannellini beans and continue to cook over medium–low heat for 5 minutes, to heat through. Season with salt and pepper, if desired.

Place the cut rolls on the lined baking sheet and spread over the goat's cheese. Spray lightly with oil spray and bake for 6–7 minutes or until lightly coloured.

To serve, ladle the soup into serving bowls and serve with the goat's cheese rolls on the side.

NOTE: Extra portions can be stored in an airtight container in the freezer. To reheat, thaw in the fridge overnight and warm through in a saucepan or in the microwave.

Spaghetti & Meatballs

SERVES 1 | **PREP TIME** 15 MINUTES | **COOKING TIME** 25 MINUTES | **DIFFICULTY** EASY

oil spray
¼ small brown onion, finely diced
1 garlic clove, crushed
¼ teaspoon dried mixed herbs
2 teaspoons salt-reduced tomato paste
2 teaspoons balsamic vinegar
5¼ oz tinned crushed tomatoes
½ cup (125 ml) salt-reduced
  vegetable stock
3 oz whole wheat spaghetti
chopped fresh basil, to taste
⅔ oz parmesan cheese, grated

MEATBALLS

3¼ oz lean ground beef
¼ small brown onion, finely diced
1 garlic clove, crushed
¼ medium zucchini, grated
1 tablespoon chopped fresh parsley
sea salt and ground black pepper,
  to taste
oil spray

Preheat the oven to 400°F (350°F convection) and line a baking sheet with baking paper.

To make the meatballs, place the ground beef, onion, garlic, zucchini, and parsley in a medium mixing bowl. Season with salt and pepper, if desired, and mix until well combined.

Using clean hands, roll heaped tablespoons of the meatball mixture into balls and place on the lined baking sheet. Spray lightly with oil spray and bake in the oven for 10–12 minutes or until they are cooked through, turning once during the cooking time.

Meanwhile, lightly spray a non-stick fry pan with oil and heat over medium heat. Add the onion and cook for 5 minutes or until soft and translucent, stirring occasionally. Add the garlic and mixed herbs and cook for 1 minute or until fragrant, stirring constantly. Add the tomato paste and balsamic vinegar and cook for a further minute, stirring constantly. Stir in the crushed tomatoes and stock and bring to a boil. Reduce the heat to medium–low and simmer for 10 minutes or until the sauce has thickened slightly, stirring occasionally.

Fill a large saucepan with water, add a pinch of salt and bring to the boil. Add the pasta and cook until al dente (see the pasta packet for the recommended cooking time). Drain and set aside.

Add the meatballs and basil to the tomato sauce and stir gently to combine. Cook for a further 5 minutes.

To serve, place the pasta in a serving bowl and top with the meatballs and tomato sauce. Sprinkle over the parmesan.

Seafood Soup

SERVES 4 | **PREP TIME** 20 MINUTES | **COOKING TIME** 35 MINUTES | **DIFFICULTY** MEDIUM

oil spray

1 small fennel bulb, sliced

1 small brown onion, sliced

3 garlic cloves, thinly sliced

¼ teaspoon dried chilli flakes

2 tablespoons salt-reduced tomato paste

16 oz tinned crushed tomatoes

3½ cups (800 ml) salt-reduced vegetable stock

1 bay leaf

8 medium mussels, scrubbed and beards removed

9 oz white fish fillet, cut into ¾ in cubes

10 medium raw shrimp, peeled and deveined, tails intact

1 medium zucchini, halved and thinly sliced

3 oz tinned cannellini beans, drained and rinsed

sea salt and ground black pepper, to taste

2 tablespoons fresh parsley leaves

3 oz parmesan cheese, grated

GARLIC PITA CRISPS

2 whole wheat pita breads, cut into wedges

1 garlic clove, halved

oil spray

Lightly spray a large saucepan with oil and heat over medium heat. Add the fennel and cook for 5 minutes, stirring occasionally. Add the onion and cook for a further 5 minutes or until the fennel and onion are soft. Add the garlic and chilli flakes and cook for 1 minute or until fragrant, stirring frequently.

Add the tomato paste, crushed tomatoes, stock, and bay leaf and bring to the boil over high heat. Reduce the heat to medium–low and simmer for 15 minutes, stirring occasionally. Increase the heat to medium–high, add the mussels, and cook, covered, for 2–3 minutes. Add the fish, shrimp, zucchini, and beans and cook, covered, for 4–5 minutes or until the seafood is cooked through and the zucchini is tender. Season with salt and pepper, if desired.

Meanwhile, to make the garlic pita crisps, preheat the oven to 400°F (350°F convection) and line a baking sheet with baking paper. Rub each side of the pita wedges with the cut side of the garlic clove. Place on the lined baking sheet and spray with oil spray. Bake in the oven for 5 minutes or until they begin to colour. Turn the wedges over and bake for a further 5–8 minutes or until both sides are lightly coloured, then set aside to cool.

To serve, ladle the soup into serving bowls and garnish with the parsley and parmesan. Serve with the garlic pita crisps on the side.

NOTE: Extra portions can be stored in an airtight container in the freezer. To reheat, thaw in the fridge overnight and warm through in a saucepan or in the microwave.

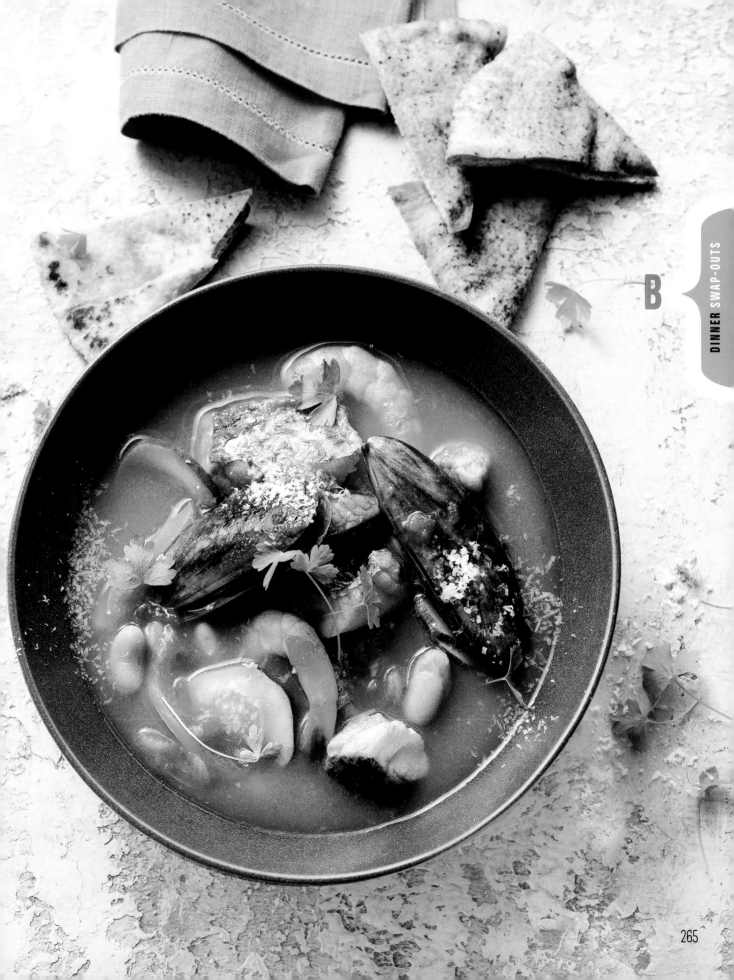

Tex-Mex Steak & Salad

SERVES 1 | **PREP TIME** 15 MINUTES, PLUS 10 MINUTES COOLING TIME
COOKING TIME 20 MINUTES | **DIFFICULTY** EASY

4½ oz lean beef steak

oil spray

¾ teaspoon sunflower oil

½ ear of corn

sea salt and ground black pepper, to taste

2 oz tinned red kidney beans, drained and rinsed

¼ small red onion, sliced

5 cherry tomatoes, halved

1 small handful baby spinach leaves

¼ medium green bell pepper, seeds removed, chopped

1 oz salt-reduced low-fat feta cheese, crumbled

½ small handful fresh cilantro leaves

lime wedges, to serve

SPICE MIX

¼ teaspoon smoked paprika

pinch of cayenne pepper

¼ teaspoon ground cumin

½ garlic clove, crushed

finely grated lime zest, to taste

DRESSING

lemon juice, to taste

¼ fresh red chilli, seeds removed, finely chopped

½ teaspoon Dijon mustard

½ teaspoon honey

To make the spice mix, whisk the paprika, cayenne pepper, cumin, garlic, and lime zest together in a bowl. Place the steak on a plate and rub both sides with the spice mix, then lightly spray each side of the steak with oil.

Heat a barbecue grill-plate or chargrill pan over medium–high heat.

Rub the sunflower oil over the ear of corn and season with salt and pepper. Grill for 10 minutes or until lightly charred and tender, turning occasionally. Remove from the heat and set aside to cool slightly. When cool enough to handle, remove the kernels by running a sharp knife down the length of the ear of corn.

Grill the steak for 4–5 minutes or until slightly charred. Turn the steak over and cook for a further 5 minutes or until cooked to your liking. Loosely cover with foil and set aside to rest for 2 minutes.

To make the dressing, whisk the lemon juice, chilli, mustard, honey, and 2 tablespoons of water together in a small bowl.

Place the corn kernels, kidney beans, onion, tomatoes, spinach, bell pepper, feta, and cilantro in a mixing bowl. Drizzle over the dressing and toss gently to combine.

To serve, place the steak on a serving plate with the corn salad and lime wedges on the side.

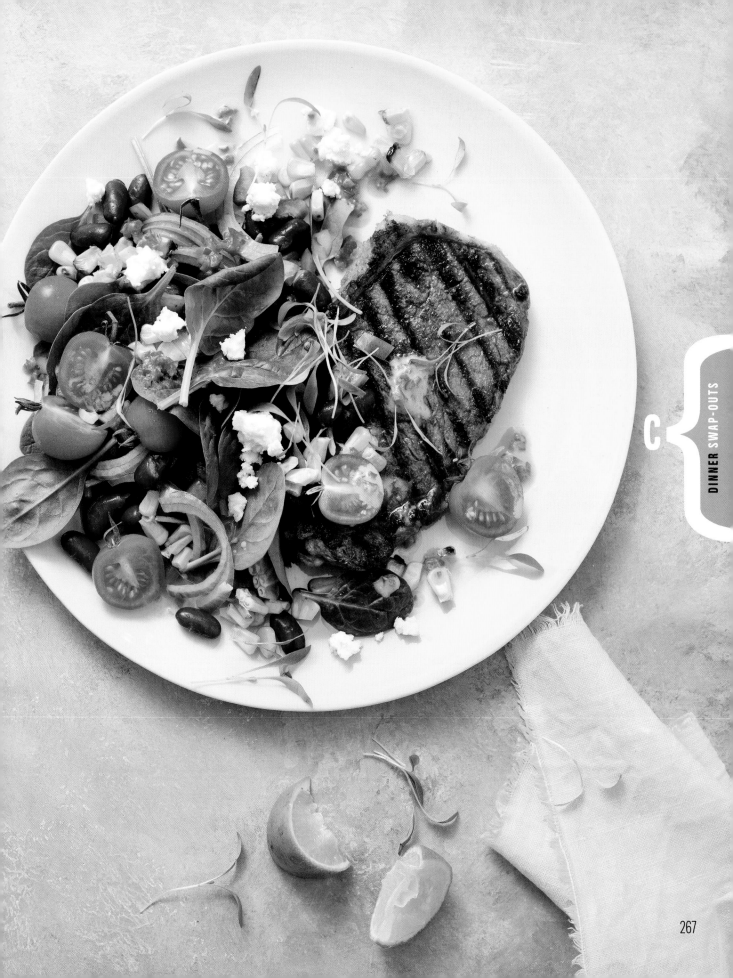

Thai Fish Cakes & Asian Slaw

SERVES 1 | **PREP TIME** 20 MINUTES, PLUS 1 HOUR CHILLING TIME
COOKING TIME 10 MINUTES | **DIFFICULTY** EASY

3 oz Chinese cabbage (wombok), shredded

1½ oz snow peas, trimmed and thinly sliced lengthways

½ medium carrot, grated

¼ medium red bell pepper, seeds removed, thinly sliced

¼ small red onion, thinly sliced

1 small handful bean sprouts

½ scallion, thinly sliced

1 tablespoon fresh cilantro leaves

FISH CAKES

6⅔ oz white fish fillet, skin removed, deboned

¼ garlic clove, crushed

2 teaspoons fresh cilantro leaves

2 teaspoons red curry paste

lime juice, to taste

sea salt, to taste

4 green beans, trimmed and finely chopped

½ scallion, thinly sliced

oil spray

DRESSING

3½ oz low-fat plain yoghurt

¾ teaspoon sesame oil

2 teaspoons chopped fresh cilantro

lime juice, to taste

1 teaspoon honey

1 teaspoon salt-reduced tamari or soy sauce

pinch of ground ginger

½ garlic clove, crushed

Line a baking sheet with baking paper.

To make the fish cakes, place the fish and garlic in a food processor and process until smooth. Add the cilantro, red curry paste, lime juice, and salt, and process until well combined. Transfer the fish mixture to a large mixing bowl. Add the beans and scallion and mix until well combined. Using damp hands, shape the mixture into three even patties and place on the lined baking sheet. Refrigerate for 1 hour if time permits.

Lightly spray a large non-stick fry pan with oil and heat over medium–high heat. Cook the fish patties for 3–4 minutes on each side or until golden brown and cooked through. Set aside on a plate lined with paper towel.

To make the dressing, place the yoghurt, sesame oil, cilantro, lime juice, honey, tamari or soy sauce, ginger, and garlic in a high-powered blender and blend until well combined.

Place the cabbage, snow peas, carrot, bell pepper, onion, bean sprouts, and scallion in a mixing bowl.

To serve, place the Thai fish cakes on a serving plate with the Asian slaw on the side. Drizzle the dressing over the slaw and garnish with the cilantro leaves. Alternatively, the dressing may be served on the side.

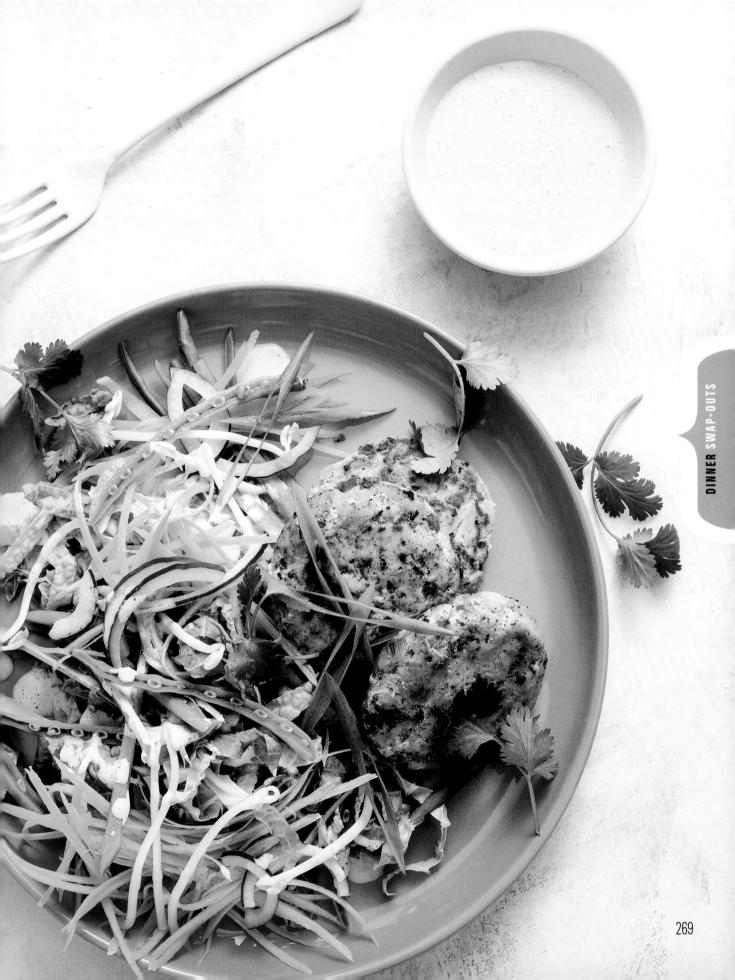

Hearty Roast

SERVES 1 | **PREP TIME** 15 MINUTES, PLUS 2 HOURS MARINATING TIME
COOKING TIME 55 MINUTES | **DIFFICULTY** MEDIUM

½ garlic clove, crushed

¼ fresh red chilli, seeds removed, finely chopped

2 teaspoons red wine vinegar

¾ teaspoon sunflower oil

1 teaspoon honey

1 teaspoon sweet paprika

sea salt and ground black pepper, to taste

2 teaspoons finely chopped fresh oregano

3½ oz boneless, skinless chicken breast

1 small beetroot, cut into wedges

½ medium sweet potato, peeled and cut into 1 in cubes

1 medium carrot, chopped

½ small red onion, cut into wedges

2¾ oz tinned chickpeas, drained and rinsed

finely grated zest of ¼ lemon

oil spray

1 oz low-fat goat's cheese, crumbled

Whisk the garlic, chilli, vinegar, oil, honey, paprika, salt, and 1 teaspoon of the oregano together in a medium bowl. Add the chicken and turn to coat. Cover with plastic wrap and refrigerate for 2 hours to marinate.

Preheat the oven to 400°F (350°F convection).

Place the beetroot, sweet potato, carrot, onion, chickpeas, and lemon zest in a roasting tin. Lightly spray the vegetables with oil, ensuring they are all lightly coated. Season with salt and pepper, if desired.

Roast the vegetables in the oven for 20 minutes. Remove from the oven and turn using tongs. Add the chicken and cook for a further 25–30 minutes or until the vegetables are tender and lightly browned and the chicken is tender and cooked through, turning halfway through the cooking time. Remove the chicken from the roasting tin and set aside on a plate. Cover loosely with foil and rest for 5 minutes.

Dot the goat's cheese over the roasted vegetables and return to the oven for 3–5 minutes or until melted.

To serve, place the roasted vegetables on a serving plate and top with the chicken. Scatter over the remaining 1 teaspoon oregano.

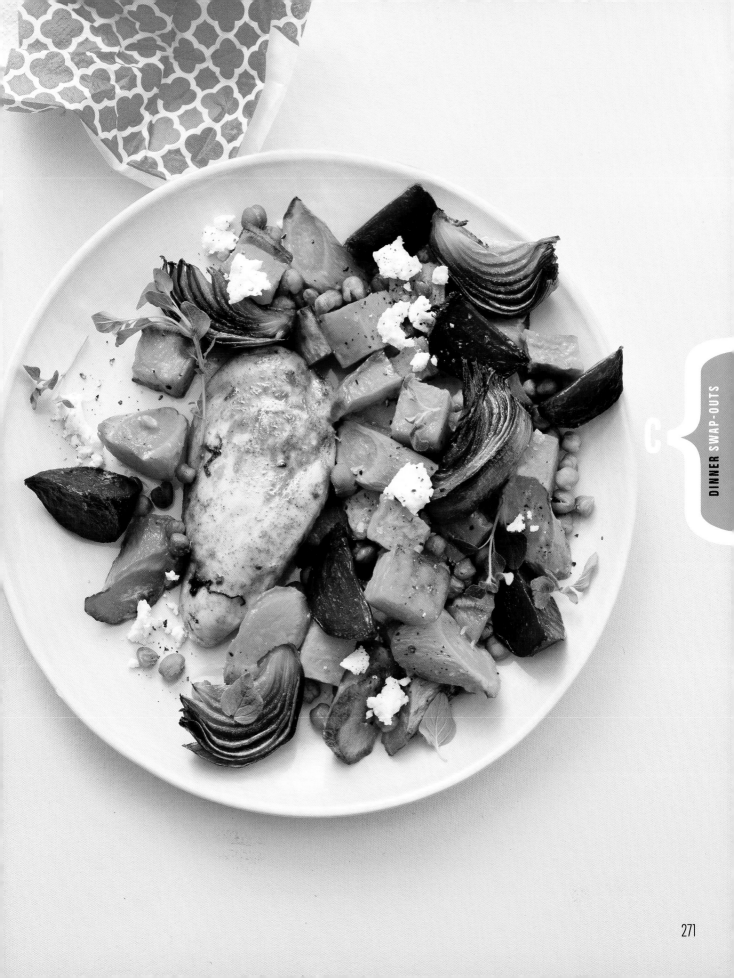

Cauliflower Pizza

SERVES 1 | **PREP TIME** 10 MINUTES, PLUS 5 MINUTES COOLING TIME
COOKING TIME 35 MINUTES | **DIFFICULTY** MEDIUM

7 oz cauliflower, cut into florets
1 large egg, lightly whisked
1 teaspoon dried oregano
3 teaspoons flaxseed (linseed) meal
sea salt and ground black pepper, to taste
⅛ medium eggplant, thinly sliced

oil spray
3½ oz boneless, skinless chicken breast
½ oz tomato passata (puree)
1¾ oz low-fat ricotta cheese
1 small handful arugula leaves

Preheat the oven to 430°F (400°F convection) and line a baking sheet with baking paper.

Place the cauliflower florets in a food processor and process until the consistency resembles rice.

Add 2 inches of water to a saucepan and insert a steamer basket. Line the steamer basket with a clean muslin cloth (this will stop any cauliflower from falling through). Cover with a lid and bring the water to the boil over high heat, then reduce the heat to medium. Add the cauliflower and steam for 5–6 minutes or until cooked. Set aside for 2 minutes to cool slightly.

Place the cooked cauliflower in a clean tea towel. Scrunch up the tea towel and squeeze out as much liquid as possible, then transfer to a mixing bowl. Add the egg, oregano, flaxseed meal, salt, and pepper and mix until well combined.

Place the cauliflower mixture in the middle of the lined baking sheet. Using your hands, firmly press the mixture to form a round pizza shape, ensuring the edges are a little thicker to create a "crust." Bake in the oven for 15–18 minutes or until golden brown and crispy.

Meanwhile, heat a chargrill pan over medium heat. Lightly spray the eggplant slices with oil and season with salt and pepper, if desired. Cook for 3–4 minutes on each side or until softened and charred. Transfer to a plate.

Lightly spray the chargrill pan with oil and reheat over medium heat. Add the chicken and cook for 3–4 minutes on each side or until cooked through. Remove from the heat and cool slightly. When cool enough to handle, cut the chicken into ¼-inch-thick slices.

Spread the passata over the cauliflower base. Top with the chicken and eggplant and dot over the ricotta. Return to the oven and cook for a further 8–10 minutes or until the toppings are hot.

To serve, slice the pizza and top with the arugula.

Spiced Chickpea Tagine with Cauliflower Rice

SERVES 1 | **PREP TIME** 10 MINUTES | **COOKING TIME** 35 MINUTES | **DIFFICULTY** EASY

oil spray

¼ small brown onion, diced

½ garlic clove, crushed

¼ teaspoon ground cumin

¼ teaspoon ground coriander

¼ teaspoon ground ginger

¼ teaspoon ground cinnamon

½ medium eggplant

½ medium sweet potato

½ cup (125 ml) salt-reduced vegetable stock

3 oz tinned crushed tomatoes

8 oz tinned chickpeas, drained and rinsed

finely grated zest and juice of ½ lemon

sea salt and ground black pepper, to taste

2 tablespoons chopped fresh cilantro

3 oz cauliflower, cut into florets

3½ oz low-fat plain yoghurt

1 teaspoon flaked almonds

Lightly spray a large saucepan with oil spray and heat over medium heat. Add the onion and cook for 3–4 minutes, stirring frequently. Add the garlic, cumin, ground coriander, ginger, and cinnamon and cook for 1 minute or until fragrant, stirring constantly.

Add the eggplant and sweet potato and cook for 5–7 minutes or until the eggplant has started to soften, stirring frequently. Add the stock, tomatoes, chickpeas, lemon zest and juice. Reduce the heat to low and cook, covered, for 12–15 minutes until the eggplant and sweet potato are tender, stirring occasionally. Season with salt and pepper, if desired. Remove from the heat and stir through half of the cilantro.

To make the cauliflower rice, place the cauliflower in a food processor and, using the grater attachment, process until the cauliflower resembles rice. Transfer the "rice" to a paper towel and press to remove any excess moisture. Lightly spray a non-stick fry pan with oil spray and heat over medium heat. Add the cauliflower and cook for 3–5 minutes until softened, stirring frequently. Season with salt and pepper, if desired, and remove from the heat.

To serve, place the cauliflower rice in a serving bowl and top with the spiced chickpea tagine and yoghurt. Sprinkle over the flaked almonds and remaining chopped cilantro.

Jambalaya

SERVES 1 | **PREP TIME** 15 MINUTES | **COOKING TIME** 45 MINUTES | **DIFFICULTY** EASY

1½ teaspoons olive oil

1¾ oz boneless, skinless chicken breast, cut into ¾ in cubes

¼ small brown onion, diced

1 garlic clove, crushed

1 teaspoon smoked paprika

¼ teaspoon dried oregano

¼ teaspoon ground cumin

pinch of cayenne pepper

1 medium tomato, diced

1 oz brown rice

½ cup (125 ml) salt-reduced chicken stock

½ celery stalk, diced

¼ medium green bell pepper, seeds removed, diced

5 medium raw shrimp, peeled and deveined

1 medium mango, peeled and sliced

2 teaspoons lime juice

sea salt and ground black pepper, to taste

3½ oz low-fat plain yoghurt

2 teaspoons finely chopped fresh parsley, plus extra to garnish

Heat the oil in a large saucepan over medium heat. Add the chicken and cook for 4–5 minutes or until lightly browned, stirring frequently. Add the onion and half the garlic and cook for 3–4 minutes or until the onion is soft and the garlic is fragrant, stirring frequently.

Add the paprika, oregano, cumin, cayenne pepper, and tomato and cook for 2–3 minutes or until the tomato starts to soften, stirring frequently. Add the rice and cook for 1 minute, stirring constantly, then add the stock. Bring to a boil, then reduce the heat to low and cook, covered, for 15 minutes.

Add the celery and bell pepper and cook, covered, for 10 minutes, stirring occasionally. Remove the lid. Add the shrimp and mango and cook for 2–3 minutes or until the shrimp are cooked, stirring occasionally. Add the lime juice and season with salt and pepper, if desired.

Meanwhile, whisk the yoghurt, parsley, and remaining garlic together in a small bowl.

To serve, place the jambalaya in a serving bowl and sprinkle over the extra parsley. Serve with the garlic yoghurt on the side.

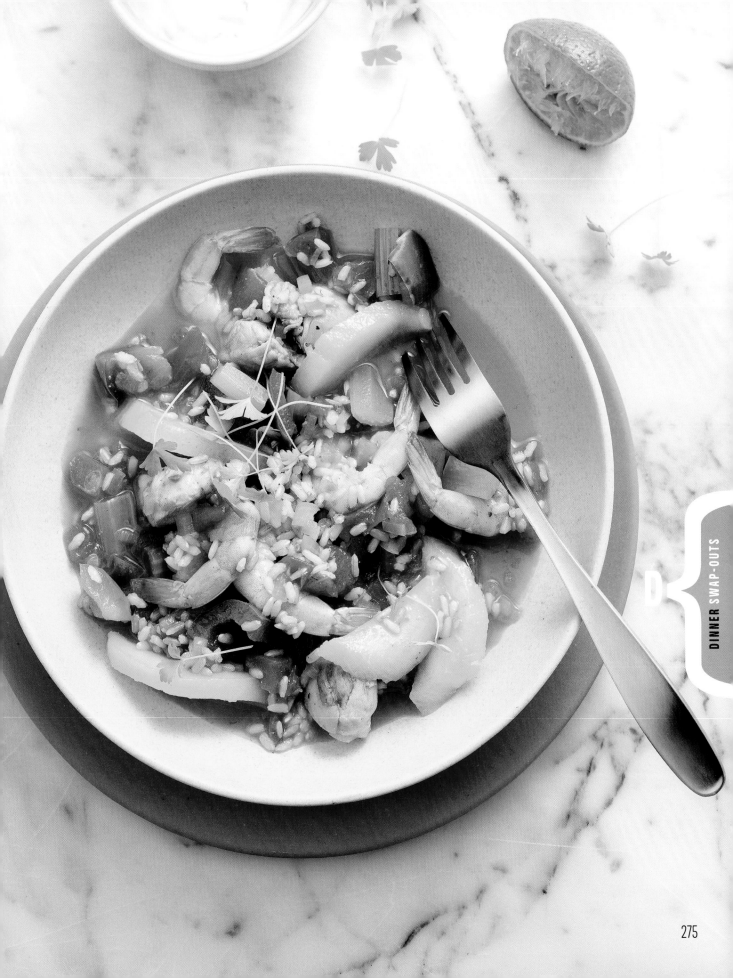

Superfood Salad

SERVES 1 | **PREP TIME** 10 MINUTES | **COOKING TIME** 20 MINUTES | **DIFFICULTY** EASY

½ medium sweet potato, peeled
  and cut into ¾ inch cubes

oil spray

pinch of cayenne pepper

pinch of ground cinnamon

sea salt and ground black pepper,
  to taste

2 large eggs

1 oz quinoa

1¾ oz broccoli, cut into florets

1 small handful kale, chopped

1 oz dried cranberries

1 oz salt-reduced low-fat feta
  cheese, crumbled

2 teaspoons pumpkin seeds (pepitas)

chopped fresh parsley, to garnish

DRESSING

juice of ¼ lemon

½ garlic clove, crushed

1 teaspoon finely chopped fresh parsley

¼ teaspoon honey

Preheat the oven to 350°F (325°F convection) and line a baking sheet with baking paper.

Place the sweet potato in a single layer on the lined baking sheet and spray lightly with oil. Season with cayenne pepper, cinnamon, salt, and black pepper, if desired. Bake in the oven for 15–20 minutes or until tender and lightly browned, using tongs to turn the sweet potato halfway through the cooking time.

Meanwhile, place the eggs in a small saucepan and fill with cold water until they are covered by ¾ inch. Bring the water to the boil over high heat. Reduce the heat to low and simmer, covered, for 7–8 minutes. Remove the eggs from the pan with a slotted spoon and place in a bowl of iced water. Leave for 1 minute. Tap the eggs gently on the bench to crack the shells and peel. Cut in half.

Bring the quinoa and ½ cup (125 ml) of water to the boil in a small saucepan over high heat, stirring occasionally. Reduce the heat to low and simmer, covered, for 10–12 minutes or until the quinoa is tender. Drain off any excess liquid. To save time, the sweet potato, eggs, and quinoa can be cooked the night before and stored in an airtight container in the refrigerator.

Add 2 inches of water to another saucepan and insert a steamer basket. Cover with a lid and bring the water to the boil over high heat, then reduce the heat to medium. Steam the broccoli for 2–3 minutes. Refresh under cold running water and drain.

To make the dressing, whisk the lemon juice, garlic, parsley, honey, and 2 teaspoons of water together in a small bowl.

Place the sweet potato, quinoa, broccoli, kale, and cranberries in a mixing bowl. Drizzle over the dressing, season with salt and black pepper, if desired, and toss gently to combine.

To serve, place the salad in a serving bowl and top with the eggs. Sprinkle over the feta, pumpkin seeds, and parsley.

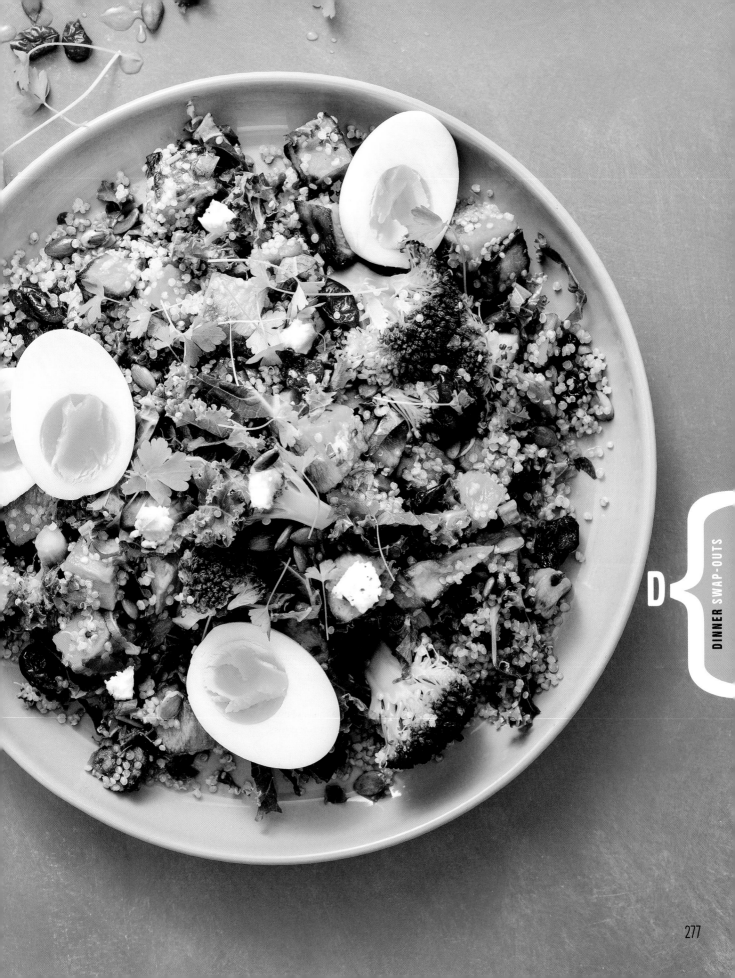

Eggplant Tagine

SERVES 1 | **PREP TIME** 10 MINUTES | **COOKING TIME** 30 MINUTES | **DIFFICULTY** EASY

oil spray

¼ small brown onion, diced

½ garlic clove, crushed

½ teaspoon ground cumin

½ teaspoon ground cinnamon

¼ teaspoon ground turmeric

¼ teaspoon smoked paprika

½ medium eggplant, cut into
 ¾ in cubes

2¾ oz tinned crushed tomatoes

½ cup (125 ml) salt-reduced
 vegetable stock

5¼ oz tinned chickpeas,
 drained and rinsed

3 medjool dates, pitted and chopped

sea salt and ground black pepper,
 to taste

2 teaspoons flaked almonds

¼ teaspoon olive oil

1½ oz couscous

1 oz salt-reduced low-fat feta
 cheese, crumbled

2 teaspoons chopped fresh parsley

Spray a large saucepan with oil and heat over medium heat. Add the onion and garlic and cook for 3–4 minutes or until the onion is soft, stirring frequently. Add the cumin, cinnamon, turmeric, and paprika and cook for 1 minute or until fragrant, stirring constantly.

Add the eggplant and cook for 5 minutes or until it starts to soften, stirring occasionally. Add the crushed tomatoes, stock, chickpeas, and dates and bring to a boil, stirring occasionally. Reduce the heat to low and cook, covered, for 15–20 minutes or until the eggplant is tender, stirring occasionally. Season with salt and pepper, if desired.

Meanwhile, heat a small non-stick fry pan over medium heat. Add the almonds and cook for 2–3 minutes or until fragrant and lightly toasted, stirring constantly.

In a small saucepan, bring the olive oil and ½ cup (125 ml) of water to the boil. Add the couscous and remove from the heat. Leave to stand, covered, for 2–3 minutes before fluffing with a fork to help separate the grains. Stir in the almonds.

To serve, place the couscous in a serving bowl and spoon over the eggplant tagine. Top with the feta and scatter over the parsley.

Persian Chicken & Rice Salad

SERVES 1 | **PREP TIME** 10 MINUTES, PLUS 15 MINUTES STANDING AND COOLING TIME
COOKING TIME 25 MINUTES | **DIFFICULTY** MEDIUM

1 oz brown rice

pinch of ground turmeric

1 cup (250 ml) salt-reduced
  chicken stock

½ garlic clove, crushed

1 sprig fresh thyme

3½ oz boneless, skinless chicken
  breast

½ medium carrot, grated

½ Lebanese cucumber, thinly sliced

1 large handful baby spinach leaves

¼ small red onion, thinly sliced

1 oz low-fat goat's cheese, crumbled

3 medjool dates, pitted and sliced

½ oz slivered almonds

1 tablespoon finely chopped fresh mint,
  plus extra to garnish

sea salt and ground black pepper,
  to taste

DRESSING

1 teaspoon lemon juice, to taste

pinch of ground cinnamon

½ teaspoon honey

Bring the rice and ½ cup (125 ml) of water to a boil in a small saucepan over high heat, stirring occasionally. Reduce the heat to low and simmer, covered, for 20–25 minutes or until the liquid has been absorbed and the rice is tender. Remove from the heat, stir through the turmeric and leave to stand, covered, for 5 minutes. Set aside to cool. To save time, the rice can be cooked the night before and stored in an airtight container in the refrigerator.

Meanwhile, place the stock, garlic, and thyme in a medium saucepan over medium–high heat and bring to a boil. Add the chicken and return to the boil. Reduce the heat to low and simmer, covered, for 12 minutes or until the chicken is cooked through. Remove from the heat and leave the chicken to stand in the stock for 5 minutes. Transfer to a plate and set aside to cool. When cool enough to handle, slice the chicken into thin strips.

To make the dressing, whisk the lemon juice, cinnamon, honey, and 1 teaspoon of water together in a small bowl.

Place the rice, chicken, carrot, cucumber, spinach, red onion, goat's cheese, dates, almonds, and mint in a mixing bowl. Drizzle over the dressing, season with salt and pepper, if desired, and toss gently to combine.

To serve, place the rice salad in a serving bowl and garnish with extra mint.

Matcha Pistachio Bliss Balls

MAKES ABOUT 8 | **PREP TIME** 10 MINUTES, PLUS 30 MINUTES
CHILLING TIME | **DIFFICULTY** EASY

1⅓ oz unsalted cashew nuts

1½ oz unsalted
  pistachio kernels

6 medjool dates, pitted

⅔ oz desiccated coconut

1 teaspoon matcha powder

½ teaspoon pure
  vanilla extract

1 tablespoon pure
  maple syrup

Line a baking sheet with baking paper.

Place the cashews and half the pistachios in a food processor and process until crumbly. Add the dates, coconut, matcha powder, vanilla extract, and maple syrup and process until well combined. The mixture should be a little sticky. If it is too thick, add 1–2 tablespoons of water.

Scoop out 1 tablespoon of the mixture and roll it into a ball using wet hands. Repeat with the remaining mixture to make about eight balls.

Place the balls on the lined baking sheet and refrigerate for 30 minutes.

Finely chop the remaining pistachios.

To serve, roll the balls through the chopped pistachio to coat. Store in an airtight container in the refrigerator for up to a week.

Peanut Butter & Chocolate Protein Balls

MAKES ABOUT 10 | **PREP TIME** 10 MINUTES, PLUS 30 MINUTES CHILLING TIME | **DIFFICULTY** EASY

1¾ oz rolled oats

2½ tablespoons sunflower seeds

6 medjool dates, pitted

2½ tablespoons 100% natural peanut butter

2½ tablespoons chocolate protein powder

¼ teaspoon ground cinnamon

2 teaspoons chia seeds

½ teaspoon pure vanilla extract

2 teaspoons pure maple syrup

2½ tablespoons desiccated coconut

Line a baking sheet with baking paper.

Place the oats and sunflower seeds in a food processor and process until crumbly.

Add the dates, peanut butter, protein powder, cinnamon, chia seeds, vanilla extract, and maple syrup and process until well combined. The mixture should be a little sticky. If it is too thick, add 1–2 tablespoons of water.

Scoop out 1 tablespoon of the mixture and roll it into a ball using wet hands. Repeat with the remaining mixture to make about 10 balls.

Place the balls on the lined baking sheet and refrigerate for 30 minutes.

To serve, roll the balls through the coconut to coat. Store in an airtight container in the refrigerator for up to a week.

Chocolate & Goji Bliss Balls

MAKES ABOUT 8 | **PREP TIME** 10 MINUTES, PLUS 30 MINUTES CHILLING TIME | **DIFFICULTY** EASY

3½ oz almond meal

5 medjool dates, pitted

2½ tablespoons raw cacao powder

1 tablespoon pure maple syrup

2 oz goji berries

Place the goji berries in a high-powered blender and blend to form a smooth "dust." Store uncovered in the freezer overnight to make it easier to handle.

The next day, line a baking sheet with baking paper.

Place the almond meal, dates, cacao powder, and maple syrup in a food processor and process until well combined. The mixture should be a little sticky. If it is too thick, add 1–2 tablespoons of water.

Scoop out 1 tablespoon of the mixture and roll it into a ball using wet hands. Repeat with the remaining mixture to make about eight balls. Place the balls on the lined baking sheet and refrigerate for 30 minutes.

To serve, roll the balls through the goji "dust" to coat. Store in an airtight container in the refrigerator for up to a week.

Chocolate & Avocado Mousse

SERVES 4 | **PREP TIME** 15 MINUTES, PLUS 1 HOUR CHILLING TIME | **DIFFICULTY** EASY

1 medium banana, peeled

1 large avocado

¼ cup (1 oz) raw cacao powder

2½ tablespoons honey or
  pure maple syrup

1 teaspoon lemon juice

1 teaspoon pure vanilla extract

4 tablespoons coconut oil, melted

raw cacao nibs, to garnish (optional)

SMASHED RASPBERRIES

4½ oz raspberries

2 teaspoons pure maple syrup

Place the banana, avocado, cacao powder, honey or maple syrup, lemon
juice, vanilla, and coconut oil in a high-powered blender or food processor
and process until smooth.

Spoon the mousse into four individual serving bowls, cover with plastic wrap,
and chill in the refrigerator for 1 hour.

To make the smashed raspberries, place the raspberries and maple syrup in
a small bowl and roughly mash with a fork.

To serve, top the mousse with the smashed raspberries and sprinkle over
the cacao nibs (if using).

Apple Pie Cookies

MAKES 12 | **PREP TIME** 10 MINUTES, PLUS 30 MINUTES CHILLING TIME
COOKING TIME 15 MINUTES | **DIFFICULTY** EASY

3½ oz rolled oats

3 oz whole wheat plain flour

1 teaspoon baking powder

1 teaspoon ground cinnamon

¼ teaspoon ground nutmeg

pinch of sea salt

2½ tablespoons coconut oil, melted and cooled slightly

1 large egg

2½ tablespoons pure maple syrup

1 medium red apple, grated

Place the oats, flour, baking powder, cinnamon, nutmeg, and salt in a large mixing bowl and mix to combine. Set aside.

In a separate bowl, whisk together the coconut oil, egg, and maple syrup. Add to the dry ingredients and stir until just combined. Don't overmix, but make sure that all the flour has been incorporated. Fold in the grated apple.

Cover the bowl with plastic wrap and refrigerate for 30 minutes.

Preheat the oven to 340°F (315°F convection) and line a baking sheet with baking paper.

Scoop out 1 heaped tablespoon of the mixture and roll it into a ball using wet hands. Place on the lined baking sheet and flatten slightly with the back of a spoon. Repeat with the remaining mixture to make 12 flattened balls. Ensure that you leave ¾ inch between each ball to allow room for spreading during baking.

Bake in the oven for 10–12 minutes or until the edges of the cookies are slightly browned. Leave to cool on the baking sheet for 5 minutes before transferring to a wire rack to cool completely.

Store in an airtight container for up to 3 days.

Chocolate & Coconut Bars

MAKES 12 | **PREP TIME** 15 MINUTES, PLUS 1 HOUR 40 MINUTES CHILLING AND FREEZING TIME
COOKING TIME 5 MINUTES | **DIFFICULTY** EASY

2½ cups (7 oz) desiccated coconut
4 tablespoons coconut oil, melted
¼ cup (60 ml) coconut milk
¼ cup (60 ml) pure maple syrup
½ teaspoon pure vanilla extract
pinch of sea salt

CHOCOLATE COATING
4¼ oz coconut oil
¼ cup (1 oz) raw cacao powder
1 tablespoon pure maple syrup

Line a 10 × 6-inch slice tin with baking paper.

Place the desiccated coconut, coconut oil, coconut milk, maple syrup, vanilla, and salt in a food processor. Pulse until the mixture forms a thick and sticky paste, but is not smooth. Ensure that you scrape down the side of the bowl occasionally.

Press the mixture firmly into the lined baking sheet so it is ½ inch thick. Don't worry if it doesn't completely fill the tin—just make sure that the mixture is pressed firmly in a neat rectangular shape. Place in the refrigerator for 30 minutes to set.

Once set, cut the mixture into 12 even bars. Return to the lined baking sheet and place in the freezer for 1 hour to harden. This will make coating the coconut bars in the chocolate easier.

To make the chocolate coating, place the coconut oil, cacao powder, and maple syrup in a small saucepan over low heat. Whisk until well combined, smooth, and shiny. Remove from the heat and set aside to cool slightly.

Remove the coconut bars from the freezer, or if time permits remove one bar at a time. Using two forks, dip one bar into the chocolate mixture and roll it over several times to cover all sides. Return to the lined baking sheet and repeat with the remaining bars. Return to the freezer for 10 minutes or until the chocolate is set.

For a thicker chocolate, dip the bars in the remaining chocolate again. Return to the freezer for 10 minutes or until the chocolate is set.

Store in an airtight container in the refrigerator for up to 2 weeks.

Chocolate Orange Tart

SERVES 12 | **PREP TIME** 15 MINUTES, PLUS OVERNIGHT CHILLING AND SETTING TIME
DIFFICULTY EASY

5 oz almond meal

4 oz coconut oil

6⅓ oz desiccated coconut

3 tablespoons honey

1 tablespoon raw cacao powder,
 plus extra for dusting

finely grated orange zest, to garnish

FILLING

10¾ oz unsalted cashew nuts

4¾ oz honey

juice of 3 oranges

finely grated zest of 1 orange

6⅓ oz coconut oil, melted

1¾ oz raw cacao powder

pinch of sea salt

Grease an 8 inch tart tin with a removable base with coconut oil.

Place the almond meal, coconut oil, desiccated coconut, honey, and cacao powder in a food processor and process until well combined. Tip the mixture into the prepared baking sheet and spread evenly over the base and up the sides. Cover with plastic wrap and place in the refrigerator for 30 minutes.

To make the filling, place all the ingredients in a high-powered blender or food processor and blend for 2–3 minutes or until smooth and creamy. Pour the chocolate orange mixture into the prepared base and place in the freezer overnight to set.

To serve, dust the chocolate orange tart with extra cacao powder and garnish with orange zest.

Store in an airtight container in the refrigerator for up to a week. Alternatively, you can freeze the whole tart or pre-slice and freeze the slices in airtight containers for up to a month.

Healthy Chocolate Crackles

MAKES 12 | **PREP TIME** 10 MINUTES, PLUS 30 MINUTES CHILLING TIME | **DIFFICULTY** EASY

4¼ oz coconut oil, melted

2½ tablespoons pure maple syrup

1 teaspoon pure vanilla extract

1 tablespoon 100% natural nut butter
  or tahini

¼ cup (1 oz) raw cacao powder

2 cups (1½ oz) puffed brown rice

1¾ oz desiccated coconut

Place 12 cupcake liners in a 12-cup muffin tin.

Whisk the melted coconut oil, maple syrup, vanilla extract, nut butter or tahini, and cacao powder together in a large mixing bowl. Ensure that the cacao powder has dissolved.

Add the puffed rice and coconut and mix until well combined.

Spoon the mixture evenly into the cupcake liners. Refrigerate for 30 minutes to set.

Serve straight from the refrigerator.

Store the remaining crackles in an airtight container in the refrigerator for up to 2 days. If the crackles are left out too long the coconut oil may melt and the crackles will soften.

Healthy Berry Crumble

SERVES 1 | **PREP TIME** 10 MINUTES, PLUS 5 MINUTES COOLING TIME
COOKING TIME 40 MINUTES | **DIFFICULTY** EASY

oil spray

3 oz rhubarb stalks, cut into
 1¼ in lengths

1½ oz frozen raspberries

1½ oz frozen blueberries

¼ teaspoon cornstarch

1 teaspoon coconut oil, melted

¾ oz rolled oats

⅓ oz almonds

pinch of ground cinnamon

¼ teaspoon honey

sea salt, to taste

VANILLA YOGHURT

1¾ oz low-fat plain yoghurt

¼ teaspoon pure vanilla extract

¼ teaspoon honey

Preheat the oven to 400°F (350°F convection) and spray a 4 inch ramekin with oil spray.

Place the rhubarb, raspberries, blueberries, and cornstarch in a mixing bowl and mix until well combined. Transfer the fruit mixture to the greased ramekin.

Place the oil, rolled oats, almonds, and cinnamon in a food processor and pulse to a crumb-like consistency. Stir in the honey and season with salt, if desired.

Sprinkle the crumble evenly over the rhubarb and berry mixture and bake for 30–40 minutes or until the crumble is golden and the rhubarb is tender. Remove from the oven and set aside for 5 minutes to settle and cool slightly.

To make the vanilla yoghurt, whisk the yoghurt, vanilla, and honey together in a small bowl.

To serve, place the rhubarb and berry crumble on a serving plate and top with the vanilla yoghurt.

Flourless Chocolate Cake

SERVES 10–12 | **PREP TIME** 10 MINUTES, PLUS 1 HOUR 20 MINUTES STANDING AND COOLING TIME
COOKING TIME 40 MINUTES | **DIFFICULTY** EASY

16 medjool dates, pitted

7 oz almond meal

2⅓ oz raw cacao powder, plus extra
 for dusting

½ teaspoon baking soda

½ teaspoon baking powder

pinch of sea salt

3 large eggs

1 teaspoon pure vanilla extract

¼ cup (60 ml) olive oil

Preheat the oven to 350°F (330°F convection) and line an 8 inch round cake tin with baking paper.

Place the dates in a heatproof bowl, cover with ¾ cup (190 ml) boiling water and leave to soak for 30 minutes to soften. Place the dates and water in a high-powered blender and blend until a smooth paste forms.

Place the almond meal, cacao powder, baking soda, baking powder, and salt in a mixing bowl and mix until well combined.

Whisk the eggs, vanilla, and oil together. Add the date paste and mix until well combined.

Add the date mixture to the dry ingredients and mix until well combined.

Pour the cake mixture into the lined tin and bake for 30–40 minutes or until a skewer inserted into the centre comes out clean.

Remove from the oven and leave to cool in the cake tin for 20 minutes. Transfer to a wire rack to cool completely.

To serve, dust with extra cacao powder.

The cake can be kept in an airtight container for up to a week.

Mug Cake

SERVES 1 | **PREP TIME** 10 MINUTES | **COOKING TIME** 5 MINUTES | **DIFFICULTY** EASY

2 tablespoons almond meal
¼ teaspoon baking powder
½ ripe banana, peeled and mashed
1 large egg, whisked
2 tablespoons low-fat milk
1 teaspoon pure vanilla extract

TOPPING

2 teaspoons chopped walnuts
pinch of ground cinnamon
2 teaspoons coconut sugar

Place the almond meal and baking powder in a small bowl and mix to combine. Add the banana, egg, milk, and vanilla and mix well to combine.

To make the topping, combine the walnuts, cinnamon, and coconut sugar in a small bowl.

Pour the cake mixture into a mug or 1 cup (250 ml) heatproof dish. Sprinkle the topping evenly over the top.

Microwave for 2–3 minutes or until a skewer inserted into the centre comes out clean. The cake should be soft and springy to the touch. If the cake is not ready, continue in 30-second increments until cooked.

(Alternatively, bake in a preheated 340°F [315°F convection] oven for 12–14 minutes or until a skewer inserted into the centre comes out clean.)

Enjoy straight from the mug or wait until the cake cools completely, then run a knife around the inside of the mug to remove the cake.

Waffles

SERVES 1 | **PREP TIME** 5 MINUTES | **COOKING TIME** 20 MINUTES
DIFFICULTY EASY

¾ oz quinoa flour

¾ oz rice flour

1½ oz whole wheat plain flour

½ teaspoon baking powder

pinch of ground cinnamon

pinch of ground nutmeg

1 large egg

2 tablespoons low-fat milk

1 teaspoon honey

¼ teaspoon pure vanilla extract

oil spray

Preheat a waffle iron on medium heat.

Place the flours, baking powder, cinnamon, and nutmeg in a mixing bowl and mix until well combined.

In a separate bowl, whisk the egg until light and fluffy. Add the milk, honey, and vanilla and whisk until well combined.

Add the wet ingredients to the dry ingredients and gently stir with a wooden spoon. Try not to overmix.

Lightly spray the waffle iron with oil.

Carefully pour the batter onto the waffle iron and cook for 3–5 minutes or until golden brown. Repeat until the batter is finished.

Serve with your choice of topping (see recipes on the next page).

Blueberry & Lemon Yoghurt Topping

SERVES 1 | **PREP TIME** 10 MINUTES
COOKING TIME 5 MINUTES | **DIFFICULTY** EASY

1½ oz blueberries

2 teaspoons pure maple syrup

finely grated zest and juice of
½ lemon, plus extra zest to
garnish (optional)

3½ oz low-fat plain yoghurt

½ teaspoon honey,
plus extra to serve

Place the blueberries, maple syrup, and 1 teaspoon of the lemon juice in a small saucepan and bring to the boil over medium–high heat. Reduce the heat to low and gently mash the blueberries with a fork. Simmer for 3 minutes, then remove from the heat.

Meanwhile, whisk the yoghurt, honey, lemon zest, and remaining lemon juice together in a small bowl.

To serve, place the waffles on a serving plate and top with the blueberry sauce and lemon yoghurt. Drizzle over extra honey and sprinkle with extra lemon zest, if desired.

Coconut Citrus Topping

SERVES 1 | **PREP TIME** 10 MINUTES **COOKING TIME** 5 MINUTES
PLUS 30 MINUTES CHILLING TIME | **DIFFICULTY** EASY

1¾ oz low-fat ricotta cheese

2 tablespoons coconut milk

1 teaspoon pure maple syrup

2 teaspoons shredded
coconut

½ medium blood orange,
segmented

½ medium grapefruit,
segmented

Place the ricotta, coconut milk, maple syrup, and shredded coconut in a small bowl and mix until well combined. Cover with plastic wrap and chill in the refrigerator for 30 minutes or overnight.

To serve, place the waffles on a serving plate and top with the coconut ricotta and blood orange and grapefruit segments.

FOOD GROUP SAMPLE SERVING SIZE

FOOD GROUP	SAMPLE SERVINGS
Grains	BREADS ½ medium whole wheat bread roll ½ medium whole wheat lavash ½ medium whole wheat pita ½ medium whole wheat wrap 1 slice raisin bread 1 slice whole wheat bread 1 whole wheat English muffin CEREALS 1 oz muesli 1 oz rolled oats CRACKERS 2 rye crispbreads 3 thin rice or corn cakes 12 rice crackers 6 plain water crackers GRAINS 3 oz cooked brown rice 3½ oz cooked couscous 3½ oz cooked hokkien noodles 3½ oz cooked pearl barley 3 oz cooked pearl couscous 4¼ oz cooked polenta 3 oz cooked quinoa 3½ oz cooked rice vermicelli noodles 3½ oz cooked spelt 3 oz cooked whole wheat pasta 8 small rice paper wraps
Fruit	1 medium apple 5 small apricots or 4 dried apricot halves 1 medium banana 6 oz frozen berries 7 oz blackberries 5¾ oz blueberries 20 cherries 1 oz dried cranberries 3 medjool dates 2 medium figs ½ cup (125 ml) 100% fruit juice 5¼ oz mixed fruit salad 1 oz goji berries 1 medium grapefruit 25 grapes 2 kiwifruit 3 lemons 2 small mandarins 1 medium mango 2 medium nectarines 1 medium orange 5 passionfruit 1 large peach 1 small pear 6 oz pineapple 3 small plums 1 pomegranate 5¾ oz raspberries 14 oz rhubarb 9 oz canteloupe ¼ oz sultanas 1 medium tangelo 9 oz watermelon

FOOD GROUP	SAMPLE SERVINGS
Vegetables & legumes	STARCHY VEGETABLES 2 oz corn kernels (frozen or tinned) ½ medium ear of corn 1 oz frozen or fresh peas ½ medium potato ½ medium sweet potato NON-STARCHY VEGETABLES 1 large handful alfalfa sprouts 1 large handful arugula leaves 6 asparagus spears 1 large handful baby spinach leaves 15 green beans 1 large handful bean sprouts 1 small beetroot 4¼ oz bok choy 3 oz broccoli florets 4 Brussels sprouts 3½ oz cabbage (white or red) ½ medium bell pepper 1 medium carrot 3½ oz cauliflower florets 2 celery stalks 10 cherry tomatoes 1 medium cucumber ½ medium eggplant 1 small fennel bulb 1 large handful kale ½ large leek 1 large handful lettuce leaves 3½ oz button/white mushrooms 1 portobello mushroom (3½ oz) 8 kalamata olives 1 small red or brown onion 1 small parsnip 4¼ oz pumpkin 4 medium radishes 2¾ oz snow peas 2 large scallions 5 pieces semi-dried tomato 5¼ oz tinned tomatoes 1 medium tomato 1 medium zucchini LEGUMES 2¾ oz cooked or tinned bean mixes 2¾ oz cooked or tinned black beans 2¾ oz cooked or tinned butter beans 2¾ oz cooked or tinned cannellini beans 2¾ oz cooked or tinned chickpeas 2¾ oz cooked or tinned kidney beans 2¾ oz cooked or tinned lentils 2¾ oz cooked or tinned split peas

FOOD GROUP	SAMPLE SERVINGS
Lean meat, seafood, eggs & meat alternatives	RED MEAT (lean cuts) 2⅓ oz cooked beef 2⅓ oz cooked lamb 1 medium lamb chop 2⅓ oz cooked pork 2⅓ oz cooked veal 2⅓ oz cooked venison POULTRY 3 oz cooked chicken breast or thigh 3 oz cooked turkey breast SEAFOOD 3½ oz cooked white fish fillet 8 medium mussels 4¼ oz cooked octopus 10 medium shrimp 2½ oz cooked, tinned, or smoked salmon 4¼ oz cooked squid 3½ oz cooked or tinned tuna ALTERNATIVES 5¼ oz cooked or tinned bean mixes 5¼ oz cooked or tinned black beans 5¼ oz cooked or tinned butter beans 5¼ oz cooked or tinned cannellini beans 5¼ oz cooked or tinned chickpeas 5¼ oz cooked or tinned kidney beans 5¼ oz cooked or tinned lentils 5¼ oz cooked or tinned split peas 2 large eggs 3 oz tempeh 6 oz plain tofu
Dairy products & alternatives	MILK 1¼ cups (300 ml) calcium-fortified almond milk 1 cup (250 ml) calcium-fortified milk alternatives 1 cup (250 ml) low-fat (cow's) milk YOGHURT 7 oz low-fat plain yoghurt 7 oz calcium-fortified soy yoghurt CHEESE 1½ oz bocconcini cheese 1½ oz camembert cheese 1½ oz reduced-fat cheddar cheese 4¼ oz low-fat cottage cheese 1¾ oz light cream cheese 2 oz salt-reduced low-fat feta cheese 1¾ oz soft goat's cheese 1¾ oz halloumi cheese 1½ oz low-fat mozzarella cheese 1½ oz low-fat parmesan cheese 3½ oz low-fat ricotta cheese 1½ oz soy cheese

FOOD GROUP	SAMPLE SERVINGS
Healthy fats	NUTS & SEEDS ⅓ oz almonds ⅓ oz brazil nuts ⅓ oz cashew nuts ⅓ oz chestnuts ⅓ oz chia seeds (2 teaspoons) ⅓ oz hazelnuts ¼ cup light coconut milk ⅓ oz macadamia nuts ⅓ oz peanuts ⅓ oz pecan nuts ⅓ oz pine nuts (2 teaspoons) ⅓ oz pistachio nuts ⅓ oz sesame seeds (2 teaspoons) ⅓ oz sunflower seeds ⅓ oz walnuts OIL 1½ teaspoons almond oil 1½ teaspoons avocado oil 1½ teaspoons canola oil 1½ teaspoons coconut oil 1½ teaspoons corn oil 1½ teaspoons linseed oil 1½ teaspoons macadamia oil 1½ teaspoons olive oil 1½ teaspoons peanut oil 1½ teaspoons rice bran oil 1½ teaspoons safflower oil 1½ teaspoons sesame oil 1½ teaspoons sunflower oil 1½ teaspoons walnut oil NUT BUTTER/SPREADS 2 teaspoons nut butter 2 teaspoons peanut butter 2 teaspoons tahini OTHER 1 oz avocado ⅔ oz dessicated, shredded, or flaked coconut ¼ cup (60 ml) light coconut milk 2 teaspoons margarine/spreads

UNCOOKED TO COOKED

Throughout this book, I have used the raw or uncooked weights for the majority of the grain and protein foods. If you are tailoring any of my recipes to suit your preferences, or creating your own recipes using the serving recommendations, it is important that you consider the change in weight of these ingredients once cooked. To help you with this, here's a handy chart giving you the cooked and uncooked weights for the most popular foods.

PROTEINS

UNCOOKED	COOKED	NUMBER OF SERVINGS
LEAN RED MEATS (beef, lamb, pork, veal, venison)		
1¾ oz	1¼ oz	½
3 oz	2⅓ oz	1
4¾ oz	3½ oz	1½
6 oz	4¾ oz	2
12 oz	9 oz	4
POULTRY (chicken breast, chicken thigh)		
1¾ oz	1½ oz	½
3½ oz	3 oz	1
5¼ oz	4¼ oz	1½
7 oz	5¾ oz	2
14 oz	11¼ oz	4
POULTRY (turkey breast)		
2 oz	1¾ oz	½
4 oz	3 oz	1
6 oz	4¾ oz	1½
8 oz	6⅓ oz	2
16 oz	12⅔ oz	4
DRIED BEANS		
1¼ oz	2¾ oz	½
2½ oz	5¼ oz	1
3⅔ oz	8 oz	1½
5 oz	10¾ oz	2
10 oz	21 oz	4

UNCOOKED	COOKED	NUMBER OF SERVINGS
SALMON FILLET		
1¾ oz	1¼ oz	½
3 oz	2½ oz	1
4½ oz	3⅔ oz	1½
6 oz	5 oz	2
12 oz	10 oz	4
WHITE FISH FILLET		
2⅓ oz	1¾ oz	½
4½ oz	3½ oz	1
6⅔ oz	5¼ oz	1½
9 oz	7 oz	2
17¾ oz	14 oz	4
SQUID, OCTOPUS		
2¾ oz	2 oz	½
5¼ oz	4¼ oz	1
8 oz	6⅓ oz	1½
10¾ oz	8½ oz	2
21 oz	17 oz	4

GRAINS

UNCOOKED	WATER NEEDED	COOKED	NUMBER OF SERVINGS
BROWN RICE			
1 oz	½ cup (125 ml)	3 oz	1
2 oz	⅞ cup (200 ml)	6⅓ oz	2
3 oz	1 cup (250 ml)	9½ oz	3
4¼ oz	1¼ cups (300 ml)	12⅔ oz	4
QUINOA			
1 oz	½ cup (125 ml)	3 oz	1
2 oz	⅔ (160 ml)	6⅓ oz	2
3 oz	¾ cup (185 ml)	9½ oz	3
4¼ oz	1⅓ cups (320 ml)	12⅔ oz	4
COUSCOUS			
1¼ oz	½ cup (125 ml)	3½ oz	1
2½ oz	¾ cup (170 ml)	7 oz	2
3½ oz	1 cup (250 ml)	10¾ oz	3
4¾ oz	1⅔ cups (375 ml)	14 oz	4
PEARL COUSCOUS			
1 oz	⅞ cup (200 ml)	3 oz	1
2 oz	1⅔ cups (400 ml)	6⅓ oz	2
3 oz	3⅓ cups (800 ml)	9½ oz	3
4¼ oz	5 cups (1.2 L)	12⅔ oz	4
PASTA			
1½ oz	2 cups (500 ml)	2¾ oz	1
2 oz	3 cups (750 ml)	4¼ oz	1½
3 oz	4¼ cups (1 L)	5¾ oz	2
4¼ oz	6⅓ cups (1.5 L)	8½ oz	2½
5¾ oz	8½ cups (2 L)	11¼ oz	4
RICE VERMICELLI NOODLES			
1 oz	1 cup (250 ml)	1¾ oz	½
1¾ oz	2 cups (500 ml)	3½ oz	1
2¾ oz	3 cups (750 ml)	5¼ oz	1½
3½ oz	4¼ cups (1 L)	7 oz	2
7 oz	8½ cups (2 L)	14 oz	4

PART 5

WORKOUTS

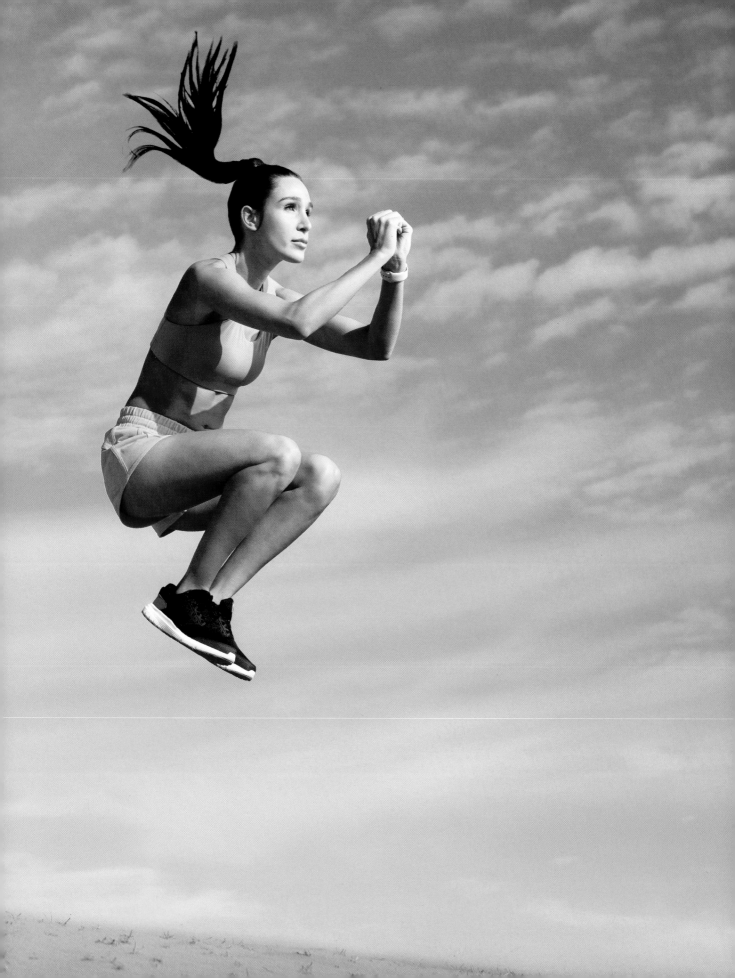

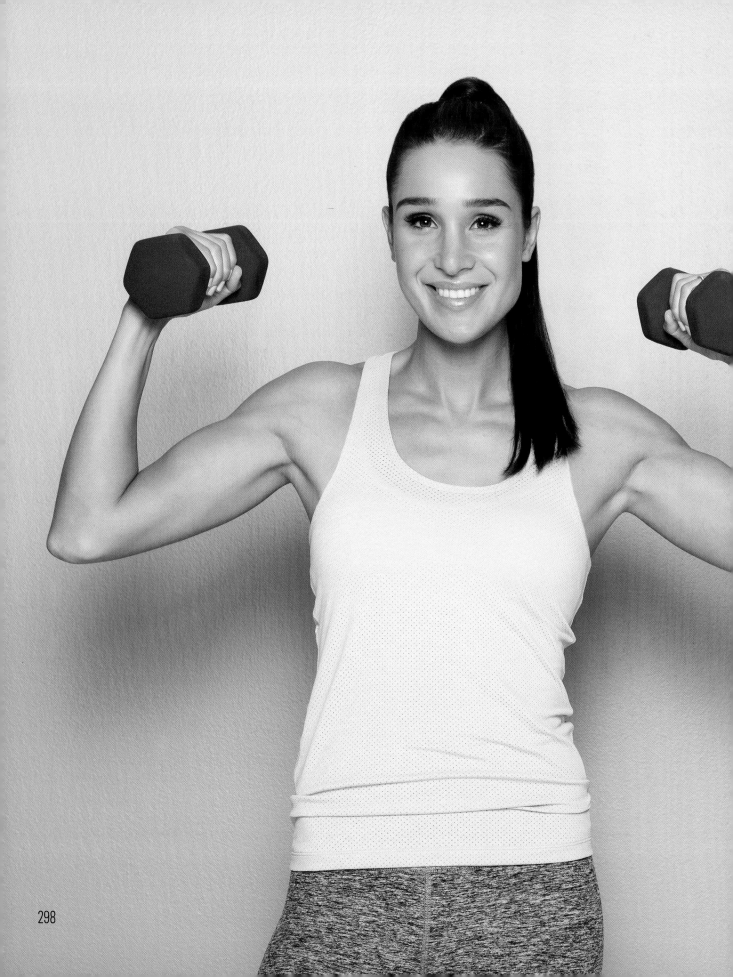

28-DAY WORKOUT GUIDE

This workout guide consists of two weeks of workouts to be completed twice. Each week includes:

■ **Three resistance workouts that focus on different areas—legs, arms & abs, and full body**
(all pictured on the poster in the front of the book)

■ **Three to four low-intensity steady state (LISS) cardio sessions**
(examples include walking, swimming, or cycling for 30–45 minutes)

■ **One rehabilitation (active recovery) session**
(a brief 5–10 minute walk followed by some foam-rolling and stretching).

It is also important that you set aside at least one day a week to give your body a chance to rest and recover. Here is a suggested timetable that incorporates all of these elements into a four-week period:

WEEK 1 (WEEKS 1 & 3)

Monday	Tuesday	Wednesday	Thursday	Friday	Saturday	Sunday
Legs	LISS	Arms & Abs	LISS	Full Body	LISS + Rehabilitation	Rest

WEEK 2 (WEEKS 2 & 4)

Monday	Tuesday	Wednesday	Thursday	Friday	Saturday	Sunday
Legs	LISS	Arms & Abs	LISS	Full Body	LISS + Rehabilitation	Rest

WEEK 3 (WEEKS 1 & 3)

Monday	Tuesday	Wednesday	Thursday	Friday	Saturday	Sunday
Legs	LISS	Arms & Abs	LISS	Full Body + LISS*	Rest	LISS + Rehabilitation

WEEK 4 (WEEKS 2 & 4)

Monday	Tuesday	Wednesday	Thursday	Friday	Saturday	Sunday
Legs	LISS	Arms & Abs	LISS	Full Body + LISS*	Rest	LISS + Rehabilitation

Using this guideline, we have provided you with a sample workout (see poster at the front of the book). To download an electronic version of the workout poster, please visit kaylaitsines.com/28dayguide/book2/workoutposter

This schedule may not suit everyone, and that's okay. The beauty of this plan is that it is **flexible** and can easily be adapted to suit any lifestyle. Just make sure that you follow these guidelines when arranging your own workout schedule:

■ Do not complete more than two workouts in any given day.

■ * If you choose to complete two workouts in the same day, avoid doing them back-to-back. Instead, do one in the morning and one in the evening.

■ Rehabilitation (active recovery) is a low-intensity form of exercise and can be done after any resistance or cardio workout.

If you wish to create your own workout schedule, you can download a free workout planner tool at kaylaitsines.com/28dayguide/book2/workoutplanner or use the 28-Day Workout Planner on page 300.

28-DAY WORKOUT PLANNER

Below is a table that can be used to create your own workout schedule from week to week, like the example provided. Just make sure you are following the guidelines on page 299. You can download a copy of this planner by visiting kaylaitsines.com/28dayguide/book2/workoutplanner

Monday	Tuesday	Wednesday	Thursday	Friday	Saturday	Sunday
Legs	LISS	Arms & Abs	LISS	Full Body	LISS and Rehab	Rest

WEEK 1 (WEEKS 1 & 3)

Monday	Tuesday	Wednesday	Thursday	Friday	Saturday	Sunday

WEEK 2 (WEEKS 2 & 4)

Monday	Tuesday	Wednesday	Thursday	Friday	Saturday	Sunday

WEEK 3 (WEEKS 1 & 3)

Monday	Tuesday	Wednesday	Thursday	Friday	Saturday	Sunday

WEEK 4 (WEEKS 2 & 4)

Monday	Tuesday	Wednesday	Thursday	Friday	Saturday	Sunday

EXERCISE GLOSSARY

Here are step-by-step instructions for each of the exercises featured in the tear-out poster at the front of the book.

BENCH HOP

1 Place a bench vertically in front of you and position yourself to the right hand side of it. Firmly grip the bench on both sides, ensuring your fingers are facing outwards.

2 Transfer your weight onto your hands and propel your feet up and over the bench. Ensure that you tuck your knees into your chest as you jump, to prevent hitting them on the bench.

3 Land on the left side of the bench, ensuring that you maintain "soft" knees to prevent injury. Repeat in the opposite direction.

4 Continue alternating from side to side for the specified number of repetitions.

BENCH JUMP

1 Place a bench horizontally in front of you and plant both feet on the floor slightly further than shoulder-width apart.

2 Looking straight ahead, bend at both the hips and knees, ensuring that your knees remain in line with your toes.

3 Continue bending your knees until your upper legs are parallel with the floor. Ensure that your back remains at a 45–90-degree angle to your hips. This is called squat position.

4 Propel your body upwards and forwards towards the bench.

5 Land in squat position on top of the bench, ensuring that you maintain "soft" knees to prevent injury.

6 Carefully jump backwards off the bench and onto the floor, landing in squat position. (You can carefully step off the bench if that is more comfortable.)

7 Repeat for the specified number of repetitions.

BENT LEG JACKKNIFE

1 Start by lying straight on your back with both arms extended above your head. This is your starting position.

2 Engage your abdominal muscles by drawing your belly button in towards your spine.

3 Keeping your feet together, contract your abdominal muscles and bend your legs to bring your knees into your chest.

4 At the same time, bring your arms forwards towards your feet, slowly lifting your head, shoulder blades, and torso off the floor.

5 Briefly hold this position and then slowly release your arms and legs back to starting position until they are both just slightly off the floor.

6 Repeat for the specified number of repetitions.

BENT OVER REVERSE FLY

1 Holding one dumbbell in each hand, plant both feet on the floor slightly further than shoulder-width apart.

2 Bend forwards from the hips until a small amount of tension is felt in your hamstrings (back of your legs) before bending your knees slightly.

3 Reposition the dumbbells so that they are together directly below your chest. This is your starting position.

4 Keeping your arms slightly bent, gently raise the dumbbells outwards and upwards from below your chest until they reach shoulder height.

5 Gently lower the dumbbells back down into starting position.

6 Repeat for the specified number of repetitions.

BURPEE

1 Plant both feet on the floor slightly further than shoulder-width apart. Bend at both the hips and knees, and place your hands on the floor directly in front of your feet.

2 Keeping your body weight on your hands, kick both of your feet backwards so that your legs are completely extended behind you, resting on the balls of your feet. Your body should be in one straight line from your head to your heels.

3 Jump both of your feet back in towards your hands, ensuring that they remain shoulder-width apart.

4 Propel your body upwards into the air. Extend your legs below you and your arms above your head.

5 Land in a neutral standing position, ensuring that you maintain "soft" knees to prevent injury.

6 Repeat for the specified number of repetitions.

COMMANDO

1 Start by placing your forearms on the floor and extending both legs behind you, resting on the balls of your feet. This is called plank position.

2 Release your right forearm and place your right hand firmly on the floor directly below your right shoulder.

3 Push up onto your right hand, followed immediately by your left in the same pattern. Ensure that you brace your abdominals to prevent your hips from swaying.

4 Return to plank position by releasing your right hand and lowering onto your forearm, before doing the same with your left hand.

5 Repeat this exercise, starting with your left hand. Continue alternating between right and left for the specified number of repetitions.

DONKEY KICK

1 Start on all fours, ensuring that your knees are directly below your hips and your hands are directly below your shoulders. This is your starting position.

2 Keeping your foot flexed and knee bent, slowly raise your right leg behind you until your upper leg is in line with your back. Ensure that you brace your abdominals to prevent your hips from swaying.

3 Slowly lower your right leg to return to the starting position.

4 Complete half of the specified number of repetitions on the same side, before completing the remaining repetitions on the other side.

DUMBBELL SQUAT

1 Holding one dumbbell in each hand on either side of your body, plant both feet on the floor slightly further than shoulder-width apart. This is your starting position.

2 Looking straight ahead, bend at both the hips and knees, ensuring that your knees remain in line with your toes. Allow the dumbbells to gently run down the outside of your legs.

3 Continue bending your knees until your upper legs are parallel with the floor. Ensure that your back remains at a 45–90-degree angle to your hips.

4 Push through your heels and extend your legs to return to the starting position.

5 Repeat for the specified number of repetitions.

DUMBBELL SQUAT & PRESS

1 Holding one dumbbell in each hand on either side of your body, plant both feet on the floor slightly further than shoulder-width apart.

2 Bend at both the hips and knees, ensuring that your knees remain in line with your toes. Allow the dumbbells to gently run down the outside of your legs.

3 Continue bending your knees until your upper legs are parallel with the floor. Ensure that your back remains at a 45–90-degree angle to your hips.

4 Push through your heels to extend your legs and bend your elbows to bring both dumbbells into your chest. Ensure that the dumbbells are parallel to (in line with) the floor.

5 Extend your arms and press both dumbbells up above your head.

6 Gently lower the dumbbells into your chest and then extend your arms down by your sides.

7 Repeat for the specified number of repetitions.

JUMP LUNGE

1 Plant both feet on the floor slightly further than shoulder-width apart and take a big step forwards with your left foot.

2 As you plant your foot on the floor, bend both knees to approximately 90 degrees. If done correctly, your front knee should be aligned with your ankle and your back knee should be hovering just off the floor. This is called a lunge position.

3 Propel your body upwards into the air.

4 Whilst in the air, extend both legs and reposition them so that you land in lunge position with your right leg forward and left leg back.

5 Continue alternating between left and right for the specified number of repetitions.

KNEE UP

1 Place the bench horizontally in front of you and plant both feet on the floor slightly further than shoulder-width apart.

2 Firmly plant your entire right foot on the bench, making sure your knee is in line with your ankle.

3 Push through your right heel to extend your right leg. Avoid pushing through your toe to prevent placing additional pressure on your shins, knees, and quadriceps.

4 As you straighten your right leg, bend your left knee and bring your left leg in towards your chest.

5 Release your left leg from your chest and place it back on the floor.

6 Repeat half of the specified number of repetitions on the same leg before completing the remaining repetitions on the other leg.

OUTWARD SNAP JUMP

1 Place both hands on the floor slightly further than shoulder-width apart and both feet together behind you, resting on the balls of your feet. This is your starting position.

2 Quickly jump both feet outwards so that they are wider than your hips.

3 Quickly jump both of your feet inwards to bring them back together into starting position.

4 Continue alternating between feet together and feet apart for the specified number of repetitions.

PUSH UP

1 Place both hands on the floor slightly further than shoulder-width apart and both feet together behind you, resting on the balls of your feet. This is your starting position.

2 Keeping a straight back and stabilising through your abdominals, bend your elbows and lower your torso towards the floor until your arms form two 90-degree angles.

3 Push through your chest and extend your arms to lift your body back into starting position.

4 Repeat for the specified number of repetitions.

REBOUND LUNGE

1 Plant both feet on the floor slightly further than shoulder-width apart. Carefully take a big step backwards with your left foot.

2 As you plant your left foot on the floor, bend both knees to approximately 90 degrees, ensuring that your weight is evenly distributed between both legs. If done correctly, your front knee should be aligned with your ankle and your back knee should be hovering just off the floor.

3 Extend both knees and transfer your weight completely onto your right foot and take a big step forwards with your left foot. As you plant your foot on the floor, bend both knees to approximately 90 degrees.

4 Extend both knees and transfer your weight completely onto your right foot.

5 Continue alternating between reverse lunge and forward lunge on the same leg until you have completed half of the specified number of repetitions before completing the remaining repetitions on the other leg.

SCISSOR KICK

1 Start by lying straight on your back and place both hands underneath your coccyx.

2 Extend both legs to approximately 45 degrees and engage your abdominal muscles by drawing in your belly button to your spine.

3 Slightly raise your right leg and slightly lower your left leg. Then slightly raise your left leg and slightly lower your right leg. This should create a "scissor-like" motion.

4 Continue alternating between right and left for the specified number of repetitions.

SIDE CRUNCH

1 Start by lying on your right side with your feet on top of each other and knees slightly bent.

2 Release your right arm from under your body and lay it straight out on the floor in front of you and place your left hand behind your earlobe.

3 Engage your abdominal muscles by drawing your belly button in towards your spine. This is your starting position.

4 Slowly raise your shoulder blades and torso off the floor to bring your left elbow to your left hip (or as far as you can).

5 Slowly release your torso and return to starting position.

6 Complete half of the specified number of repetitions on the same side, before completing the remaining repetitions on the other side.

SIDE RAISE

1 Holding one dumbbell in each hand on either side of your body, plant both feet on the floor slightly further than shoulder-width apart. This is your starting position.

2 Keeping your arms slightly bent, gently raise the dumbbells outwards and upwards from the sides of your body until they reach shoulder height.

3 Gently lower the dumbbells to return to starting position.

4 Repeat for the specified number of repetitions.

SIT SQUAT

1 Place a bench horizontally behind you.

2 Plant both feet on the floor slightly further than shoulder-width apart. This is your starting position.

3 Looking straight ahead, bend at both the hips and knees, ensuring that your knees remain in line with your toes.

4 Continue bending your knees until you are able to sit on the bench behind you. Lean back slightly to sit up tall.

5 Push through your heels and extend your legs to return to starting position.

6 Repeat for the specified number of repetitions.

SNAP JUMP

1 Plant both feet on the floor slightly further than shoulder-width apart. Bend at both the hips and knees, and place your hands on the floor directly in front of your feet.

2 Keeping your body weight on your hands, kick both of your feet backwards so that your legs are completely extended behind you, resting on the balls of your feet.

3 Jump both of your feet back in towards your hands, ensuring that they remain shoulder-width apart.

4 Repeat for the specified number of repetitions.

STAR JUMP

1 With your arms by your sides, plant both feet together on the floor. This is your starting position.

2 Quickly jump both feet outwards so that they are spread slightly further than your hips. At the same time, raise your arms upwards and outwards from the sides of your body so that your hands almost meet directly above your head.

3 Quickly jump both of your feet inwards to bring them back together while lowering your arms downwards and in towards your body to return to starting position.

4 Repeat for the specified number of repetitions.

STEP UP

1 Start by placing the bench horizontally in front of you and plant both feet on the floor slightly further than shoulder-width apart.

2 Firmly plant your entire left foot on the bench, making sure your knee is in line with your toes.

3 Push through your left heel to extend your left leg. Avoid pushing through your toes to prevent placing additional pressure on your shins, knees, and quadriceps.

4 As you straighten your left leg, release your right leg and step up onto the bench.

5 Reverse this pattern back to the floor, starting with your left leg.

6 Repeat starting with your right foot on the bench. Continue alternating between left and right for the specified number of repetitions.

STRAIGHT LEG RAISE

1 Start by lying straight on your back and place both hands underneath your coccyx.

2 Engage your abdominal muscles by drawing your belly button in towards your spine.

3 Keeping your feet together, slowly raise your legs off the floor.

4 Continue raising your legs until they form a 90-degree angle with your hips.

5 Slowly lower your legs until they are slightly off the floor.

6 Repeat for the specified number of repetitions.

STRAIGHT LEG SIT UP & TWIST

1 Start by lying straight on your back. Place both hands behind your earlobes.

2 Engage your abdominal muscles by drawing your belly button in towards your spine. This is your starting position.

3 Keeping your heels firmly planted on the floor, slowly lift your head, shoulder blades, and torso off the floor. Ensure that it is your abdominals that initiate the movement, and that you do not "swing" your torso up.

4 As you sit up, extend your left arm and twist over the right side of your body.

5 Slowly untwist and lower your torso back into starting position.

6 Repeat using your right arm and twisting over the left side of your body. Continue alternating between left and right for the specified number of repetitions.

SUMO SQUAT

1 Plant both feet on the floor further than shoulder-width apart. Point both feet slightly outwards. This is your starting position.

2 Looking straight ahead, bend at both the hips and knees, ensuring that your knees point towards your toes.

3 Continue bending your knees until your upper legs are parallel with the floor, ensuring that your back remains between 45–90 degrees of your hips.

4 Push through your heels and extend your legs to return to starting position.

5 Repeat for the specified number of repetitions.

TOE TAP

1 Start by lying straight on your back. Place both hands behind your earlobes.

2 Gently raise your legs off the floor so that they form a 90-degree angle at your hips. Engage your abdominal muscles by drawing your belly button in towards your spine. This is your starting position.

3 Bring your hands up towards your feet—slowly lifting your head, shoulder blades, and torso off the floor. Allow your hands to meet your toes (or as far as you can) before releasing your torso and laying back to return to starting position.

4 Repeat for the specified number of repetitions.

TRICEP DIP

1 Start seated on a bench and position your hands under your glutes and directly below your shoulders. Ensure that your fingers are facing forwards.

2 Shift your glutes forwards off the bench. This is your starting position.

3 Lower your body by bending at the elbows to create two 90-degree angles with your arms. Ensure that your shoulders, elbows, and wrists remain in line with one another at all times.

4 Push through the heel of your hand and extend your arms to return to starting position. Avoid using your legs to assist you and always try to maintain an upright position.

5 Repeat for the specified number of repetitions.

TUCK JUMP

1 Plant both feet on the floor slightly further than shoulder-width apart.

2 Looking straight ahead, bend at both the hips and knees, ensuring that your knees remain in line with your toes. This is your starting position.

3 Continue bending your knees until your upper legs are parallel with the floor. Ensure that your back remains at a 45–90-degree angle to your hips.

4 Propel your body upwards into the air and tuck in both your elbows and knees.

5 Extend both your legs and arms to land in starting position. When landing, ensure that you maintain "soft" knees to prevent injury.

6 Repeat for the specified number of repetitions.

WALKING LUNGE

1 With your hands on your hips, plant both feet on the floor slightly further than shoulder-width apart.

2 Take a big step forwards with your left foot. As you plant your foot on the floor, bend both knees to approximately 90 degrees. If done correctly, your front knee should be aligned with your ankle and your back knee should be hovering just off the floor. This is called a lunge position.

3 Extend both knees and transfer your weight completely onto your left foot and take a big step forwards with your right foot. As you plant your foot on the floor, bend both knees to approximately 90 degrees.

4 Continue alternating between left and right for the specified number of repetitions.

X MOUNTAIN CLIMBER

1 Place both hands on the floor shoulder-width apart and both feet together behind you, resting on the balls of your feet. This is your starting position.

2 Keeping your left foot on the floor, bend your right leg and bring your right knee in towards your left elbow.

3 Extend your right leg and return to starting position.

4 Keeping your right foot on the floor, bend your left leg and bring your left knee in towards your right elbow.

5 Extend your left leg and return to starting position.

6 Continue alternating between right and left for the specified number of repetitions. Gradually increase your speed, ensuring that the leg that is moving does not touch the floor.

X PLANK

1 Place both hands on the floor shoulder-width apart and both feet apart behind you, resting on the balls of your feet. This is your starting position.

2 Whilst maintaining a straight back and stabilising through your abdominals, release your left hand and reach towards your right foot (or as far as you can).

3 Release your right hand and return to starting position. Repeat, reaching your right hand towards your left foot (or as far as you can).

4 Continue alternating between left and right for the specified amount of repetitions. Each repetition is equivalent to one touch of your hand to your foot.

INDEX

Thank you

to the Pan Macmillan team:

Ross Gibb, Ingrid Ohlsson, Virginia Birch, Megan Pigott, and Charlotte Ree. The support you have provided throughout this journey is second only to your enthusiasm! A huge thank you to Trisha Garner, for making everything beautiful. To photography superstar Jeremy Simons, stylist Michelle Noerianto, and chef Tammi Kwok, thank you! The creativity and dedication you bring to each shoot is why these photos look so incredible. Thanks also to editors Rachel Carter and Ariane Durkin. Thank you to every single member of the BBG Community for your ongoing motivation, support, and encouragement. To the best, most dynamic team in the world: thank you a thousand times. You are amazing and I'm so glad to have you as part of this journey. A special thank you to my family: my mum, dad, Leah (my sister), yiayia, and papou. You are a constant source of encouragement and support in my life and I cannot thank you enough for always having faith in me. Finally, to Tobi, thank you for showing me that everything we dreamed of is possible! I will be forever grateful for your belief in me and in our message. Working alongside you is truly a dream come true and I cherish every moment.

Kayla

ABOUT THE AUTHOR

KAYLA ITSINES is a personal trainer and global fitness phenomenon. She has created the world's largest and most supportive online female fitness community, and the successful BBG and BBG Stronger Workout and Eating Guides, all hosted in the renowned women's fitness app, SWEAT. Kayla was recently named the world's number one fitness influencer in the 2017 *Forbes Influencer List*. She lives with her partner Tobi Pearce in Adelaide, Australia.

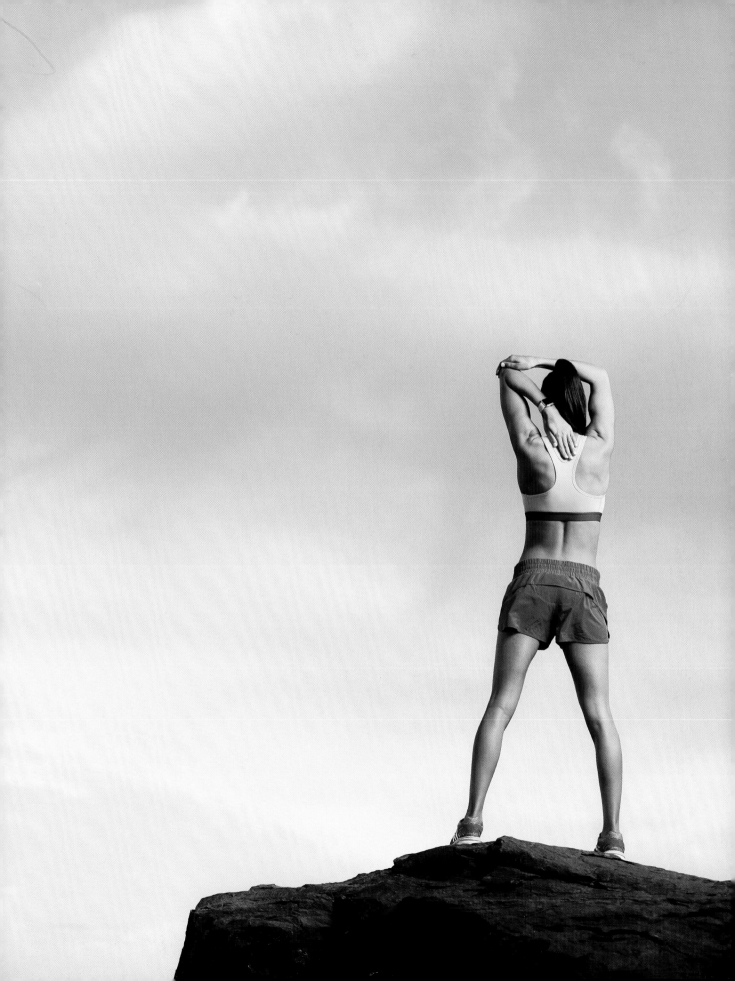

Photo of Kayla's record-breaking bootcamp, held in Melbourne, Australia, in November 2016. Kayla and the BBG Community broke five separate Guinness World Records, including:

- Most people performing star jumps: 2192 participants
- Most people running in place simultaneously: 2195 participants
- Most people doing sit ups simultaneously: 2005 participants
- Most people performing lunges: 2146 participants
- Most people performing squats: 2201 participants